Akinori Akaike • Shun Shimohama
Yoshimi Misu
Editors

Nicotinic Acetylcholine Receptor Signaling in Neuroprotection

Editors
Akinori Akaike
Department of Pharmacology, Graduate School of Pharmaceutical Sciences
Kyoto University
Kyoto, Japan

Wakayama Medical University
Wakayama, Japan

Yoshimi Misu
Graduate School of Medicine
Yokohama City University
Yokohama, Kanagawa, Japan

Shun Shimohama
Department of Neurology, School of Medicine
Sapporo Medical University
Sapporo, Hokkaido, Japan

https://doi.org/10.1007/978-981-10-8488-1

Preface

Nicotinic acetylcholine receptors (nAChRs) are typical ligand-gated ion channels that evoke cation-selective currents across the plasma membrane. On exposure to agonists, nAChR exists in an active, open state, and elicits rapid depolarization of neurons. In addition to acute ionic responses, it has been widely recognized that nAChRs mediate long-term modification of cell functions. Persistent stimulation of nAChRs for a longer period occurs during habitual tobacco smoking as well as during acetylcholinesterase (AChE) inhibitor therapy for Alzheimer's disease. Long-term tobacco smoking, nicotine application, or exposure to AChE inhibitors induces upregulation of nAChRs and, in most cases, facilitates cellular responses. Such long-term nAChR stimulation contributes to the elaboration of complex intracellular signals, resulting in functional changes in cells expressing nAChRs in the central nervous system (CNS). The concept of nAChRs as ligand-gated ion channels generating rapid ionic currents is likely to be supplemented with more complex mechanisms, in which nAChRs are important elements triggering intracellular signaling toward gradual alteration of cellular functions. Neuroprotection is one of the major effects of gradual functional modification induced by nicotine and AChE inhibitors including donepezil, which is used in the treatment of Alzheimer's disease.

The goal of this book is to describe current knowledge on roles and mechanisms of signal transduction triggered by nAChR stimulation in neuroprotection against toxic effects of risk factors of neurodegenerative diseases. The major topic of this book is neuroprotection mediated by nAChRs in neurodegenerative diseases such as Alzheimer's disease. Authors of this book are members of research projects supported by the Smoking Research Foundation (SRF), Japan. The SRF project titles are "Functional changes induced by long-term stimulation of nAChRs," "Brain nicotinic acetylcholine receptors and Alzheimer's disease – for the proposal of innovative therapeutic strategies," and "Smoking and nervous system." The authors acknowledge support over many years from SRF.

In response to rapidly evolving areas in clinical and laboratory neuropharmacology and neurochemistry, we provide an in-depth coverage of nAChR-mediated neuroprotection in basic research and of future developments in clinical application of effective neuroprotective strategies in neurodegenerative diseases. We hope that our work will result in an increased interest in the fascinating subject of nicotinic neuroprotection signaling in the CNS.

Kyoto, Japan	Akinori Akaike
Sapporo, Japan	Shun Shimohama
Yokohama, Japan	Yoshimi Misu

Acknowledgement

We appreciate the kind support of grants listed below.

Chapter 1, a Grant-in-Aid for Scientific Research (KAKENHI) from the Japan Society for the Promotion of Science (JSPS) and a grant from the Smoking Research Foundation (SRF), Japan.

Chapter 2, a Grant-in-Aid for center of excellence (COE) projects by Ministry of education, culture, sports, science and technology (MEXT), Japan titled "Center of excellence for molecular and gene targeting therapies with micro-dose molecular imaging modalities", KAKENHI from JSPS, a grant from SRF and Nagai Memorial Research Scholarship from the Pharmaceutical Society of Japan.

Chapter 3, support of the Life Science Research Laboratory, University of Fukui, KAKENHI from JSPS and a grant from SRF.

Chapter 4, KAKENHI from JSPS, a grant from SRF and a grant from the Naito Foundation of Japan.

Chapter 5, a grant from SRF. The authors of this chapter also thank Dr. Aldric T. Hama for his careful editing of the manuscript.

Chapter 6, KAKENHI from JSPS, a Challenging Exploratory Research grant from the JSPS, a Research on Regulatory Science of Pharmaceuticals and Medical Devices grant from the Japan Agency for Medical Research and Development (AMED), a grant from SRF and a grant from the Kobayashi International Foundation.

Chapter 7, KAKENHI from JSPS and a grant from SRF.

Chapter 8, KAKENHI from JSPS and a grant from SRF.

Chapter 9, KAKENHI from JSPS, a Project of Translational and Clinical Research Core Centers from AMED and a grant from SRF.

Chapter 10, KAKENHI from JSPS and a grant from SRF.

Many sincere thanks to Emmy Lee and Selvakumar Rajendran, editors at Springer Nature.

Contents

Chapter 1
Overview

Akinori Akaike and Yasuhiko Izumi

Abstract The nicotinic acetylcholine receptor (nAChR) is a typical ion channel type receptor. nAChR agonists such as nicotine evoke rapid excitatory responses in order of milliseconds. In addition to acute responses, sustained stimulation of nAChRs induces delayed cellular responses leading to neuroprotection via intracellular signal pathways probably triggered by Ca^{2+} influx. The most predominant subtypes of nAChRs expressed in the central nervous system (CNS) are α4 (known as α4β2) and α7 nAChRs. Long-term exposure to nicotine or acetylcholinesterase (AChE) inhibitors exerts protection against neurotoxicity induced by glutamate, β-amyloid, and other toxic insults. Nicotinic neuroprotection is mediated by α7 nAChR which shows high Ca^{2+} permeability, though contribution of α4 nAChR to nicotinic neuroprotection has also been suggested. Agonist stimulation of these receptors leads to activation of the phosphoinositide 3-kinase (PI3K)-Akt signaling pathway, downstream of neurotrophin receptors. AChE inhibitors including donepezil which is used for treatment of Alzheimer's disease, also activate PI3K-Akt pathway via nAChRs. Neuroprotective effects induced by long-term nAChR stimulation indicate that CNS nAChRs play important roles in promotion of neuronal survival under pathophysiological conditions such as brain ischemia and neurodegenerative diseases. Elucidation of neuroprotective mechanisms of nAChRs may enable development of novel therapies for neurodegenerative diseases.

Keywords Acetylcholine · Acetylcholinesterase · Neuroprotection · Nicotine · Nicotinic

---

A. Akaike (✉)
Department of Pharmacology, Graduate School of Pharmaceutical Sciences, Kyoto University, Kyoto, Japan

Wakayama Medical University, Wakayama, Japan
e-mail: aakaike@ps.nagoya-u.ac.jp

Y. Izumi
Department of Pharmacology, Graduate School of Pharmaceutical Sciences, Kyoto University, Kyoto, Japan

Department of Pharmacology, Kobe Pharmaceutical University, Kobe, Japan

A. Akaike et al. (eds.), *Nicotinic Acetylcholine Receptor Signaling in Neuroprotection*, https://doi.org/10.1007/978-981-10-8488-1_1

1.1 Introduction

Acetylcholine (ACh) is a small molecule with a simple chemical structure comprising an ester of choline and acetic acid. This molecule plays a crucial role in maintaining homeostasis and brain functions by acting as a neurotransmitter in the peripheral nervous system including motor nerves and the autonomic and the central nervous system (CNS). ACh is synthetized by choline acetyltransferase with choline and acetyl coenzyme A as substrates (Fig. 1.1). ACh released from nerve endings upon nerve excitation is rapidly degraded by acetylcholinesterase (AChE) into choline and acetic acid. ACh released in the synaptic cleft acts as an agonist to its specific receptors to evoke various cellular responses. ACh receptors are divided into two major classes, nicotinic ACh receptors (nAChRs) and muscarinic ACh receptors (mAChRs). The names of these receptors are derived from their specific agonists; nicotine contained in tobacco leaves and muscarine isolated from poisonous mushrooms, *Amanita muscaria*. nAChRs are ligand-gated ion channels, which evoke rapid depolarization responses to elicit neuronal excitation or skeletal muscle contraction. On the other hand, mAChRs are representative G-protein-coupled receptors classified as M_1–M_5 (Caulfield and Birdsall 1998). M_1, M_3, and M_5 receptors interact with Gq-type G proteins and primarily cause excitatory responses, whereas M_2 and M_4 receptors interact with Gi/Go type G proteins and cause suppressive responses such as hyperpolarization. Responses mediated by mAChRs are relatively slow whereas opening of ligand-gated channels of nAChRs induces rapid cellular responses in the order of milliseconds.

nAChRs are highly expressed in skeletal muscle and the nervous system. Recently, expression of nAChRs in immune cells and glial cells has also attracted attention for potential therapeutic targeting in inflammation and neurodegenerative diseases (de Jonge and Ulloa 2007; Fujii et al. 2017; Jurado-Coronel et al. 2016).

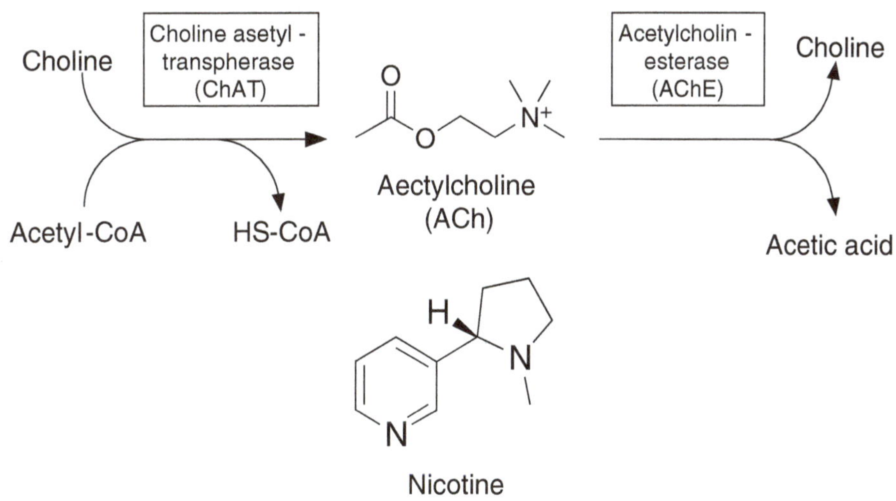

Fig. 1.1 Synthesis and metabolism of acetylcholine (ACh). Choline acetyltransferase (ChAT) and acetylcholinesterase (AChE) are involved in synthesis and metabolism of ACh. ACh is synthesized from Acetyl coenzyme A (Acetyl-CoA) and Choline, releasing Coenzyme A (HS-CoA)

nAChRs are grouped into muscle-type (N_m), peripheral neuronal-type (N_n), and central neuronal-type (CNS) based on their distribution, subunit composition, and selective antagonists, as per the classification in Goodman & Gilman's "The Pharmacological Basis of Therapeutics" (12th Edition, 2011). In their classification, CNS AChRs are further divided into two subtypes: $(\alpha4)_2(\beta2)_3$ (α-bungarotoxin-insensitive) and $(\alpha7)_5$ (α-bungarotoxin-sensitive). N_n AChRs are widely expressed in autonomic ganglia and the adrenal medulla. CNS AChRs are expressed in neurons and glia of various brain areas. One of the typical antagonists of N_m AChRs is *d*-tubocurarine, a toxic alkaloid derived from an arrow poison and clinically used as a non-depolarizing blocking agent of the neuromuscular junction. Hexamethonium and mecamylamine are selective antagonists of N_n and CNS AChRs.

In all types of nAChRs, agonists such as ACh itself or nicotine-induced ion channel opening and evoke influx of Na^+ and Ca^{2+}. This triggers cell depolarization and turns on various functional switches (Albuquerque et al. 2009). Nicotinic cholinergic responses correlated with fast neurotransmission are easily detected in the endplate at the neuromuscular junction and ganglion cells of the sympathetic nerves. By contrast, it is relatively difficult to detect postsynaptic nicotinic responses of neurons in the CNS because most neuronal nAChRs quickly desensitized when exposed to nicotinic agonists (Albuquerque et al. 2009; Alkondon et al. 1998; Frazier et al. 1998). Development of drug-delivery devices that allow fast drug delivery and removal has made it possible to detect fast responses mediated by functional CNS nAChRs. While peripheral nAChRs are involved in rapid responses such as skeletal muscle contraction, nAChRs expressed in the CNS tend to be involved in relatively slow functional changes. For example, in the cerebral cortex, persistent nAChR stimulation triggers signals to the phosphoinositide 3-kinase (PI3K) cascade, which contributes to neuroprotection (Kihara et al. 2001; Dajas-Bailador and Wonnacott 2004). In the hippocampal neurons, nAChRs induce long-term potentiation of synaptic transmission (Kenney and Gould 2008). nAChRs regulate dopamine release in the striatum (Exley and Cragg 2008). Moreover, nAChRs are one of the important factors regulating memory and addiction (Molas et al. 2017; Nees 2015). Thus, in addition to rapid responses such as membrane depolarization induced by inward currents via ion channels, nAChR can generate longer-lasting effects in the CNS neurons, where rapid cation influx may trigger activation of complex intracellular signaling pathways.

1.2 Structural and Pharmacological Characterization of Nicotinic Acetylcholine Receptors

nAChRs are classified as members of the cysteine-loop (Cys-loop) family of ligand-gated ion channels (Sine and Eagle 2006; Tsetlin et al. 2011). The Cys-loop ligand-gated channels, also known as Cys-loop receptors, play prominent roles in generating excitatory and inhibitory postsynaptic potentials in the nervous system. nAChRs,

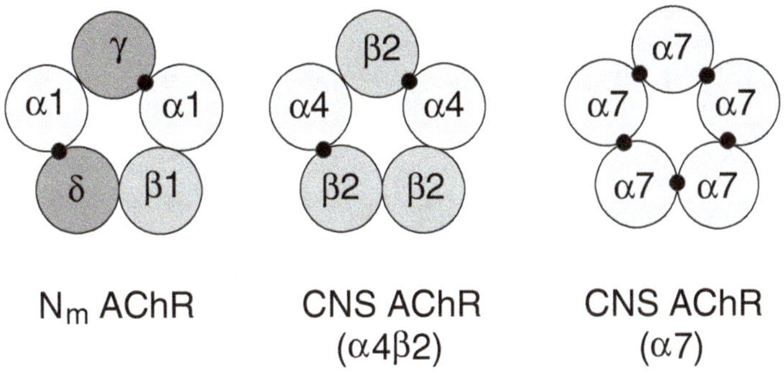

Fig. 1.2 Examples of subunit assembly and location of agonist-binding sites. Large circles indicate subunits of nicotinic acetylcholine receptor (nAChR). Small filled circles indicate binding sites of acetylcholine. Muscle-type AChR (N_m AChR), central nervous system AChR (CNS AChR)

γ-aminobutyric acid type A ($GABA_A$) receptors, glycine receptors, and 5-hydroxytryptamine type-3 ($5\text{-}HT_3$) receptors are classified as Cys-loop receptors. These receptors are composed of five subunits, forming a pentameric conformation around a central water-filled pore. The Cys-loop receptors have structurally common features with a characteristic loop formed by a disulfide bond between two cysteine residues. In nAChRs, the two cysteine residues separate 13 highly conserved amino acids located in the extracellular N-terminal domain of the α-subunit. The four hydrophobic transmembrane domains are estimated to form α-helices that make up the ion channel pore. The channel pore is lined with residues from the second transmembrane domain (TM2) from each of the five subunits of the receptors. The extracellular domain is largely composed of the N-terminus with binding sites for agonists.

The International Union of Basic and Clinical Pharmacology Committee on Receptor Nomenclature and Drug Classification (NC-IUPHAR, URL: http://www.guidetopharmacology.org/nciuphar.jsp) recommends a nomenclature and classification scheme for nAChRs based on subunit composition of known, naturally occurring and/or heterologously-expressed nAChR subtypes. A total of 17 subunits (α1–10, β1–4, γ, δ, and ε) have been identified in nAChRs. All subunits except α8, which is present in avian species, have been identified in mammals. ACh-binding sites are found at interfaces of the α subunit and the δ or γ subunit in N_m AChRs, and at interfaces of the α subunit and β subunit or two adjacent α subunits in N_n and CNS AChRs (Fig. 1.2). All α subunits possess two tandem cysteine residues near the ACh-binding site. By contrast, β, γ, δ, and ε subunits lack these cysteine residues. N_m AChRs of adult animals possess the stoichiometry $(\alpha1)_2\beta1\delta\varepsilon$ while N_m AChRs expressed in embryonic muscles and denervated adult muscles possess the stoichiometry $(\alpha1)_2\beta1\gamma\delta$ (Lukas et al. 1999). Other types of nAChRs are predominantly expressed in neurons (Table 1.1). They are assembled as combinations of α2–α6 and β2–β4 subunits or α7, α8, and α9 subunits forming functional homo-oligomers. N_m AChRs and some subtypes of CNS AChRs (α7, α8, α9, and α10) are sensitive to α-bungarotoxin, a well-known neurotoxic protein derived from the venom of kraits.

Table 1.1 Characteristics of nAChR

Subtype	Primary subunit composition	Ca^{2+} permeability	Major location	α-Bungarotoxin sensitivity
α1	$(\alpha1)_2\beta1\gamma\delta$, $(\alpha1)_2\beta1\delta\varepsilon$	Low	Neuromuscular junction	Sensitive
α2	α2β2, α2β4	Low	CNS	Insensitive
α3	α3β2, α3β4	Low	Autonomic ganglion, CNS	Insensitive
α4	$(\alpha4)_3(\beta2)_2$, $(\alpha4)_2(\beta2)_3$	Low	CNS	Insensitive
α5	α3β2α5, α3β4α5, $(\alpha4)_2(\beta2)_2\alpha5$	High	Autonomic ganglion, CNS	Insensitive
α6	α6β2β3, α6α4β2β3	High	CNS	Insensitive
α7	$(\alpha7)_5$	High	CNS, Non-neuronal cells	Sensitive
α8 (avian only)	$(\alpha8)_5$	High	CNS	Sensitive
α9	$(\alpha9)_5$, α9α10	High	Mechanosensory hair cells	Sensitive
α10	α9α10	High	Mechanosensory hair cells	Sensitive

For α2, α3, α4, and β2 and β4 subunits, pairwise combinations of α and β (e.g., α3β4 and α4β2) are sufficient to form a functional receptor in vitro, but more complex isoforms may exist in vivo. Among those subunit combinations, the α3β4 subunit combination is dominant in nAChRs of autonomic ganglia neurons. The α5 and β3 subunits participate in formation of functional hetero-oligomeric receptors when they are expressed as a third subunit with another α and β pair such as α4α5αβ2, α4αβ2β3, and α5α6β2. The α6 subunit can form a functional receptor when co-expressed with β4 in vitro. The α7 subunit forms functional homo-oligomers. This subunit can also combine with a β subunit to form a hetero-oligomeric assembly such as α7β2. The α8 and α9 subunits show similar properties to the α7 subunit. For functional expression of the α10 subunit, co-assembly with α9 is necessary.

Subtypes of nAChRs can be classified based on the predominant α-subunits (α1–α10) because the α subunit plays a key role in agonist binding to trigger ion channel opening, and subtype-selective antagonists like α-bungarotoxin distinguish receptors based on the α subunit combination (see Table 1.1). As per this receptor classification, N_m AChRs can be defined as α1 nAChRs, because the α1 subunit is highly expressed only in skeletal muscle and other α subunits are not detected in this tissue. N_n and CNS AChRs can be broadly classified into two subgroups, α2–α6 nAChRs, formed from the combination of α- and β-subunits, and α7–α9 nAChRs, forming homo-oligomers. The former subgroup, α2–α6 nAChRs, is insensitive to α-bungarotoxin whereas the latter subgroup, α7–α9 nAChRs, is sensitive to the toxin. Ion channels of homo-oligomeric receptors α7–α9 show high Ca^{2+} permeability. The α5 and α6 hetero-oligomeric receptors also show high Ca^{2+} permeability.

Table 1.2 Distribution of nAChR in CNS

α2	α3	α4	α5	α6	α7
Cortex		Cortex	Cortex		Cortex
Hippocampus	Hippocampus	Hippocampus	Hippocampus		Hippocampus
		Striatum	Striatum	Striatum	
Amygdala		Amygdala			Amygdala
		Thalamus			
Hypothalamus		Hypothalamus			Hypothalamus
	Substantia nigra	Substantia nigra	Substantia nigra	Substantia nigra	Substantia nigra
	Cerebellum	Cerebellum			Cerebellum
	Spinal cord	Spinal cord			Spinal cord

Among those neuronal receptors, α3 nAChR is highly expressed in autonomic ganglia though this subtype is also expressed in CNS. The most predominant subtypes of nAChRs expressed in CNS are α4, known as α4β2 and α7 nAChRs (Dani 2015). Expression of both subunits is detected across wide areas of the CNS (Table 1.2). In the cerebral cortex, α2 and α5 subunits are also detected. Accumulating evidence also suggests anti-inflammatory and neuroprotective roles of α7 nAChR expressed in immune cells and glial cells (Egea et al. 2015; Morioka et al. 2015).

1.3 Neuroprotection Mediated by Nicotinic Acetylcholine Receptors

It is widely recognized that glutamate acts as an excitatory neurotransmitter but also exerts excitatory neurotoxicity in pathological conditions such as ischemia (Meldrum and Garthwaite 1990; Duggan and Choi 1994; Brassai et al. 2015). In addition to cerebral ischemia, glutamate neurotoxicity is also considered as one of the risk factors for neurodegenerative diseases, such as Alzheimer's disease and Parkinson's disease. Involvement of the cholinergic system in glutamate neurotoxicity was first reported in Mattson's study (1989), showing that glutamate neurotoxicity in the hippocampus was enhanced by mAChR stimulation. Olney et al. (1991) showed evidence suggesting that *N*-methyl-D-aspartate (NMDA) receptor blockade by MK801 induces disinhibition of the central cholinergic system and causes excessive stimulation of mAChRs. They hypothesized that MK801 occasionally induces neurotoxicity instead of neuroprotection due to such an indirect mAChR stimulation. Thus, it is likely that mAChRs facilitate neuronal death in pathological states where glutamate neurotoxicity causes neurodegeneration.

On the other hand, accumulating evidence has suggested that nAChRs play a protective role in glutamate neurotoxicity. Approximately two decades ago, Akaike et al. (1994) and Kaneko et al. (1997) reported that glutamate neurotoxicity in the cerebral cortex was suppressed by nicotine and other nAChR agonists. Because NMDA receptors are acknowledged as a predominant route of glutamate cytotoxicity in the cerebral cortex, nicotine was suggested to prevent glutamate neurotoxicity by exerting a protective action against NMDA receptor-mediated intracellular responses to induce neuronal death. The neuroprotective effect of nicotine was antagonized by hexamethonium and mecamylamine, which are N_n and CNS nAChR antagonists, respectively, indicating that nicotine induces neuroprotection by its selective action on nAChRs. To our knowledge, our study (Akaike et al. 1994) was the first evidence for the neuroprotective role of nAChRs in the CNS. In this study, nicotine markedly reversed glutamate cytotoxicity, whereas muscarine exacerbated it. Carbachol, which acts on both nicotinic and muscarinic receptors, reduced glutamate cytotoxicity although its effect was less potent than that of nicotine. These observations indicate that nAChRs and mAChRs exert opposing effects on glutamate cytotoxicity. Moreover, findings of nAChR-mediated neuroprotection suggested a role of nicotinic cholinergic system in promoting neuronal survival under pathological conditions such as brain ischemia. A characteristic feature of the neuroprotective action of nicotine was that long-term exposure of more than an hour was necessary to ameliorate glutamate neurotoxicity. Following our findings in the cerebral cortex, neuroprotective effects mediated by nAChRs have been detected in various areas of the brain, including the hippocampus (Dajas-Bailador et al. 2000; Liu and Zhao 2004), the striatum (Ohnishi et al. 2009), dopaminergic neurons in the substantia nigra (Takeuchi et al. 2009), and the spinal cord (Nakamizo et al. 2005; Toborek et al. 2007). Nicotinic neuroprotection detected in those studies is estimated to be mediated by nAChR expressed in neurons though contribution of microglia activation by α7 nAChR in nicotinic neuroprotection is also suggested (Morioka et al. 2015).

It is unlikely that nicotine-induced protection against glutamate neurotoxicity is due to its direct action on NMDA receptors though there are some reports indicating that nicotine partially inhibits NMDA receptors. Aizenman et al. (1991) have demonstrated that nicotinic agonists partially inhibit whole cell NMDA-induced responses in cultured cortical neurons. Akaike et al. (1991) also reported modulatory action of cholinergic drugs on NMDA responses in the nucleus basalis of Meynert neurons. These studies suggest that nicotinic agonists have properties to directly interact with NMDA receptors and modulate their function. In this case, concomitant application of nicotine and glutamate or short-term nicotine exposure should affect glutamate neurotoxicity by direct modification of NMDA receptors. However, as described above, long-term exposure for more than an hour is necessary to detect nicotinic neuroprotection (Akaike et al. 1994; Kaneko et al. 1997). Moreover, nicotine-induced protection against glutamate cytotoxicity was antagonized by CNS nAChR antagonists. Therefore, persistent stimulation of nAChRs, but not direct inhibition of NMDA receptors is estimated to be the major route of nicotine-induced neuroprotection though direct interaction of nicotine with NMDA receptors may potentiate nicotine-induced neuroprotection.

In the forebrain including the cerebral cortex, α7 nAChRs, homo-oligomers of α7 subunits and α4β2 nAChRs, hetero-oligomers of α4 and β2 subunits are the major subtypes among CNS nAChRs (Albuquerque et al. 2009; Zoli et al. 2015). It has been reported that nicotine-induced protection against glutamate neurotoxicity was antagonized by selective α7 nAChR antagonists α-bungarotoxin and methyllycaconitine, as well as by the selective α4β2 nAChR antagonist dihydro-β-erythroidine (Kaneko et al. 1997). The α7 nAChR has attracted more attention because its mechanisms are thought to be involved in Alzheimer's disease and β-amyloid (Aβ), a well-known risk factor of Alzheimer's disease, is bound to α7 nAChRs under several conditions including in post-mortem Alzheimer's disease brains (Wang et al. 2000; Parri et al. 2011). A selective α7 nAChR agonist, 3-(2,4)-dimethoxybenzylidene anabaseine (DMXB), exhibits potent neuroprotective action on glutamate neurotoxicity in vitro and brain ischemia in vivo (Shimohama et al. 1998). Aβ-induced neurotoxicity was suppressed by nicotine and DMXB (Kihara et al. 1997). Protective effects of nicotine and DMXB against Aβ-induced toxicity were antagonized by α-bungarotoxin, indicating that stimulation of α7 nAChRs is essential in suppressing Aβ-induced neurotoxicity. It is widely accepted that the β sheet conformation of Aβ is necessary in eliciting its neurotoxicity (Fändrich et al. 2011). Nicotine might influence the β sheet conformation of Aβ to attenuate its toxicity or to modulate survival signals. However, it has been reported that neither nicotine nor DMXB influences the β sheet conformation (Kihara et al. 1999). Thus, signal transduction downstream of α7 nAChRs is likely to be involved in the protective effect of nicotine against Aβ neurotoxicity.

1.4 Intracellular Signal Transduction Triggered by Nicotinic Acetylcholine Receptors

On exposure to agonists, nAChR exists in an active, open state, and elicits rapid depolarization in order of milliseconds. Thus, nAChR is classified as an excitatory receptor that evokes rapid excitation in neuronal, muscular, and secreting cells. Progressive decline of agonist-evoked current indicates closure of the channel. Upon further exposure to agonists, nAChRs exist in desensitized, non-functional states. Besides such short-term response, it is also recognized that nAChRs mediate long-term modification of cell functions via specific signaling pathways (Dajas-Bailador and Wonnacott 2004). nAChRs, especially α7 nAChRs, generate specific and complex Ca^{2+} signals that include adenylyl cyclase, protein kinase A, protein kinase C, Ca^{2+}-calmodulin-dependent kinase, and phosphatidylinositol 3-kinase (PI3K) (Fig. 1.3). These phosphorylated downstream targets activate cellular signaling related to exocytosis and extracellular signal-regulated mitogen-activated protein kinase (ERK)-linked neuronal functions. Kihara et al. (2001) showed that α7 nAChR stimulation promoted PI3K-Akt signal transduction and inhibited Aβ neurotoxicity.

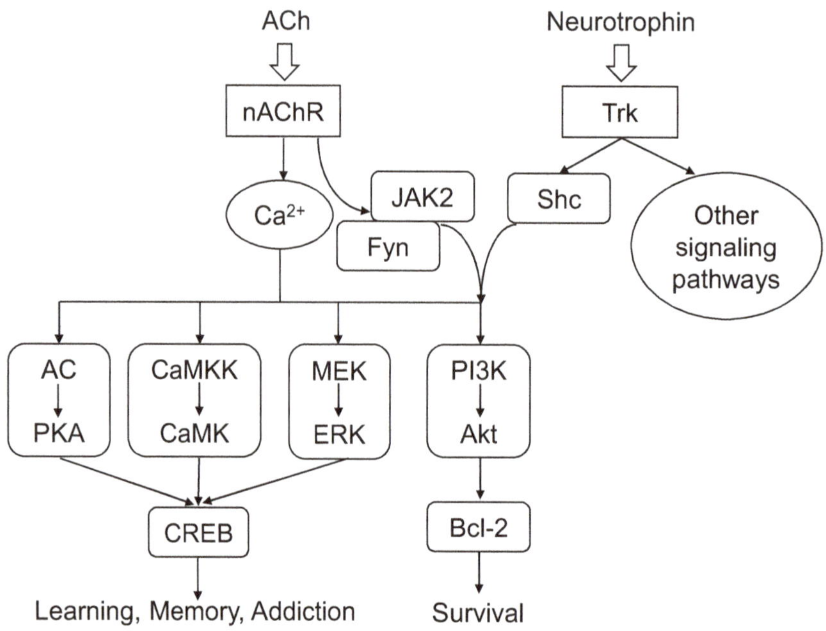

Fig. 1.3 Nicotinic acetylcholine receptor (nAChR)-mediated signaling pathway in the brain. Adenylate cyclase (AC), acetylcholine (ACh), nAChR, AKT8 virus oncogene cellular homolog (Akt), B-cell lymphoma 2 (Bcl-2), calcium/calmodulin-dependent protein kinase (CaMK), calcium/calmodulin-dependent protein kinase kinase (CaMKK), cAMP-responsive element binding protein (CREB), extracellular signal-regulated kinase (ERK), Fgr/Yes-related novel protein (Fyn), Janus-activated kinase (JAK), MAPK/ERK kinase (MEK), nicotinic acetylcholine receptor (nAChR), phosphoinositide 3-kinase (PI3K), protein kinase A (PKA), SH2-containing collagen-related proteins (Shc), tropomyosin receptor kinase (Trk)

PI3K phosphorylates Akt (or known as protein kinase B), a serine/threonine kinase. Activation of PI3-Akt cascade stimulates B-cell lymphoma 2 (Bcl-2) family members, which act as anti-apoptotic factors. It has been shown that Fyn, a member of the non-receptor type Src tyrosine kinase family, is associated with α7 nAChRs, though it is not clear whether other Src family members are involved in the cascade downstream of nAChRs. A relationship between nAChRs and Fyn was also implicated in a study, showing that catecholamine release induced by nicotine was dependent on the presence of Fyn and extracellular Ca^{2+} (Allen et al. 1996). In the study by Kihara et al. (2001), an inhibitor of Src tyrosine kinase reduced Akt phosphorylation. In addition, PI3K and Fyn were physically associated with α7 nAChRs. These findings suggest that nAChR stimulation causes Akt phosphorylation via signal transduction through Fyn to PI3K. Ca^{2+} influx through the α7 nAChR ion channels might contribute to this process. It has been proposed that PI3K-Akt activation leads to up-regulation of Bcl-2 to promote neuronal survival (Matsuzaki et al. 1999; Kihara et al. 2001).

The intracellular signal pathway downstream of CNS nAChRs is known as a major pathway of neuroprotective action of neurotrophins including nerve growth factor (NGF) and brain-derived neurotrophic factor (BDNF) (Dajas-Bailador and Wonnacott 2004; Lim et al. 2008). NGF and BDNF are known to affect survival and differentiation of central and peripheral neurons. The PI3K/Akt signaling cascades play a key role in neuronal survival due to neurotrophins (Chan et al. 2014). It has been reported that NGF and BDNF prevent glutamate neurotoxicity in a time-dependent manner, exhibiting significant neuroprotection in a period >1 h (Shimohama et al. 1993a, b; Kume et al. 1997, 2000). Each neurotrophin interacts with specific tropomyosin receptor kinase (Trk) receptors. Trk receptors show selectivity to members of the neurotrophin family. TrkA, TrkB, and TrkC serve as preferential receptors for NGF, BDNF, and neurotrophin-3, respectively (Kalb 2005). In contrast to these high-affinity receptors, the low-affinity neurotrophin receptor, p75, interacts with all neurotrophin members. BDNF promotes survival of neurons via TrkB in several brain regions including the cerebral cortex. Moreover, nAChRs appear to transduce survival signals similar to signals downstream of the Trk receptors of neurotrophins (Dajas-Bailador and Wonnacott 2004). Thus, nicotine and neurotrophins show similar properties in terms of time-course and signal pathways of neuroprotection.

1.5 Acetylcholinesterase Inhibitors Used for Treatment of Alzheimer' Disease

The finding that glutamate neurotoxicity is suppressed by continuous stimulation of nAChRs suggests a possible function of the nicotinic cholinergic system as a factor promoting neuron survival in the CNS. AChE inhibitors including donepezil, which easily permeates the blood–brain barrier, are used for Alzheimer's disease. Takada et al. (2003) reported that in cultured cortical neurons, AChE inhibitors including donepezil, galantamine, and tacrine inhibited glutamate neurotoxicity, though concomitant addition of AChE inhibitors and glutamate did not exhibit neuroprotection. Neuroprotective effects of AChE inhibitors were antagonized by N_n and CNS AChR antagonists including mecamylamine and methyllycaconitine, but not by a mAChR antagonist, scopolamine. Thus, AChE inhibitors appeared to possess neuroprotective effects similar to properties of nicotinic neuroprotection. AChE inhibitors such as donepezil remarkably suppress apoptosis of neurons induced by long-term administration of low concentrations of glutamate. Investigation of the involvement of PI3K on the protective action of AChE inhibitors revealed that the neuroprotective action of donepezil and galantamine is associated with Fyn, Janus Activating Kinase 2 (JAK2), and PI3K (Takada-Takatori et al. 2006; Akaike et al. 2010). In addition, these central AChE inhibitors promoted phosphorylation of Akt and increased the expression level of Bcl-2 protein. These results indicate that the PI3K-Akt signaling pathway is important for protection mechanisms of AChE inhibitors.

nAChRs are also recognized as major functional molecules mediating pharmacological action of tobacco smoking. Nicotine is a major ingredient of tobacco and stimulates all subtypes of nAChRs, though nicotine induces more rapid desensitization of nAChRs than ACh (Albuquerque et al. 2009). Several clinical studies have shown a negative correlation between prevalence of sporadic Parkinson's disease and smoking history in relation to nAChR and neurodegenerative diseases, although no clear conclusion can be reached as to the relationship between Alzheimer's disease and smoking (Godwin-Austen et al. 1982; Tanner et al. 2002; Ulrich et al. 1997). Moreover, galantamine, possessing allosteric potentiating action on α7 nAChR, is used as a treatment for Alzheimer's disease (Albuquerque et al. 2001; Santos et al. 2002). Interestingly, long-term tobacco smoking or nicotine application induces up-regulation of nAChRs and, in most cases, facilitates their functions (Brody et al. 2013; Govind et al. 2009). This phenomenon is quite unique because, in most neuronal receptors including mAChRs, long-term receptor stimulation by specific agonists usually induces down-regulation of receptors and reduction of receptor functions. Moreover, AChE inhibitors including donepezil induce significant up-regulation of nAChRs (Kume et al. 2005; Takada-Takatori et al. 2010). Activation of the PI3-Akt pathway is necessary for nAChR up-regulation following long-term donepezil exposure. Receptor up-regulation following long-term exposure to nicotine and AChE inhibitors may be linked to diverse properties of nAChRs, from enhancement of learning and memory to addiction and neuroprotection, although precise mechanisms of up-regulation are not fully understood.

1.6 Conclusion

Nicotine induces fast nAChR currents of the order of milliseconds, while sustained nicotine exposure induces delayed intracellular responses. Neuroprotection is one of the dominant delayed responses mediated by CNS nAChRs. Mechanisms of neuroprotective effects exerted by persistent nAChR stimulation cannot be described only by simple excitatory reactions following depolarization induced by ion channel openings, but rather by activation of the intracellular PI3K-Akt signaling pathway leading to up-regulation of the anti-apoptotic protein Bcl-2. α7 nAChR, which shows high Ca^{2+} permeability, plays a crucial role in nicotinic neuroprotection. The metabolic change with Ca^{2+} as the second messenger may play an important role in triggering signals downstream of nAChRs. Therefore, it can be proposed that nAChRs are apparently implicated in two types of cellular functions; one for fast depolarization and the other for slow intracellular responses leading to neuroprotection (Fig. 1.4). Nicotine and other nAChR agonists evoke both acute and delayed responses; the former involves receptor desensitization and the latter involves receptor up-regulation. On the other hand, AChE inhibitors directly or indirectly stimulate nAChRs without evoking apparent acute responses (Akaike et al. 2010; Takada-Takatori et al. 2010). Neuroprotection and nAChR up-regulation by long-term exposure to AChE inhibitors, used in treatment of Alzheimer's disease, suggest that CNS nAChRs are an important component of defense mechanisms of neurons

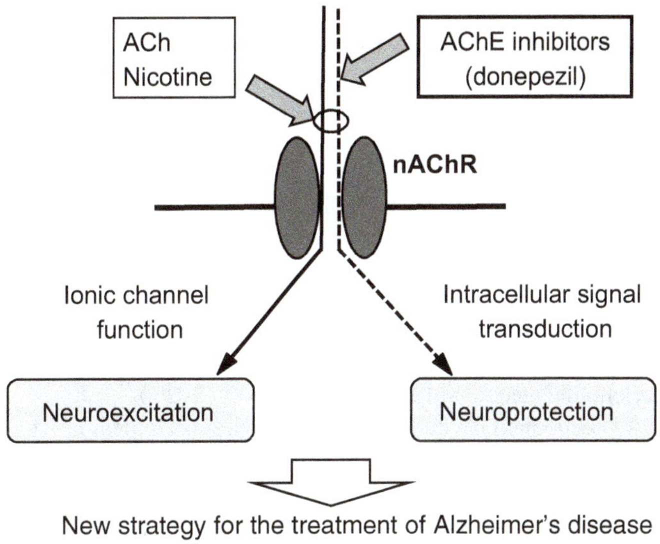

Fig. 1.4 Schematic representation of presumed roles of the nicotinic acetylcholine receptor (nAChR) in the central nervous system (CNS). Acetylcholine (ACh) and nicotine act on CNS nAChR to exert both neuroexcitation via ionic channel function and neuroprotection via intracellular signal transduction. Acetylcholinesterase (AChE) inhibitors such as donepezil exert neuroprotection without exhibiting neuroexcitation

against risk factors of neurodegeneration in pathophysiological conditions. Manipulation of neuroprotective properties of nAChRs may be a novel therapeutic approach for treatment of neurodegenerative diseases including Alzheimer's disease.

References

Aizenman E, Tang LH, Reynolds IJ (1991) Effects of nicotinic agonists on the NMDA receptor. Brain Res 551:355–357

Akaike N, Harata N, Tateishi N (1991) Modulatory action of cholinergic drugs on *N*-methyl-D-aspartate response in dissociated rat nucleus basalis of Meynert neurons. Neurosci Lett 130:243–247

Akaike A, Tamura Y, Yokota T et al (1994) Nicotine-induced protection of cultured cortical neurons against *N*-methyl-D-aspartate receptor-mediated glutamate cytotoxicity. Brain Res 644:181–187

Akaike A, Takada-Takatori Y, Kume T et al (2010) Mechanisms of neuroprotective effects of nicotine and acetylcholinesterase inhibitors: role of α4 and α7 receptors in neuroprotection. J Mol Neurosci 40:211–216. https://doi.org/10.1007/s12031-009-9236-1

Albuquerque EX, Santos MD, Alkondon M (2001) Modulation of nicotinic receptor activity in the central nervous system: a novel approach to the treatment of Alzheimer disease. Alzheimer Dis Assoc Disord 5(Suppl 1):S19–S25

Albuquerque EX, Pereira FR, Alkondon M et al (2009) Mammalian acetylcholine receptors: from structure to function. Physiol Rev 89:73–120

Alkondon M, Pereira EF, Albuquerque EX (1998) α-bungarotoxin- and methyllycaconitine-sensitive nicotinic receptors mediate fast synaptic transmission in interneurons of rat hippocampal slices. Brain Res 810:257–263

Allen CM, Ely CM, Juaneza MA et al (1996) Activation of Fyn tyrosine kinase upon secretagogue stimulation of bovine chromaffin cells. J Neurosci Res 44:421–429

Brassai A, Suvanjeiev RG, Bán E et al (2015) Role of synaptic and nonsynaptic glutamate receptors in ischemia induced neurotoxicity. Brain Res Bull 112:1–6. https://doi.org/10.1016/j.brainresbull.2014.12.007

Brody AL, Mukhin AG, La Charite J et al (2013) Up-regulation of nicotinic acetylcholine receptors in menthol cigarette smokers. Int J Neuropsychopharmacol 16:957–966. https://doi.org/10.1017/S1461145712001022

Caulfield MP, Birdsall NJ (1998) International Union of Pharmacology. XVII. Classification of muscarinic acetylcholine receptors. Pharmacol Rev 50:279–290

Chan KM, Gordon T, Zochodne DW et al (2014) Improving peripheral nerve regeneration: from molecular mechanisms to potential therapeutic targets. Exp Neurol 261:826–835. https://doi.org/10.1016/j.expneurol.2014.09.006

Dajas-Bailador F, Wonnacott S (2004) Nicotinic acetylcholine receptors and the regulation of neuronal signaling. Trends Pharmacol Sci 25:317–324

Dajas-Bailador FA, Lima PA, Wonnacott S (2000) The α7 nicotinic acetylcholine receptor subtype mediates nicotine protection against NMDA excitotoxicity in primary hippocampal cultures through a Ca^{2+} dependent mechanism. Neuropharmacology 39:2799–2807

Dani JA (2015) Neuronal nicotinic acetylcholine receptor structure and function and response to nicotine. Int Rev Neurobiol 124:3–19. https://doi.org/10.1016/bs.irn.2015.07.001

de Jonge WJ, Ulloa L (2007) The α7 nicotinic acetylcholine receptor as a pharmacological target for inflammation. Br J Pharmacol 151:915–929

Duggan LL, Choi DW (1994) Excitotoxicity, free radicals, and cell membrane changes. Ann Neurol 35(Suppl):S17–S21

Egea J, Buendia I, Parada E et al (2015) Anti-inflammatory role of microglial α7 nAChRs and its role in neuroprotection. Biochem Pharmacol 97:463–472. https://doi.org/10.1016/j.bcp.2015.07.032

Exley R, Cragg SJ (2008) Presynaptic nicotinic receptors: a dynamic and diverse cholinergic filter of striatal dopamine neurotransmission. Br J Pharmacol 153(Suppl 1):S283–S297

Fändrich M, Schmidt M, Grigorieff N (2011) Recent progress in understanding Alzheimer's β-amyloid structures. Trends Biochem Sci 36:338–345. https://doi.org/10.1016/j.tibs.2011.02.002

Frazier CJ, Buhler AV, Weiner JL et al (1998) Synaptic potentials mediated via α-bungarotoxin-sensitive nicotinic acetylcholine receptors in rat hippocampal interneurons. J Neurosci 18:8228–8235

Fujii T, Mashimo M, Moriwaki Y et al (2017) Expression and function of the cholinergic system in immune cells. Front Immunol 8:1085. https://doi.org/10.3389/fimmu.2017.01085

Godwin-Austen RB, Lee PN, Marmot MG, Stern GM (1982) Smoking and Parkinson's disease. J Neurol Neurosurg Psychiatry 45:577–581

Govind AP, Vezina P, Green WN (2009) Nicotine-induced upregulation of nicotinic receptors: underlying mechanisms and relevance to nicotine addiction. Biochem Pharmacol 78:756–765. https://doi.org/10.1016/j.bcp.2009.06.011

Jurado-Coronel JC, Avila-Rodriguez M, Capani F et al (2016) Targeting the nicotinic acetylcholine receptors (nAChRs) in astrocytes as a potential therapeutic target in Parkinson's disease. Curr Pharm Des 22:1305–1311

Kalb R (2005) The protean actions of neurotrophins and their receptors on the life and death of neurons. Trends Neurosci 28:5–11

Kaneko S, Maeda T, Kume T et al (1997) Nicotine protects cultured cortical neurons against glutamate-induced cytotoxicity via α7-neuronal receptors and neuronal CNS receptors. Brain Res 765:135–140

Kenney JW, Gould TJ (2008) Modulation of hippocampus-dependent learning and synaptic plasticity by nicotine. Mol Neurobiol 38:101–121. https://doi.org/10.1007/s12035-008-8037-9

Kihara T, Shimohama S, Sawada H et al (1997) Nicotinic receptor stimulation protects neurons against β-amyloid toxicity. Ann Neurol 42:159–163

Kihara T, Shimohama S, Akaike A (1999) Effects of nicotinic receptor agonists on β -amyloid beta-sheet formation. Jpn J Pharmacol 79:393–396

Kihara T, Shimohama S, Sawada H et al (2001) α7 nicotinic receptor transduces signals to phosphatidylinositol 3-kinase to block A β-amyloid-induced neurotoxicity. J Biol Chem 276:13541–13546

Kume T, Kouchiyama H, Kaneko S et al (1997) BDNF prevents NO mediated glutamate cytotoxicity in cultured cortical neurons. Brain Res 765:200–204

Kume T, Nishikawa H, Tomioka H et al (2000) p75-mediated neuroprotection by NGF against glutamate cytotoxicity in cortical cultures. Brain Res 852:279–289

Kume T, Sugimoto M, Takada Y et al (2005) Up-regulation of nicotinic acetylcholine receptors by central-type acetylcholinesterase inhibitors in rat cortical neurons. Eur J Pharmacol 527:77–85

Lim JY, Park SI, Oh JH (2008) Brain-derived neurotrophic factor stimulates the neural differentiation of human umbilical cord blood-derived mesenchymal stem cells and survival of differentiated cells through MAPK/ERK and PI3K/Akt-dependent signaling pathways. J Neurosci Res 86:2168–2178. https://doi.org/10.1002/jnr.21669

Liu Q, Zhao B (2004) Nicotine attenuates beta-amyloid peptide-induced neurotoxicity, free radical and calcium accumulation in hippocampal neuronal cultures. Br J Pharmacol 141:746–754

Lukas RJ, Changeux J-P, Novere NL (1999) International Union of Pharmacology. XX. Current status of the nomenclature for nicotinic acetylcholine receptors and their subunits. Pharmacol Rev 51:397–401

Matsuzaki H, Tamatani M, Mitsuda N (1999) Activation of Akt kinase inhibits apoptosis and changes in Bcl-2 and Bax expression induced by nitric oxide in primary hippocampal neurons. J Neurochem 73:2037–2046

Mattson MP (1989) Acetylcholine potentiates glutamate-induced neurodegeneration in cultured hippocampal neurons. Brain Res 497:402–406

Meldrum B, Garthwaite J (1990) Excitatory amino acid neurotoxicity and neurodegenerative disease. Trends Pharmacol Sci 11:379–387

Molas S, DeGroot SR, Zhao-Shea R et al (2017) Anxiety and nicotine dependence: emerging role of the habenulo-interpeduncular axis. Trends Pharmacol Sci 38:169–180. https://doi.org/10.1016/j.tips.2016.11.001

Morioka N, Harano S, Tokuhara M et al (2015) Stimulation of α7 nicotinic acetylcholine receptor regulates glutamate transporter GLAST via basic fibroblast growth factor production in cultured cortical microglia. Brain Res 1625:111–120. https://doi.org/10.1016/j.brainres.2015.08.029

Nakamizo T, Kawamata J, Yamashita H et al (2005) Stimulation of nicotinic acetylcholine receptors protects motor neurons. Biochem Biophys Res Commun 330:1285–1289

Nees F (2015) The nicotinic cholinergic system function. Neuropharmacology 96(Pt B):289–301. https://doi.org/10.1016/j.neuropharm.2014.10.021

Ohnishi M, Katsuki H, Takagi M et al (2009) Long-term treatment with nicotine suppresses neurotoxicity of, and microglial activation by, thrombin in cortico-striatal slice cultures. Eur J Pharmacol 602:288–293. https://doi.org/10.1016/j.ejphar

Olney JW, Labruyere J, Wang G et al (1991) NMDA antagonist neurotoxicity: mechanism and prevention. Science 254:1515–1518

Parri HR, Hernandez CM, Dineley KT (2011) Research update: α7 nicotinic acetylcholine receptor mechanisms in Alzheimer's disease. Biochem Pharmacol 82:931–942. https://doi.org/10.1016/j.bcp.2011.06.039

Santos MD, Alkondon M, Pereira EF et al (2002) The nicotinic allosteric potentiating ligand galantamine facilitates synaptic transmission in the mammalian central nervous system. Mol Pharmacol 61:1222–1234

Shimohama S, Ogawa N, Tamura Y et al (1993a) Protective effect of nerve growth factor against glutamate-induced neurotoxicity in cultured cortical neurons. Brain Res 632:269–302

Shimohama S, Tamura Y, Akaike A et al (1993b) Brain-derived neurotrophic factor pretreatment exerts a partially protective effect against glutamate-induced neurotoxicity in cultured rat cortical neurons. Neurosci Lett 164:55–58

Shimohama S, Greenwald DL, Shafron DH et al (1998) Nicotinic α7 receptors protect against glutamate neurotoxicity and neuronal ischemic damage. Brain Res 779:359–363

Sine SM, Eagle AG (2006) Recent advances in Cys-loop receptor structure and function. Nature 440:448–455. https://doi.org/10.1038/nature04708

Takada Y, Yonezawa A, Kume T et al (2003) Nicotinic acetylcholine receptor-mediated neuroprotection by donepezil against glutamate neurotoxicity in rat cortical neurons. J Pharmacol Exp Ther 306:722–727

Takada-Takatori Y, Kume T, Sugimoto M et al (2006) Acetylcholinesterase inhibitors used in treatment of Alzheimer's disease prevent glutamate neurotoxicity via nicotinic acetylcholine receptors and phosphatidylinositol 3-kinase cascade. Neuropharmacology 51:474–486

Takada-Takatori Y, Kume T, Izumi Y et al (2010) Mechanisms of chronic nicotine treatment-induced enhancement of the sensitivity of cortical neurons to the neuroprotective effect of donepezil in cortical neurons. J Pharmacol Sci 112:265–272

Takeuchi H, Yanagida T, Inden M et al (2009) Nicotinic receptor stimulation protects nigral dopaminergic neurons in rotenone-induced Parkinson's disease models. J Neurosci Res 87:576–585. https://doi.org/10.1002/jnr.21869

Tanner CM, Goldman SM, Aston DA et al (2002) Smoking and Parkinson's disease in twins. Neurology 58:581–588

Toborek M, Son KW, Pudelko A et al (2007) ERK 1/2 signaling pathway is involved in nicotine-mediated neuroprotection in spinal cord neurons. J Cell Biochem 100:279–292

Tsetlin V, Kuzmin D, Kasheverov I (2011) Assembly of nicotinic and other Cys-loop receptors. J Neurochem 116:734–741. https://doi.org/10.1111/j.1471-4159.2010.07060

Ulrich J, Johannson-Locher G, Seiler WO et al (1997) Does smoking protect from Alzheimer's disease? Alzheimer-type changes in 301 unselected brains from patients with known smoking history. Acta Neuropathol 94:450–454

Wang HY, Lee DH, D'Andrea MR et al (2000) β-Amyloid$_{1-42}$ binds to α7 nicotinic acetylcholine receptor with high affinity. Implications for Alzheimer's disease pathology. J Biol Chem 275:5626–5632

Zoli M, Pistillo F, Gotti C (2015) Diversity of native nicotinic receptor subtypes in mammalian brain. Neuropharmacology 96(Pt B):302–311. https://doi.org/10.1016/j.neuropharm.2014.11.003

Chapter 2
In Vivo Imaging of Nicotinic Acetylcholine Receptors in the Central Nervous System

Masashi Ueda, Yuki Matsuura, Ryosuke Hosoda, and Hideo Saji

Abstract Nicotinic acetylcholine receptors (nAChRs) in the central nervous system are involved in higher brain function, i.e., memory, cognition, learning, among others. These receptors also exert various pharmacological effects, such as neuroprotection and antinociception. Therefore, elucidating the localization and/or expression level of nAChRs in the brain is useful to clarify functions regulated by nAChRs, under physiological and pathological conditions. "Molecular imaging" is a powerful tool that enables one to noninvasively obtain information from living subjects. Many signal types, such as, radiation, nuclear magnetic resonance, fluorescence, bioluminescence, and ultrasound, are commonly used for molecular imaging. Among them, nuclear medical molecular imaging, which uses radioactive imaging probes, has a great advantage due to its high sensitivity and the fact that it is a quantitative approach. Many nuclear medical imaging probes targeting nAChRs have been developed and some of them have successfully visualized nAChRs in the animal and human brain. Moreover, changes in nAChR density under pathological conditions have been detected in patients. This chapter summarizes the history and recent advance of nAChR imaging.

Keywords Molecular imaging · Radioactive probe · Positron emission tomography (PET) · Single-photon emission computed tomography (SPECT) · Nicotinic acetylcholine receptor · A-85380 · Alzheimer's disease

M. Ueda · Y. Matsuura · R. Hosoda
Graduate School of Medicine, Dentistry, and Pharmaceutical Science, Okayama University, Okayama, Japan
e-mail: mueda@cc.okayama-u.ac.jp; ph422132@s.okayama-u.ac.jp; p53u2dzh@s.okayama-u.ac.jp

H. Saji (✉)
Graduate School of Pharmaceutical Sciences, Kyoto University, Kyoto, Japan
e-mail: hsaji@pharm.kyoto-u.ac.jp

A. Akaike et al. (eds.), *Nicotinic Acetylcholine Receptor Signaling in Neuroprotection*, https://doi.org/10.1007/978-981-10-8488-1_2

2.1 Introduction

Nicotinic acetylcholine receptors (nAChRs) are pentameric ligand-gated ion channels. To date, a total of 17 subunits (α1–α10, β1–β4, γ, δ, and ε) have been identified (Nemecz et al. 2016) and nAChRs are formed from various combinations of these subunits. nAChRs are located in the central and peripheral nervous systems. In the central nervous system (CNS), nAChRs not only play a role in higher brain function, but also exert various pharmacological effects (Graef et al. 2011). The two major subtypes of nAChRs found in the mammalian CNS are heteromeric α4β2 nAChRs and homomeric α7 nAChRs (Terry et al. 2015). Therefore, assessing the localization and/or expression level of both subtypes in the CNS is of great interest since it enables us to elucidate the functions they regulate, under physiological and pathological conditions.

Molecular imaging is defined as the visualization, characterization, and measurement of biological processes at the molecular and cellular levels in humans and other living systems (Mankoff 2007). The localization and/or density of nAChRs in the human brain can be evaluated in a noninvasive way using molecular imaging techniques that specifically target nAChRs. Several imaging techniques, such as nuclear medical imaging, magnetic resonance imaging, optical imaging, and ultrasound, are commonly used for molecular imaging. Among them, nuclear medical molecular imaging, which uses radioactive imaging probes, is greatly advantageous due to its high sensitivity and the fact that it is a quantitative approach. The following imaging modalities are used for nuclear medical molecular imaging: positron emission tomography (PET) and single-photon emission computed tomography (SPECT). The principles and characteristics of PET and SPECT are summarized in the next section. Many probes for nAChR imaging using PET and SPECT have been developed. Some of them have successfully visualized nAChRs in the animal and human brain. Moreover, changes in nAChR density under pathological conditions have been detected in patients. The history and recent advances in molecular imaging that target nAChRs are summarized in later sections.

2.2 Nuclear Medical Imaging Modality

2.2.1 *Positron Emission Tomography (PET)*

PET is a nuclear medical imaging technique used to noninvasively acquire images that correspond to physiological and pathological functions in a living body.

Image acquisition using PET is initiated with the injection or inhalation of a positron-emitting radiopharmaceutical. The scan is started after a delay ranging from seconds to minutes to allow the transport to or uptake by the organ of interest. When the positron-emitting radioisotope decays, it emits a positron, which travels a

Table 2.1 Major radioisotopes used for positron emission tomography (PET) in a clinical setting

Radionuclide	Half-life
^{11}C	20.4 min
^{13}N	9.97 min
^{15}O	122 s
^{18}F	110 min

short distance before an electron-positron annihilation event occurs. This annihilation event produces two high-energy photons (511 keV) propagating in nearly opposite directions. Therefore, a PET detector targets the detection of this annihilation radiation of 511 keV. If two photons are detected within a short (~10 ns) time-window, an event is recorded along the line connecting the two detectors. Summing many such events results in quantities that approximate line integrals through the radioisotope distribution. No collimator is required for the PET scanner because collimation is done electronically, leading to relatively high sensitivity. If they are suitably calibrated, PET images yield quantitative estimates of the concentration of the radioactive imaging probe at specific locations within the body.

Non-radioactive carbon, nitrogen, oxygen, and fluorine generally consist in many compounds of biological interest and/or pharmaceuticals. Positron-emitting radionuclides of carbon, nitrogen, oxygen, and fluorine also exist, and can therefore be readily incorporated into a wide variety of useful radioactive imaging probes. Table 2.1 outlines several positron-emitting radioisotopes. This is, however, not an exhaustive list of positron-emitting radioisotopes, since many other positron-emitters have been recently produced on small medical cyclotrons with 10–20 MeV protons (Nickles 1991, 2003). The major disadvantage of PET is its cost. The short half-life of most positron emitting isotopes requires an on-site cyclotron, and the scanners themselves are significantly more expensive than single-photon cameras. Nevertheless, PET is widely used in research studies and there is growing clinical acceptance of its findings, primarily for the diagnosis and staging of cancer.

2.2.2 *Single-Photon Emission Computed Tomography (SPECT)*

Most of the clinical procedures using tracers to visualize specific tissue binding sites is performed using planar gamma-camera imaging, SPECT, and PET. Even after the recent explosive growth of clinical PET, the imaging of single-photon emitting radiopharmaceuticals with gamma cameras, both in planar mode or with SPECT, constitutes the largest fraction of clinical nuclear medicine. Many clinically established radiopharmaceuticals for SPECT are commercially available and are commonly used in imaging departments. Single-photon emitting radionuclides that are used as labels for tracer molecules often have sufficiently long half-lives to

Table 2.2 Major radioisotopes used for single-photon emission computed tomography (SPECT) in a clinical setting

Radionuclide	Half-life (h)	Gamma ray energy (keV)
^{67}Ga	78.3	93, 185, 300
^{99m}Tc	6.01	141
^{111}In	67.3	171, 245
^{123}I	13.3	159

allow the long-distance transportation. Alternatively, they can be obtained on site via generator systems. Tracers for SPECT can often be readily prepared on site using commercial reagents and kits. Therefore, in contrast with PET, the infrastructure associated with cyclotron production is not required.

A key element of the SPECT camera is its collimator design, which eliminates all photons that are not traveling normal to the detector surface. The presence of a collimator limits the direction of the incoming photons. Without this, it becomes extremely difficult to determine the origin of detected photons. The collimator design largely determines not only the overall spatial resolution but also the radiation count efficiency of the system. The challenge, however, is that increasing the efficiency by expanding hole size of the collimator, will result in a low resolution. Further, the low sensitivity and efficiency mean that studies must be acquired for a relatively long time to accumulate sufficient counts. The only alternative would be to increase the administered activity, but this is limited by the radiation dose administered to the patient.

Radionuclides for SPECT have a relatively longer half-life than those for PET. It is preferential to have medium gamma ray energy (100–200 keV) for SPECT imaging. It is well recognized that PET has a higher resolution, higher sensitivity, and a better quantitation capability than SPECT. However, more hospitals are equipped with SPECT scanners, making the use of SPECT as a routine procedure more practical. Commonly used radionuclides for SPECT imaging are listed in Table 2.2.

2.3 Imaging Probes for Nicotinic Acetylcholine Receptors

2.3.1 Imaging Probes for the α4β2 Subtype

Many efforts have been dedicated to the development of PET and SPECT probes targeting α4β2 nAChRs. Several probes have been successfully used to noninvasively image α4β2 nAChRs in the brains of healthy people and also detect changes in the expression of α4β2-nAChR in the brains of patients with various diseases. Based on the structure of the parent compound, the probes can roughly be classified as follows: nicotine, A-85380, and epibatidine. The characteristics of these probes are summarized in this section and their chemical structures are shown in Fig. 2.1.

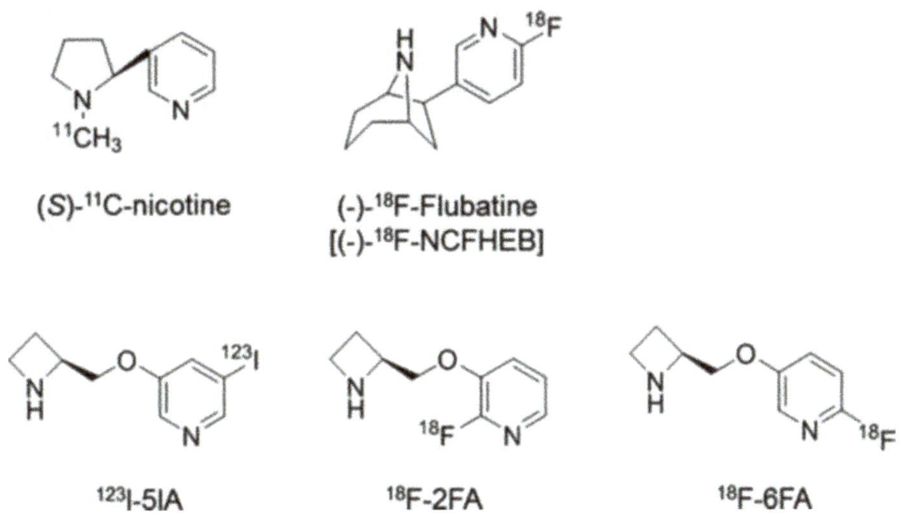

Fig. 2.1 Chemical structures of imaging probes targeting α4β2 nicotinic acetylcholine receptors (nAChRs)

2.3.1.1 Nicotine Derivatives

Nicotine was firstly selected as a parent backbone to visualize nAChRs. Saji et al. synthesized (*S*)- and (*R*)-^{11}C-nicotine by methylation of (*S*)- and (*R*)-nornicotine, respectively, using ^{11}C-methyl iodide. They then evaluated its biodistribution in mice. After an injection of (*S*)-^{11}C-nicotine, the order of regional uptake of radioactivity was as follows: cortex > thalamus > striatum > cerebellum. This uptake was displaced by the treatment of excess amount of unlabeled (*S*)-nicotine, but not by (*R*)-nicotine. (*R*)-^{11}C-nicotine showed less uptake and regional differences in the brain than (*S*)-^{11}C-nicotine (Saji et al. 1992). Nordberg et al. reported similar results using PET imaging in the rhesus monkey. After an injection of (*S*)-^{11}C-nicotine, the radioactivity in the brain peaked within 1–2 min and then rapidly declined. The highest accumulation of the probe was found in the occipital cortex and thalamus, while an intermediate and low accumulation of probe was found in the frontal cortex and white matter, respectively. Pretreatment with (*S*)-nicotine decreased the uptake of (*S*)-^{11}C-nicotine by 30%. In contrast, there was no regional difference in the distribution of (*R*)-^{11}C-nicotine (Nordberg et al. 1989). These findings indicated the specific binding of (*S*)-^{11}C-nicotine to nAChRs in vivo. However, it the amount of specific binding is low and results of (*S*)-^{11}C-nicotine in human PET studies are controversial.

2.3.1.2 A-85380 Derivatives

A-85380 [3-(2(*S*)-azetidinylmethoxy)pyridine] was developed in Abbott Laboratories. It showed 25-fold greater affinity to α4β2 nAChRs than nicotine did. The affinity of A-85380 to α4β2 nAChRs was comparable to that of epibatidine.

However, compared to the affinity of epibatidine, the affinities of A-85380 to other nicotinic receptor subtypes, such as α3β4, α7, and muscle type, were tenfold or less (Sullivan et al. 1996; Rueter et al. 2006). Therefore, A-85380 is a more α4β2-nAChR specific ligand than epibatidine. To date, radioiodinated and radiofluorinated A-85380 derivatives have been developed as SPECT and PET imaging probes, respectively, targeting α4β2 nAChRs.

A-85380-Derived SPECT Probe

The introduction of ^{123}I into five-position of pyridine ring of A-85380 yielded 5-[^{123}I]iodo-A-85380 (^{123}I-5IA) for SPECT imaging of α4β2 nAChRs. The affinity of $^{123/125}$I-5IA for α4β2 nAChRs was as extremely high (Ki = 10 pM) as that of epibatidine (Ki = 8 pM), when evaluated using rat brain homogenates. In contrast, the Ki values of 5IA for α3β4, α7, and muscle-type were 51, 250, and 1400 nM, respectively. Thus, the affinity ratios of α4β2-to-other subtype were calculated with 5100, 25,000, and 140,000, respectively (Mukhin et al. 2000). These results indicated that, despite the introduction of iodine to the parent backbone, ^{123}I-5IA maintained both the affinity and selectivity to α4β2 nAChRs.

In a biodistribution study in mice, the highest amount of ^{125}I-5IA accumulated in the thalamus (14.9% injected dose per gram of tissue [ID/g] at 60 min), while the accumulation was moderate in the cortex (8.5%ID/g at 60 min) and lowest in the cerebellum (2.4%ID/g at 60 min). Pretreatment with nAChR agonists (A-85380, (*S*)-nicotine, or cytisine) significantly reduced the accumulation of ^{125}I-5IA in the brain (Musachio et al. 1998). Saji et al. reported similar results in a study using rats. After injection of ^{125}I-5IA, the order of regional accumulation of radioactivity was followed: thalamus > cortex > striatum > cerebellum. This regional distribution was highly correlated with the nAChR density, which was determined using in vitro [^{3}H]cytisine binding. Further, SPECT imaging with ^{123}I-5IA clearly visualized the common marmoset brain. The radioactivity accumulation in the thalamus, which was higher than that in the cerebellum, decreased to the cerebellar level after the administration of cytisine (Saji et al. 2002). SPECT imaging of α4β2 nAChRs in the baboon brain was also successfully performed (Musachio et al. 1999; Fujita et al. 2000).

For the toxicity assessment of 5IA, behavior and physiological parameters (i.e., respiratory rate, heart rate, arterial blood pressure, and blood gas parameters) were examined. ICR mice that were injected intravenously 10 μg/kg of 5IA showed transient decrease in spontaneous locomotion. SD rats intravenously injected 5IA at 2 μg/kg and 5 μg/kg tended to have an increased respiratory rate. Conversely, no abnormal behavior was observed in mice injected 1 μg/kg of 5IA and their physiological parameters were maintained at normal levels. Therefore, the no observed effect level (NOEL) of 5IA was considered as 1 μg/kg (Ueda et al. 2004).

A-85380-Derived PET Probes

Two types of A-85380-based PET probes have been developed, i.e., 2-[^{18}F]fluoro-A-85380 (^{18}F-2FA) and 6-[^{18}F]fluoro-A-85380 (^{18}F-6FA). Both probes show promising properties for in vivo imaging of $\alpha4\beta2$ nAChRs.

The Ki value of ^{18}F-2FA, which was determined in rat brain homogenates, using in vitro competitive binding assay with ^{3}H-epibatidine, was 46 pM (Koren et al. 1998). The radioactivity accumulation in the thalamus and cerebellum, at 60 min after intravenous injection of ^{18}F-2FA, was approximately 6%ID/g and 1%ID/g, respectively, (Horti et al. 1998). These values were approximately half a degree of ^{125}I-5IA, indicating lower brain penetration of ^{18}F-2FA compared to $^{123/125}$I-5IA. An in vivo blocking study performed in rats revealed that pretreatment with $\alpha4\beta2$-nAChR ligands (nicotine, epibatidine, cytisine, or non-radioactive 2FA) reduced regional brain uptake of ^{18}F-2FA by 45–85%. Conversely, pretreatment with $\alpha7$-nAChR ligand (methyllycaconitine) and 5-hydroxytryptamine-3 (5-HT_3)-receptor ligand (granisetron) did not affect the accumulation of ^{18}F-2FA (Doll et al. 1999). Therefore, it was proved that ^{18}F-2FA specifically bound to $\alpha4\beta2$ nAChRs in vivo. Approximately twofold higher radioactivity was accumulated in the thalamus compared to the cerebellum in a PET imaging study performed using baboons (Valette et al. 1999). A toxicological study showed that intravenous injection of 2FA (0.8–10 μmol/kg) caused abnormal behavior in mice. However, a tracer dose (approximately 1 nmol/kg) of ^{18}F-2FA did not show signs of toxicity (Horti et al. 1998). Moreover, 2FA demonstrated no mutagenic properties evaluated by micronucleus and Ames tests (Valette et al. 2002).

The Ki value of ^{18}F-6FA was 25 pM determined by in vitro competitive binding assay using ^{3}H-epibatidine and rat brain homogenates (Koren et al. 1998). The brain uptake of ^{18}F-6FA was slight higher than that of ^{18}F-2FA. The radioactivity accumulation in the thalamus and cerebellum was approximately 8%ID/g and 1.5%ID/g, respectively, at 60 min after intravenous injection. Pretreatment with $\alpha4\beta2$-nAChR ligands (nicotine and cytisine) reduced regional brain uptake of ^{18}F-6FA by 44–92% (Scheffel et al. 2000). There was a higher accumulation of ^{18}F-6FA in the thalamus than the cerebellum on PET imaging of the baboon brain. Compared with ^{18}F-2FA, the peak uptake was similar for both tracers. However, compared to ^{18}F-2FA, ^{18}F-6FA showed slightly faster kinetics (peak uptake in the thalamus was at 55–65 min and 60–80 min after the injection of ^{18}F-6FA and ^{18}F-2FA, respectively) and better contrast (thalamus-to-cerebellum ratio at 180 min was 2.5–3.5 and 1.9–2.1 for ^{18}F-6FA and ^{18}F-2FA, respectively) (Ding et al. 2000). However, one drawback of ^{18}F-6FA compared to ^{18}F-2FA may be its associated toxicity. Although a tracer dose (0.3 nmol/kg) of ^{18}F-6FA showed no signs of toxicity, higher doses (1.3 μmol/kg) of it induced increase in breathing and heart rate and severe seizures, while doses of 2.0 μmol/kg led to certain, immediate death. The approximate LD_{50} dose for intravenously injected 6FA was estimated to be 1.74 μmol/kg, which was approximately one-ninth that of 2FA (15 μmol/kg) in mice (Scheffel et al. 2000).

2.3.1.3 Epibatidine Derivatives

Epibatidine is an alkaloid that was isolated from the Ecuadorian poison frog *Epipedobates anthonyi* in 1992 (Fitch et al. 2010). It is one of the most potent nAChR agonists. Its agonistic potency is greater than that of A-85380 and nicotine (Anderson et al. 2000). Several epibatidine-based imaging probes have been developed, and one of them, (−)-^{18}F-flubatine, was recently applied in a first-in-human study.

(−)-^{18}F-flubatine is formally known as (−)-^{18}F-norchloro-fluoro-homoepibatidine [(−)-^{18}F-NCFHEB]. This probe was first reported in 2004. The binding affinity of (+)-enantiomer (Ki = 64 pM) and (−)-enantiomer (Ki = 112 pM) to human α4β2 nAChRs was five to ten times lower than that of epibatidine (Ki = 14 pM). However, given that the affinity of both enantiomers to human α3β4 nAChR was 65 times lower than that of epibatidine, this resulted in a 14-fold increase in α4β2 nAChR-specificity of flubatine compared to epibatidine (Deuther-Conrad et al. 2004). In a biodistribution study in mice, the brain uptake of (+)-^{18}F-flubatine (7.45%ID/g at 20 min) and (−)-^{18}F-flubatine (5.60%ID/g at 20 min) was greater than that of ^{18}F-2FA (3.20%ID/g at 20 min). Pre- and co-injection of 2FA decreased the brain uptake of (−)-^{18}F-flubatine by approximately 60%, indicating specific binding of (−)-^{18}F-flubatine to α4β2 nAChRs in vivo (Deuther-Conrad et al. 2008). The results of PET imaging with ^{18}F-flubatine in the porcine brain corroborated with the results of a biodistribution study performed in mice. The brain uptake was highest for (+)-^{18}F-flubatine, intermediate for (−)-^{18}F-flubatine, and lowest for ^{18}F-2FA, in all the examined regions (i.e., the thalamus, caudate/putamen, and cerebellum). Among these three probes, (−)-^{18}F-flubatine showed the fastest equilibrium of specific binding (Brust et al. 2008). Since the drawback of using ^{18}F-2FA in clinical PET studies is its slow kinetics, (−)-^{18}F-flubatine has the potential to overcome this challenge. PET imaging in the rhesus monkey revealed that the regional distribution of (−)-^{18}F-flubatine (i.e., thalamus > cortex/striatum > cerebellum) corroborated with the known distribution of α4β2 nAChRs: (Hockley et al. 2013). The toxicological effects of flubatine were evaluated by extended single dose toxicity studies. Wistar rats were intravenously injected with (−)-flubatine, at a dose of 24.8 μg/kg or more, and with (+)-flubatine, at a dose of 12.4 μg/kg or more, presented with symptoms that included tachypnea, labored breathing, and cyanosis. However, no symptoms were detected in rats injected (−)-flubatine and (+)-flubatine, at a dose of 6.2 μg/kg and 1.55 μg/kg, respectively. Therefore, the NOEL of (−)- and (+)-flubatine was considered as 6.2 and 1.55 μg/kg, respectively (Smits et al. 2014).

2.3.2 *Imaging Probes for the α7 Subtype*

Compared to α4β2-nAChR imaging probes, several promising probes were not as effective at targeting α7 nAChRs. However, the chemical structure of some probes that reached first-in-human studies is outlined in Fig. 2.2.

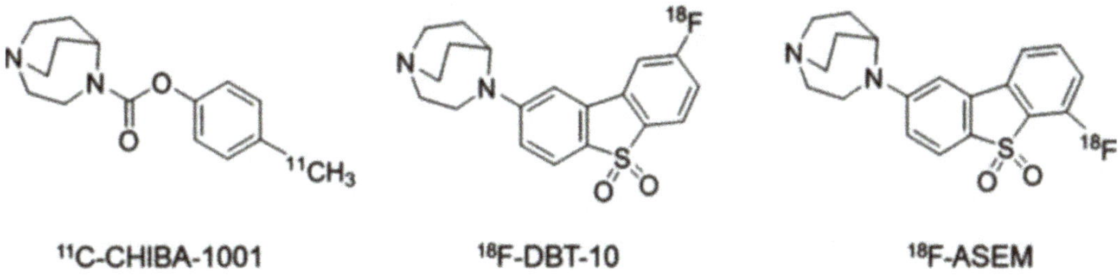

Fig. 2.2 Chemical structures of imaging probes targeting α7 nicotinic acetylcholine receptors (nAChRs)

^{11}C-CHIBA-1001 is the first α7-nAChR imaging probe to be used in humans (Toyohara et al. 2009). The IC_{50} value of CHIBA-1001 for ^{125}I-α-bungarotoxin, which is a selective antagonist for α7 nAChRs binding to rat brain homogenates, was 45.8 nM, indicating the high affinity of CHIBA-1001 to α7 nAChRs. The distribution of radioactivity matched the regional distribution of α7 nAChRs in a PET imaging study using ^{11}C-CHIBA-1001 in a conscious monkey. Moreover, the uptake of ^{11}C-CHIBA-1001 in the brain was inhibited by pretreatment with SSR180711, a selective α7-nAChR agonist, in a dose-dependent manner. It was however, not affected by A-85380, a selective α4β2-nAChR agonist (Hashimoto et al. 2008). The percentage of inhibition after treatment of SSR180711 (5 mg/kg) was approximately 40%.

Two dibenzothiophene-based probes that show a high affinity to α7 nAChRs were recently developed. These probes are ^{18}F-ASEM and ^{18}F-DBT-10, which is a *para*-isomer of ^{18}F-ASEM. The Ki value of ASEM for ^{125}I-α-bungarotoxin binding to the HEK293 cells stably expressing α7 nAChRs was 0.3 nM. A PET imaging study of the baboon clearly demonstrated its highest uptake in the thalamus and the lowest in the cerebellum. The uptake of ^{18}F-ASEM in the baboon brain was inhibited by the injection of SSR180711, in a dose-dependent manner (Horti et al. 2014). The percentage of inhibition following SSR180711 (5 mg/kg) treatment was approximately 80%, which was greater than that of ^{11}C-CHIBA-1001.

In a binding assay using SH-SY5Y cells stably expressing α7 nAChRs and ^{3}H-methyllycaconitine, ^{18}F-DBT-10 demonstrated a high affinity (Ki = 0.60 nM) for α7 nAChRs, which was comparable to ^{18}F-ASEM (Ki = 0.84 nM). PET imaging of the rhesus monkey brain clearly revelated its highest uptake in the thalamus and lowest update in the cerebellum. The brain uptake of ^{18}F-DBT-10 was inhibited by the administration of ASEM, in a dose-dependent manner (Hillmer et al. 2016b). Hillmer et al. directly compared the in vivo kinetic properties of ^{18}F-ASEM and ^{18}F-DBT-10 in identical rhesus monkeys and concluded that the two radiotracers were highly similar (Hillmer et al. 2017).

2.4 Nicotinic Acetylcholine Receptor Imaging in Human Brain

2.4.1 (S)-^{11}C-Nicotine

There are contrary reports regarding whether (*S*)-^{11}C-nicotine show specific binding to nAChRs in the human brain. Nybäck et al. performed (*S*)- and (*R*)-^{11}C-nicotine-PET in healthy male smokers and nonsmokers. Although (*S*)-^{11}C-nicotine demonstrated a higher uptake than (*R*)-^{11}C-nicotine, the co-administration of nonradioactive (*S*)-nicotine did not affect the time-activity curves of (*S*)-^{11}C-nicotine. A kinetic analysis based on a two-compartment model revealed that the brain uptake of (*S*)-^{11}C-nicotine was mainly determined using cerebral blood flow (CBF) (Nyback et al. 1994). Muzic et al. performed a similar study and demonstrated that the pharmacokinetics of (*S*)-^{11}C-nicotine could be well described using a two-compartment model, which was in accordance with the findings of Nybäck et al. Although the (*S*)-nicotine challenge induced a significant decrease in the distribution volume (DV) of (*S*)-^{11}C-nicotine, this decrease was small (Muzic et al. 1998). Therefore, both research groups concluded that (*S*)-^{11}C-nicotine was not a suitable tracer for PET studies of nAChRs in the human brain.

In contrast, Nordberg et al. developed a method for kinetic analysis of (*S*)-^{11}C-nicotine including compensation for the influence of CBF. They determined the CBF of each participant using ^{11}C-butanol- or ^{15}O-water-PET and compensated the rate constant of (*S*)-^{11}C-nicotine transport from tissue to blood using the CBF. In this analysis, a low rate constant corresponded to high (*S*)-^{11}C-nicotine binding in the brain. They revealed that the CBF-compensated rate constants were significantly and negatively correlated with cognitive function of patients with Alzheimer's disease (Nordberg et al. 1995; Kadir et al. 2006).

2.4.2 ^{123}I-5IA

Fujita et al. performed SPECT imaging and quantified the α4β2 nAChRs in the human brain using ^{123}I-5IA. A total of six healthy nonsmokers (two men and four women) participated in both a bolus and bolus-plus-constant infusion (B/I) study. Although the B/I study was not successfully applied, due to the slow kinetics of ^{123}I-5IA, regional DV values were successfully measured in the bolus study. The researchers applied one- and two-tissue compartment models to determine kinetic parameters of ^{123}I-5IA. The two-tissue compartment model provided better goodness-of-fit than the one-tissue compartment model, but the difference in the goodness-of-fit was relatively small. The obtained DV values were well-correlated between the two models. The DV values determined by two-tissue compartment model were highest in the thalamus (51 mL/cm^3), intermediate in putamen (27 mL/cm^3) and pons (32 mL/cm^3), slightly lower in cortical regions (17–20 mL/cm^3) (Fujita et al. 2003b).

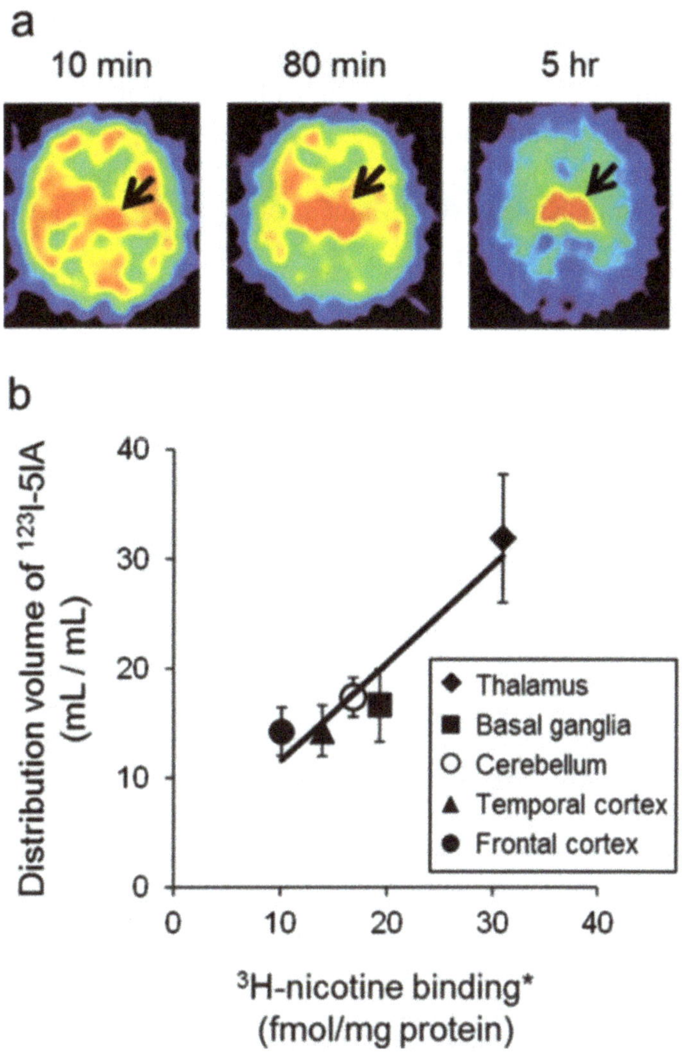

Fig. 2.3 Typical single-photon emission computed tomography (SPECT) images with ^{123}I-5IA and the correlation between distribution volumes of ^{123}I-5IA and reported nicotinic acetylcholine receptor (nAChR) density in the human brain. **(a)** Serial SPECT images obtained from a healthy human following the ^{123}I-5IA injection. Although blood flow-dependent distribution of radioactivity was observed at 10 min, the specificity of the radioactivity distribution for α4β2-nAChR in the thalamus (*the arrows*) could be distinguished in a time-dependent manner. **(b)** Correlation between distribution volumes (DV) of ^{123}I-5IA estimated using one-tissue compartment analysis and the reported nAChR density in the human brain. The Y-axis indicate DV values of ^{123}I-5IA and X-axis represent the α4β2 nAChR density in postmortem brains determined by ^{3}H-nicotine binding assay (Shimohama et al. 1986). The correlation coefficient was 0.95, indicating a highly significant correlation between the two parameters ($P < 0.05$)

Our research group also performed a similar study. Data from six healthy non-smokers (five men and one woman), imaged using ^{123}I-5IA-SPECT, were analyzed with kinetic (one- and two-tissue compartment models) and Logan graphical tests (Logan et al. 1990). Figure 2.3a shows representative serial SPECT images. In contrast to the study performed by Fujita et al., two-tissue compartment analysis could not provide adequate rate constants. However, one-tissue compartment analysis could fit the data appropriately and regional DV values were successfully determined.

The obtained DV values were the highest in the thalamus (34 mL/g), intermediate in basal ganglia (17 mL/g) and brain stem (25 mL/g), and slightly lower in cortical regions (13–14 mL/g). These data correlated well with the nAChR densities, which was measured using ^{3}H-nicotine (Fig. 2.3b, R = 0.95, $P < 0.05$), indicating the validity of the analysis method. Moreover, similar DV values were successfully estimated using a graphical analysis (Mamede et al. 2004).

2.4.3 ^{18}F-2FA

Data from seven healthy male volunteers were compared using a compartmental kinetic analysis and Logan graphical analysis to quantify regional cerebral DV values of ^{18}F-2FA. PET scans were performed up to 240 min after the administration of ^{18}F-2FA, but the maximal concentration could not always be observed in the thalamus due to the slow kinetics of ^{18}F-2FA. Kinetic analysis revealed that the two-tissue compartment model was more accurate than the one-tissue compartment model to describe the PET data. The obtained DV values were the highest in the thalamus (15 mL/mL), and lower in the cerebellum, striatum, and cortical regions (5–7 mL/mL). These data were consistent with the known densities of nAChRs in the human brain that were measured using ^{3}H-epibatidine. The DV values obtained by the Logan graphical analysis were slightly lower than those obtained by the two-tissue compartmental kinetic analysis. This could be attributed to noise-induced bias. Therefore, the two-tissue compartmental kinetic analysis seems a more reliable method to estimate regional DV values of ^{18}F-2FA (Gallezot et al. 2005).

A simplified analysis method has been developed to easily quantify $\alpha4\beta2$ nAChRs with ^{18}F-2FA-PET. Ten normal volunteers (six men and four women) were recruited for 2-h PET scan. Simplified DV values were defined as the ratio of radioactivity in the brain to that in arterial plasma at 90–120 min post-injection. Two-tissue compartment and Logan graphical analyses were also conducted on the data. DV values in the frontal cortex and cerebellum determined using the simplified method were significantly correlated with those calculated using the two-tissue compartment analysis and Logan graphical analysis ($r > 0.88$). Therefore, this simplified approach may be useful for quantifying cortical nAChRs and suitable for routine clinical application (Mitkovski et al. 2005).

2.4.4 (−)-^{18}F-Flubatine

A first-in-human PET study with (−)-^{18}F-Flubatine was reported in 2015 (Sabri et al. 2015). Dynamic PET imaging, lasting 270 min, was performed on 12 healthy male non-smoking participants, following a bolus injection of (−)-^{18}F-Flubatine intravenously. In humans, (−)-^{18}F-Flubatine is very stable against metabolism. Radiometabolite analysis of plasma demonstrated that almost 90% and 85% of

(−)-^{18}F-Flubatine existed in an intact form, at 90 min and 270 min after the injection, respectively. The tracer kinetics were well-described by both the one-tissue compartment and two-tissue compartment analyses, though the relative standard deviation of DV values determined by the two-tissue compartment analysis was much larger. The DV values were the highest in the thalamus (27 mL/cm^3), intermediate in regions like midbrain, striatum, and cerebellum (11–14 mL/cm^3), slightly lower in cortical regions (8–10 mL/cm^3), and lowest in the corpus callosum (6 mL/cm^3). These values were highly correlated with in vitro measurements of regional nAChR densities in the postmortem human brain using (±)-^{3}H-epibatidine (Marutle et al. 1998). DV values could be reliably estimated within 90 min for all the regions examined, demonstrating the faster kinetic property of (−)-^{18}F-Flubatine in humans.

Another research group performed (−)-^{18}F-Flubatine-PET in humans using a bolus-plus-infusion (B/I) paradigm, which could establish the true equilibrium between a probe in the plasma and at nAChRs in the brain. The DV values in the extrathalamic grey matter regions obtained from the B/I study corroborated well with those estimated by the two-tissue compartment analysis and multilinear analysis of the bolus data. The equilibrium in the thalamus, however, could not established under the B/I paradigm adopted in this study. The research group also assessed the probe's sensitivity to ACh fluctuations following physostigmine treatment in humans. PET acquisition with the B/I paradigm was performed and 1.5 mg of physostigmine was infused from 125 to 185 min. The DV values of (−)-^{18}F-Flubatine in the cortex, striatum, and cerebellum decreased by 2.8–6.5%. This difference was small since only a low dose to avoid peripheral side effects. However, this finding suggested that (−)-^{18}F-Flubatine is probably sensitive to changes in acetylcholine levels in humans (Hillmer et al. 2016a).

2.4.5 α7-nAChR Imaging Probes

^{11}C-CHIBA-1001 is the first α7-nAChR imaging probe to be used in humans. In the human brain, ^{11}C-CHIBA-1001 was widely distributed in all brain regions, including the cerebellum where uptake was low like in the monkey brain. This discrepancy could be attributed to species difference since it was in line with the result of a postmortem study, which demonstrated that the level of ^{125}I-α-bungarotoxin binding in the cerebellum was comparable to that in the cortex (Toyohara et al. 2009). Thus, this probe can be used to measure the occupancy rate of α7 nAChRs in the human brain. Ishikawa et al. examined the effect of tropisetron and ondansetron on PET imaging with ^{11}C-CHIBA-1001 in healthy non-smoking male participants. Tropisetron has a high affinity for both 5-HT$_3$ receptors and α7 nAChRs, while ondansetron only has a high affinity for 5-HT$_3$ receptors. Two serial PET scans were performed before and after an oral administration of these medications. Tropisetron decreased the total distribution volume of ^{11}C-CHIBA-1001 in the human brain, in a dose-dependent manner, while ondansetron had no effect (Ishikawa et al. 2011).

^{18}F-ASEM is another α7-nAChR imaging probe used in human PET imaging. The regional distribution of ^{18}F-ASEM in the brain was consistent with the expression of α7-nAChR in the post-mortem human brain. The cerebral cortex and putamen showed higher DV values (>20 mL/mL), while the caudate, cerebellum, and corpus callosum showed lower DV values (<15 mL/mL). Both one-tissue compartment and two-tissue compartment analyses fitted the data well and provided similar DV values. The average test-retest variability was 10.8%, indicating accurate estimation of DV values. However, this study was only performed on a limited number of participants (n = 2) (Wong et al. 2014). Another research group performed a ^{18}F-ASEM-PET in humans in 2017. In this study, one-tissue compartment analysis, rather than two-two compartment analysis, was the more suitable analysis method for the quantification of ^{18}F-ASEM kinetic parameters. However, since the one-tissue compartment analysis could produce a biased result in regions with high uptake of the probe, the authors finally chose a multilinear analysis method. The calculated DV values were higher in the cerebral cortex and putamen (>25 mL/cm^3) and lower in the caudate and cerebellum (19–21 mL/cm^3). The test-retest variability between the four participants was 11.7 ± 9.8% (Hillmer et al. 2017).

2.5 Alteration of Nicotinic Acetylcholine Receptor Density

2.5.1 Alzheimer's Disease (AD)

Memory impairment is the main symptom of AD, which is a progressive neurodegenerative disorder. Since nAChRs play a role in higher brain functions, such as cognition and memory, changes in the expression of nAChRs in AD is of great interest. Postmortem studies have demonstrated reduced activity of α4β2 nAChRs in patients with AD (Martin-Ruiz et al. 2000). O'Brien et al. recruited patients with AD, at the mild–moderate stages of illness and normal elderly controls, for a ^{123}I-5IA-SPECT study. Compared to that in the controls, significant reductions in ^{123}I-5IA binding were identified in the frontal cortex, striatum, and pons in patients with AD. There were no significant correlations with clinical or cognitive measures, which could be attributed to homogeneous stages of illness of the patients (O'Brien et al. 2007). In our study, DV values of ^{123}I-5IA in the cortical regions and thalamus in patients with AD were also decreased compared to that in age-matched healthy participants (Fig. 2.4) (Hashikawa et al. 2002; Ueda 2016).

AD is a progressive neurodegenerative disorder. The symptoms of AD are preceded by years of neurodegeneration in the brain. Mild cognitive impairment (MCI) is a clinically detectable initial stage of cognitive deficits and is considered as an intermediate state between healthy aging and AD. Therefore, if an nAChR abnormality is detected in patients with MCI, it will be an important biomarker at the earliest stage of the disease. It could consequently be used as a predictive biomarker to determine patients with MCI who are at risk for developing AD. Using ^{18}F-2FA-PET, Sabri et al. demonstrated a significant reduction in α4β2-nAChR availability

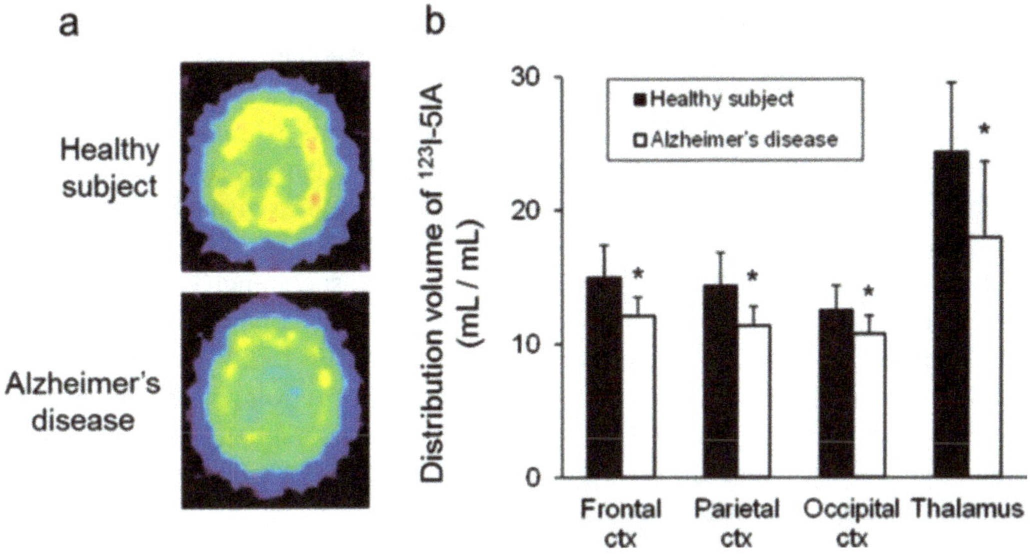

Fig. 2.4 Typical single-photon emission computed tomography (SPECT) images and mean distribution volumes of ^{123}I-5IA in age-matched healthy participant and patients with Alzheimer's disease (AD). (**a**) Representative ^{123}I-5IA SPECT images of an age-matched healthy participant and a patient with AD. (**b**) Mean distribution volumes of ^{123}I-5IA in age-matched healthy participants and patients with AD. Each bar represents an average of ten healthy participants and eight patients, and each error bar represents the SD (*$P < 0.05$ vs. healthy subject). *ctx* cortex

in the cortical regions, caudate head, and hippocampus, in patients with AD and MCI (Sabri et al. 2008). Kendziorra et al. also performed a ^{18}F-2FA-PET study on patients with MCI and AD, and age-matched healthy controls. The availability of α4β2-nAChR in the cortical regions, caudate, and hippocampus in patients with AD and MCI significantly decreased. More interestingly, compared to controls, patients with MCI who converted to AD showed a significantly low α4β2-nAChR availability in the above three regions. In contrast, the α4β2-nAChR availability of patients with MCI with stable cognitive course was also lower than that of controls, but the difference was not statistically significant (Kendziorra et al. 2011). However, other studies report conflicting results. The availability of α4β2 nAChRs in patients with MCI and at an early stage of AD were demonstrated to be maintained at a control level, using ^{123}I-5IA-SPECT (Mitsis et al. 2009) and ^{18}F-2FA-PET (Ellis et al. 2008).

2.5.2 *Other Causes of Dementia*

Although vascular dementia (VaD) is one of the most common causes of dementia in older people, the cholinergic involvement in VaD remains controversial. Some studies reported cholinergic loss (Gottfries et al. 1994), while others failed to demonstrate a cholinergic deficit in patients with VaD (Perry et al. 2005). Using ^{123}I-5IA-SPECT imaging, Colloby et al. demonstrated reductions in uptake of ^{123}I-5IA in the dorsal thalamus and right caudate of patients with VaD, compared to that in age-matched healthy participants (Colloby et al. 2011). Another study revealed that, overall, ^{125}I-5IA binding in postmortem brains did not significantly differ between patients with VaD and age-matched healthy participants (Pimlott et al. 2004). However, an 11% reduction in ^{125}I-5IA binding was also demonstrated in the dorsal thalamus of patients with VaD. Nonetheless, the small sample size may have reduced statistical power.

Dementia with Lewy bodies (DLB) is the second most common cause of degenerative dementia in older people. It is well-known that cholinergic deficits are involved in DLB. O'Brien et al. performed a ^{123}I-5IA-SPECT study in patients with DLB and similarly aged controls. Compared to that in controls, the uptake of ^{123}I-5IA were significantly reduced in the frontal, striatal, temporal, and cingulate regions of patients with DLB (O'Brien et al. 2008). These findings were consistent with the findings obtained by a ^{125}I-5IA binding study using postmortem brains, where a significant reduction of ^{125}I-5IA binding was also observed in the striatum, entorhinal cortex, and substantia nigra (Pimlott et al. 2004).

2.5.3 Parkinson's Disease (PD)

In addition to the dopaminergic system, cholinergic neurons also play an important role in PD. Postmortem studies demonstrated widespread decrease in the expression of nAChR in the cortical and striatal regions of patients with PD (Rinne et al. 1991). Fujita et al. successfully detected this decrease in living patients with PD using ^{123}I-5IA-SPECT. A decrease of 3–9% and 15% in DV values was found in the cortical regions and thalamus, respectively, in patients with PD. However, this decrease was small and not statistically significant compared to healthy participants (Fujita et al. 2006). Oishi et al. also reported similar results using ^{123}I-5IA-SPECT. Patients with PD demonstrated a statistically significant decrease (20–25%) in the brainstem and frontal cortex, compared with that in the control group (Oishi et al. 2007). The difference in the SPECT scan procedure and/or withdrawal duration of antiparkinsonian medication may account for the discrepancy of the results obtained by the two studies.

Using ^{18}F-2FA PET, Meyer et al. estimated DV values in each brain region of patients with PD and healthy volunteers. They used the corpus callosum as a reference region, and the binding potential (BP) was calculated as follows: BP = (DV value in each brain region)/(DV value in the corpus callosum) − 1 (Brody et al. 2006). The BP values in patients with PD were significantly decreased (30–50%) in broad brain regions, such as cortical regions, caudate nucleus, midbrain, and cerebellum (Meyer et al. 2009).

2.5.4 Other Diseases

2.5.4.1 Alcohol Abuse

Although ethanol binding sites have not been identified in nAChRs, prolonged alcohol exposure reportedly increased agonist binding to α4β2 nAChRs (Robles and Sabria 2006). Therefore, Esterlis et al. examined α4β2-nAChR availability in heavy drinking nonsmokers and age- and sex-matched control nonsmokers (Esterlis et al. 2010). The nine participants who met the criteria for current alcohol abuse and two subjects who met criteria for current alcohol dependence were included in the ^{123}I-5IA-SPECT study. There were no significant differences in the availability of α4β2-nAChR between the two groups. However, as the authors noted, a larger study is warranted to explore effects of heavy alcohol drinking. In fact, recent PET and SPECT studies performed in nonhuman primates indicated a decrease in α4β2-nAChR availability after chronic ethanol consumption (Cosgrove et al. 2010; Hillmer et al. 2014).

2.5.4.2 Autosomal Dominant Nocturnal Frontal Lobe Epilepsy

Nocturnal frontal lobe epilepsy is a common non-lesional focal epilepsy (Provini et al. 1999). There are more than a hundred families with autosomal dominant nocturnal frontal lobe epilepsy (ADNFLE) and mutations in the genes encoding the α4 or β2 subunit of nAChR have been identified in several ADNFLE families (Picard and Scheffer 2005). Therefore, Picard et al. performed ^{18}F-2FA-PET imaging to measure the density of α4β2 nAChRs in eight ADNFLE patients and seven age-matched participants (Picard et al. 2006). Participants in both groups were non-smokers. The DV values in patients with ADNFLE significantly increased in the epithalamus, ventral mesencephalon, and cerebellum, but decreased in the right dorsolateral prefrontal region. The downregulation of nAChR density in the prefrontal cortex is consistent with focal epilepsy involving the frontal lobe. The upregulation of nAChR density in the midbrain may be involved in the pathogenesis of ADNFLE through the role of cholinergic neurons ascending from the brainstem.

2.5.4.3 Major Depressive Disorders

Since hyperactivity of cholinergic neurons plays a pathophysiological role in depression (Dilsaver 1986), Saricicek et al. performed a ^{123}I-5IA-SPECT study in 23 non-smoking, medication-free patients with recurrent major depressive disorders (MDD) and 23 age- and sex-matched healthy controls (Saricicek et al. 2012). Compared to that in controls, patients with MDD had significantly lower availability of α4β2 nAChRs, across all the brain regions that were analyzed. However, there was no difference in the density of α4β2 nAChRs between patients with MDD and healthy controls in the human postmortem brain. This discrepancy could be attributed to the competitive inhibition of excess amount of endogenous ACh, which could have resulted from the effect of cholinergic hyperactivity on ^{123}I-5IA accumulation.

2.5.5 Smokers

Many studies have demonstrated the upregulation of nAChRs occurred in both nicotine-treated animals (Yates et al. 1995) and postmortem brains of smokers (Buisson and Bertrand 2002). This upregulation is transient, however, and the nAChR density returns to baseline level after a period of abstinence from nicotine treatment (Pietila et al. 1998). Thus, the non-invasive detection of nAChR in smokers is important to monitor the dynamics of nAChR expression, i.e., upregulation during smoking and downregulation after smoking cessation.

Staley et al. were the first to noninvasively detect higher levels of α4β2 nAChRs in smokers (Staley et al. 2006). They performed ^{123}I-5IA-SPECT imaging and demonstrated an approximate 30% increase in DV values in the cortex and striatum of smokers after 7 days of abstinence. A similar upregulation was observed in ^{18}F-2FA-PET studies; the amount of increase, however, varied and could be attributed to differences in the extent of smoking and/or duration of smoking cessation before the imaging studies (Mukhin et al. 2008; Brody et al. 2013). Brody et al. reported an interesting finding that the upregulation of nAChRs was more pronounced in menthol cigarette smokers compared to non-menthol cigarette smokers (Brody et al. 2013). Heavy use of caffeine (i.e., an average of four cups of coffee per day) or marijuana (i.e., an average of 22 days of use per month) also affected the α4β2-nAChR density in smokers. An approximate 20–40% increase in DV values was observed in the prefrontal cortex, thalamus, and brainstem in smokers with heavy caffeine or marijuana use compared to smokers who were non-users (Brody et al. 2016). However, it is possible that the findings were independent of smoking, because the changes were not examined in nonsmokers with heavy caffeine or marijuana use.

Our research group successfully imaged the dynamic changes of nAChR expression during smoking cessation. We performed ^{123}I-5IA-SPECT imaging on six nonsmokers and ten smokers who had quit smoking for 4 h, 10 days, and 21 days. Five smokers in the 4-h group were included in either the 10-day or 21-day group. Compared to the DV values in nonsmokers, those in the brains of smokers decreased by approximately 35% in the 4-h group, but increased by approximately 25% in the 10-day group. The DV values in the 21-day group were comparable to those of nonsmokers, indicating that the density of α4β2 nAChRs had returned to the baseline level (Fig. 2.5) (Mamede et al. 2007). The decrease in the DV values in the 4-h

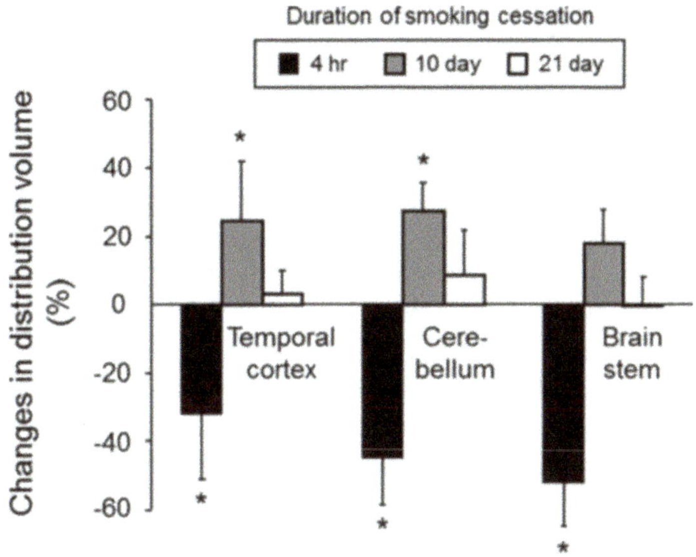

Fig. 2.5 Changes in the distribution volume of ^{123}I-5IA after smoking cessation. Compared to nonsmokers, the distribution volumes (DV) of ^{123}I-5IA of smokers at 4 h after ceasing smoking were significant lower, while those after 10-day cessation were significantly higher ($^{*}P < 0.05$ vs. nonsmoker). The increased DV values returned to nonsmoker levels 21 days after ceasing smoking

group could be attributed to competitive inhibition of nicotine derived from tobacco on the binding of ^{123}I-5IA to nAChRs. A ^{18}F-2FA-PET study demonstrated that just one to two puffs of smoking resulted in 50% occupancy of α4β2 nAChRs for 3.1 h after smoking (Brody et al. 2006). Another study demonstrated the upregulation of α4β2-nAChR (approximately 25%) in smokers after 1 week of abstinence. The upregulation was maintained up to 4 weeks of abstinence (approximately 15% increase), but the DV values then returned to nonsmoker level by 6–12 weeks of abstinence (Cosgrove et al. 2009). Differences in the study cohorts could be a possible reason for discrepancy, since only men were included in the study performed by Mamede et al., while both men and women were included the study performed by Cosgrove et al.

The degree of upregulation of nAChRs in smokers is sex-dependent. Cosgrove et al. performed a ^{123}I-5IA-SPECT study on 26 male and 28 female smokers, and 26 male and 30 female age-matched nonsmokers. The availability of α4β2 nAChRs was significantly higher in the cortex, striatum, and cerebellum of male smokers compared to that in male nonsmokers. In contrast, there was no difference in α4β2-nAChR availability between female smokers and nonsmokers. The cortical and cerebellar α4β2-nAChR availability showed a significant negative correlation with the progesterone level in a SPECT imaging day. Therefore, female sex steroid hormones may have a role in the regulation of α4β2-nAChR availability (Cosgrove et al. 2012).

2.6 Nicotinic Acetylcholine Receptor Imaging in Mouse Brain

The recent availability of many transgenic mice lines that model human diseases have enabled researchers to better elucidate disease mechanisms and drug development. However, since many studies on imaging nAChRs have been performed in nonhuman primates and humans, technical issues have hampered imaging studies of nAChRs in the brain of small animals, especially mice. Mouse brains are too small to image clearly using PET and SPECT that are used clinically. However, recent advances have improved the sensitivity and spatial resolution of PET and SPECT, enabling small animal imaging, which has allowed researchers to clearly visualize organs of small rodents. Thus, nuclear medical translational research using transgenic mice has become possible and has aided elucidation of human disease pathology. We provided the first evaluation of SPECT imaging of α4β2 nAChRs in the mouse brain (Matsuura et al. 2016). A 60-min dynamic SPECT imaging session of α4β2 nAChRs in the mouse brain was performed using ^{123}I-5IA. For the accurate definition of regions of interest (ROIs), each mouse underwent magnetic resonance (MR) brain imaging prior to SPECT imaging. The ROIs were then positioned on the MR images prior to their application to SPECT images. The mean radioactivity for each ROI (i.e., cerebral cortex, striatum, hippocampus, thalamus, and cerebellum) was expressed as standardized uptake values (SUVs) and compared to the known distribution of α4β2 nAChRs in the mouse brain. ^{123}I-5IA-SPECT allowed clear visualization of the mouse brain. A significant positive correlation was observed between the SPECT signal intensity and the reported distribution of nAChRs, which was measured using [^{3}H]epibatidine (Marks et al. 1998) (Fig. 2.6, R = 0.81, $P < 0.0001$ at 30 min; R = 0.72, $P < 0.0001$ at 60 min). The accumulation of ^{123}I-5IA was significantly inhibited by pretreatment with (−)-nicotine. These findings indicated that ^{123}I-5IA SPECT images were α4β2 nAChR-specific, and that the signal intensity of the SPECT images can be used as an index of α4β2 nAChR density.

The binding of ^{123}I-5IA decreased after the administration of acetylcholinesterase inhibitors in the baboon (Fujita et al. 2003a) and human brain (Esterlis et al. 2013). Therefore, the sensitivity of ^{123}I-5IA-SPECT to changes in the amount of endogenous acetylcholine in the mouse brain was assessed. First, the effect of different concentrations of physostigmine on the cerebral accumulation of ^{125}I-5IA was analyzed using the evisceration method. Physostigmine reduced the accumulation of ^{125}I-5IA accumulation in all nAChR-rich regions, in a dose-dependent manner. Conversely, radioactivity levels in the blood increased in a dose-dependent manner. Physostigmine at a concentration of 0.75 mg/kg reduced the uptake of ^{125}I-5IA in the thalamus by 51% (Fig. 2.7a, $P < 0.01$). Next, ^{123}I-5IA-SPECT imaging was performed twice, i.e., before and after physostigmine pretreatment (0.75 mg/kg). Compared to the baseline measurements, SUVs in the thalamus was significantly reduced (by 38%) with the physostigmine pretreatment (Fig. 2.7b, $P < 0.05$).

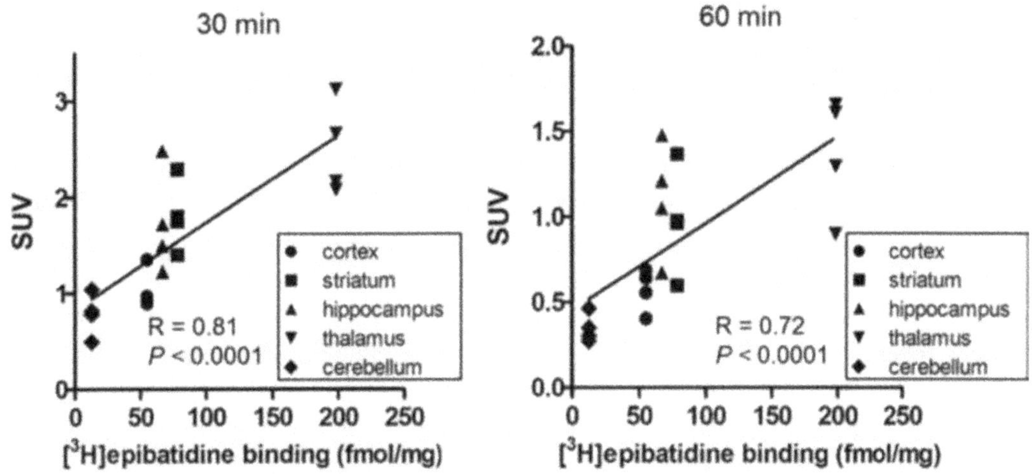

Fig. 2.6 Comparison of in vivo single-photon emission computed tomography (SPECT) analysis with the reported α4β2 nAChR density in the mouse brain. Correlation between in vivo radioactivity determined using SPECT/CT imaging and the reported α4β2 nAChR density in mouse brain. The Y-axis indicates the standardized uptake values (SUVs) in each brain region obtained at 30 min and 60 min after the ^{123}I-5IA injection. The X-axis represents the α4β2 nAChR density determined using [^{3}H]epibatidine binding assay (Marks et al. 1998). The correlation coefficient (R) was 0.81 and 0.72, at 30 min and 60 min, respectively, indicating a highly significant correlation between the two parameters ($P < 0.0001$)

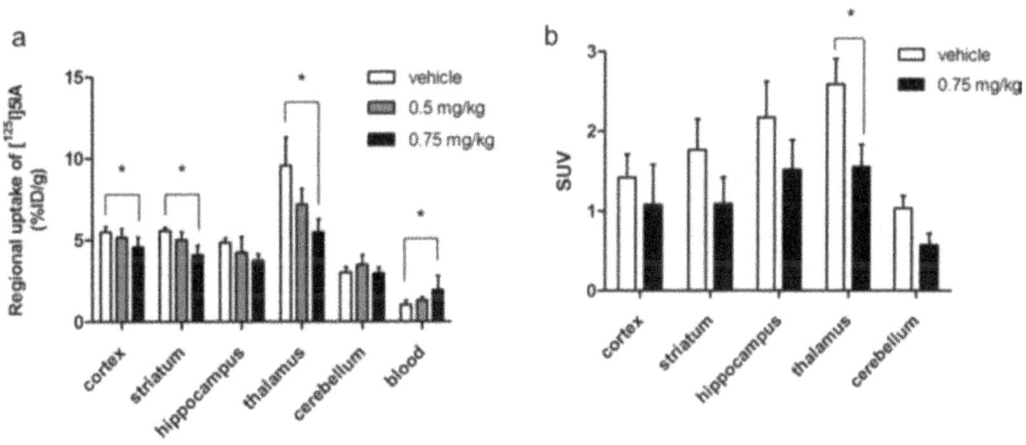

Fig. 2.7 The effect of physostigmine pretreatment on $^{123/125}$I-5IA accumulation. (**a**) The effect of different doses of physostigmine on ^{125}I-5IA accumulation in each brain region, as determined using the evisceration method. Each column represents average data from four mice and *error bars* represent the standard deviation (SD) ($*P < 0.05$, $**P < 0.01$ vs. vehicle). (**b**) The effect of physostigmine (0.75 mg/kg) on ^{123}I-5IA accumulation in each brain region was determined using the region of interest (ROI) analyses. Each *bar* represents the average of four mice and *error bars* represent the SD ($*P < 0.05$ vs. vehicle)

This suggested that SPECT images were affected by the increase in endogenous acetylcholinesterase caused by the administration of physostigmine. Therefore, ^{123}I-5IA-SPECT imaging may also be useful to evaluate the in vivo efficacy of acetylcholinesterase inhibitors in the mouse brain.

We also successfully detected the changes in nAChR density using ^{123}I-5IA-SPECT in the brains of frequently used mouse models of AD, i.e., the Tg2576 and APP/PS2 mice. Tg2576 mice overexpress human β-amyloid precursor protein (APP) with a familial AD gene mutation (Frautschy et al. 1998), while APP/PS2 mice are produced by crossbreeding Tg2576 mice with PS2 mice that overexpress human presenilin-2 (PS2) proteins carrying the Volga German Kindred mutation (N141I). The PS2 mutation reportedly accelerates AD-like phenotypes, such as the elevation of $A\beta_{1-40/1-42}$ levels, presence of amyloid plaques, and memory and learning defects, by several months, in Tg2576 mice (Toda et al. 2011). Consistent with the report by Toda et al. (2011), a novel object recognition (NOR) test demonstrated that the levels of cognition of APP/PS2 mice decreased at younger ages than those in Tg2576 mice. This test is based on the spontaneous tendency of rodents to spend more time exploring a novel object than a familiar one, and allows for the evaluation of cognition and recognition memory. The NOR test did not show significant differences in the cognitive ability between Tg2576 and wild-type mice at 13 months of age. Conversely, compared to wild-type mice, 12-month-old APP/PS2 mice exhibited a clear cognitive deficit. At first, ^{123}I-5IA-SPECT imaging was performed in Tg2576 and wild-type mice at 13 months of age. A 60-min dynamic SPECT/CT imaging was conducted following injection of ^{123}I-5IA into each mouse, via the tail vein. The distribution of radioactivity in each brain region was determined by ROI analysis and data were compared between Tg2576 and wild-type mice. ^{123}I-5IA-SPECT showed a higher signal in brains of Tg2576 mice than that in wild-type mice (Fig. 2.8a). SUVs in the thalamus were significantly higher than those in wild-type mice (22%, $P < 0.05$). SUVs in the cortex and hippocampus also tended to increase by 15% and 30%, respectively, although these differences were not statistically significant. [^{3}H]nicotine binding, which was evaluated in vitro using autoradiographic analysis at 7 days after SPECT/CT imaging, was also increased in Tg2576 mice compared to that in wild-type mice (Matsuura et al. 2016). These results suggested that nAChRs are upregulated in the Tg2576 mice at the age of 13 months.

Next, ^{123}I-5IA-SPECT imaging was performed in APP/PS2 and wild-type mice at the age of 12 months. In contrast to Tg2576 mice, the ^{123}I-5IA accumulation in APP/PS2 mice decreased in the cortex, hippocampus, and thalamus compared to that in wild-type mice ($P < 0.05$, Fig. 2.8b). The decrease in the nAChR density in the brains of APP/PS2 mice was supported by the reduction of α4 nAChRs protein levels, which was detected using Western blotting. These findings corroborated with a former study, which reported the loss of nAChRs in the cortex and hippocampus of patients with advanced AD (Guan et al. 2000). The reason for the discrepancy in α4β2 nAChR expression between Tg2576 and APP/PS2 mice, however, is unclear. It is possible that the pathology of Tg2576 mice at the age of 13 months represents a pre-AD state, while 12-month-old APP/PS2 mice might have the same extent of pathology seen in patients with AD. In fact, NOR memory and plaque deposition

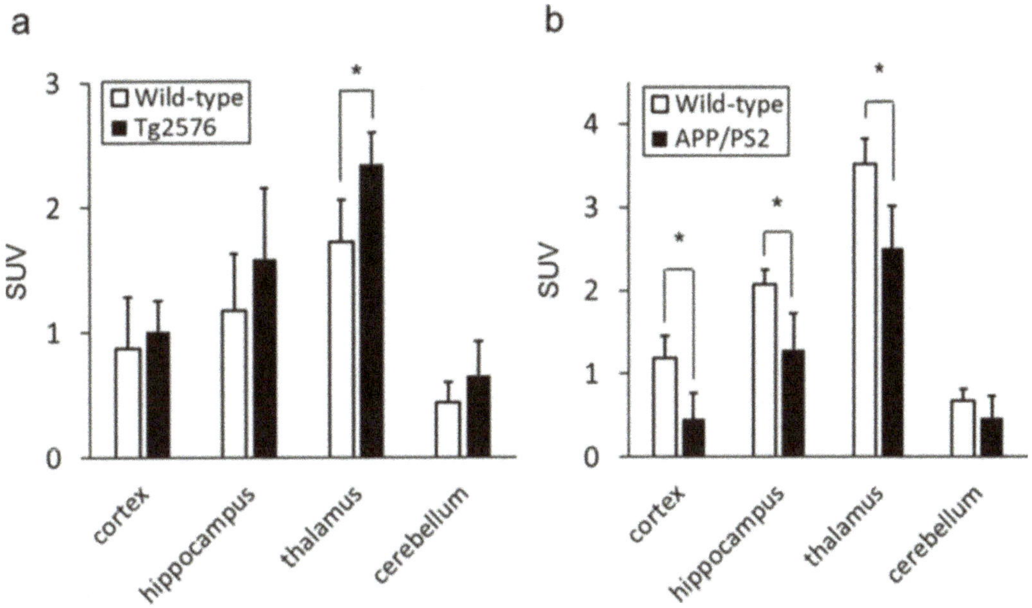

Fig. 2.8 Changes in the ^{123}I-5IA accumulation in brains of Tg2576 and APP/PS2 mice in vivo. In vivo ^{123}I-5IA-SPECT signal in brain regions of 13-month-old Tg2576 mice (**a**), 12-month-old APP/PS2 mice (**b**), and age-matched wild-type mice. ^{123}I-5IA accumulation was significantly increased in the thalamus of Tg2576 mice ($*P < 0.05$ vs. wild-type) and significantly decreased in the cortex, hippocampus, and thalamus of APP/PS2 mice ($*P < 0.05$ vs. wild-type). Each column represents averaged data from 4 to 5 mice and error bars represent the standard deviation

was not significantly different between Tg2576 and wild-type mice at the age of 13 months (Jacobsen et al. 2006). APP/PS2 mice, however, exhibited a clear cognitive deficit and severe plaque deposition in the cerebral cortex, at the age of 12 months. This hypothesis is also supported by the observation of the increase in ^{125}I-5IA accumulation in the hippocampus of APP/PS2 mouse at 6 months of age when the cognitive ability is still normal. These results suggested that the upregulation of α4β2 nAChRs might play a role in the mechanisms underlying neurodegeneration in patients with early-stage AD, who show increased Aβ expression. The discrepancy in the density of nAChR between several mouse models of AD would be an interesting focal point for research on AD pathology.

References

Anderson DJ, Puttfarcken PS, Jacobs I, Faltynek C (2000) Assessment of nicotinic acetylcholine receptor-mediated release of [^{3}H]-norepinephrine from rat brain slices using a new 96-well format assay. Neuropharmacology 39(13):2663–2672

Brody AL, Mandelkern MA, London ED et al (2006) Cigarette smoking saturates brain alpha 4 beta 2 nicotinic acetylcholine receptors. Arch Gen Psychiatry 63(8):907–915

Brody AL, Mukhin AG, La Charite J et al (2013) Up-regulation of nicotinic acetylcholine receptors in menthol cigarette smokers. Int J Neuropsychopharmacol 16(5):957–966

Brody AL, Hubert R, Mamoun MS et al (2016) Nicotinic acetylcholine receptor availability in cigarette smokers: effect of heavy caffeine or marijuana use. Psychopharmacology 233(17):3249–3257

Brust P, Patt JT, Deuther-Conrad W et al (2008) In vivo measurement of nicotinic acetylcholine receptors with [^{18}F]norchloro-fluoro-homoepibatidine. Synapse 62(3):205–218

Buisson B, Bertrand D (2002) Nicotine addiction: the possible role of functional upregulation. Trends Pharmacol Sci 23(3):130–136

Colloby SJ, Firbank MJ, Pakrasi S et al (2011) Alterations in nicotinic alpha4beta2 receptor binding in vascular dementia using ^{123}I-5IA-85380 SPECT: comparison with regional cerebral blood flow. Neurobiol Aging 32(2):293–301

Cosgrove KP, Batis J, Bois F et al (2009) Beta2-nicotinic acetylcholine receptor availability during acute and prolonged abstinence from tobacco smoking. Arch Gen Psychiatry 66(6):666–676

Cosgrove KP, Kloczynski T, Bois F et al (2010) Decreased Beta(2)*-nicotinic acetylcholine receptor availability after chronic ethanol exposure in nonhuman primates. Synapse 64(9):729–732

Cosgrove KP, Esterlis I, McKee SA et al (2012) Sex differences in availability of beta2*-nicotinic acetylcholine receptors in recently abstinent tobacco smokers. Arch Gen Psychiatry 69(4):418–427

Deuther-Conrad W, Patt JT, Feuerbach D, Wegner F, Brust P, Steinbach J (2004) Norchloro-fluoro-homoepibatidine: specificity to neuronal nicotinic acetylcholine receptor subtypes in vitro. Farmaco 59(10):785–792

Deuther-Conrad W, Patt JT, Lockman PR et al (2008) Norchloro-fluoro-homoepibatidine (NCFHEB) – a promising radioligand for neuroimaging nicotinic acetylcholine receptors with PET. Eur Neuropsychopharmacol 18(3):222–229

Dilsaver SC (1986) Pathophysiology of "cholinoceptor supersensitivity" in affective disorders. Biol Psychiatry 21(8–9):813–829

Ding Y, Liu N, Wang T et al (2000) Synthesis and evaluation of 6-[^{18}F]fluoro-3-(2(*S*)-azetidinylmethoxy)pyridine as a PET tracer for nicotinic acetylcholine receptors. Nucl Med Biol 27(4):381–389

Doll F, Dolci L, Valette H et al (1999) Synthesis and nicotinic acetylcholine receptor in vivo binding properties of 2-fluoro-3-[2(S)-2-azetidinylmethoxy]pyridine: a new positron emission tomography ligand for nicotinic receptors. J Med Chem 42(12):2251–2259

Ellis JR, Villemagne VL, Nathan PJ et al (2008) Relationship between nicotinic receptors and cognitive function in early Alzheimer's disease: a 2-[^{18}F]fluoro-A-85380 PET study. Neurobiol Learn Mem 90(2):404–412

Esterlis I, Cosgrove KP, Petrakis IL et al (2010) SPECT imaging of nicotinic acetylcholine receptors in nonsmoking heavy alcohol drinking individuals. Drug Alcohol Depend 108(1–2):146–150

Esterlis I, Hannestad JO, Bois F et al (2013) Imaging changes in synaptic acetylcholine availability in living human subjects. J Nucl Med 54(1):78–82

Fitch RW, Spande TF, Garraffo HM, Yeh HJ, Daly JW (2010) Phantasmidine: an epibatidine congener from the ecuadorian poison frog Epipedobates anthonyi. J Nat Prod 73(3):331–337

Frautschy SA, Yang F, Irrizarry M et al (1998) Microglial response to amyloid plaques in APPsw transgenic mice. Am J Pathol 152(1):307–317

Fujita M, Tamagnan G, Zoghbi SS et al (2000) Measurement of alpha4beta2 nicotinic acetylcholine receptors with [^{123}I]5-I-A-85380 SPECT. J Nucl Med 41(9):1552–1560

Fujita M, Al-Tikriti MS, Tamagnan G et al (2003a) Influence of acetylcholine levels on the binding of a SPECT nicotinic acetylcholine receptor ligand [^{123}I]5-I-A-85380. Synapse 48(3):116–122

Fujita M, Ichise M, van Dyck CH et al (2003b) Quantification of nicotinic acetylcholine receptors in human brain using [^{123}I]5-I-A-85380 SPET. Eur J Nucl Med Mol Imaging 30(12):1620–1629

Fujita M, Ichise M, Zoghbi SS et al (2006) Widespread decrease of nicotinic acetylcholine receptors in Parkinson's disease. Ann Neurol 59(1):174–177

Gallezot JD, Bottlaender M, Gregoire MC et al (2005) In vivo imaging of human cerebral nicotinic acetylcholine receptors with 2-^{18}F-fluoro-A-85380 and PET. J Nucl Med 46(2):240–247

Gottfries CG, Blennow K, Karlsson I, Wallin A (1994) The neurochemistry of vascular dementia. Dementia 5(3–4):163–167

Graef S, Schonknecht P, Sabri O, Hegerl U (2011) Cholinergic receptor subtypes and their role in cognition, emotion, and vigilance control: an overview of preclinical and clinical findings. Psychopharmacology 215(2):205–229

Guan ZZ, Zhang X, Ravid R, Nordberg A (2000) Decreased protein levels of nicotinic receptor subunits in the hippocampus and temporal cortex of patients with Alzheimer's disease. J Neurochem 74(1):237–243

Hashikawa K, Yoshida H, Inoue G et al (2002) Evaluation of nicotinic cholinergic receptors in the patients with Alzheimer disease by SPECT. J Nucl Med 43(5):63p–63p

Hashimoto K, Nishiyama S, Ohba H et al (2008) [^{11}C]CHIBA-1001 as a novel PET ligand for alpha7 nicotinic receptors in the brain: a PET study in conscious monkeys. PLoS One 3(9):e3231

Hillmer AT, Tudorascu DL, Wooten DW et al (2014) Changes in the alpha4beta2* nicotinic acetylcholine system during chronic controlled alcohol exposure in nonhuman primates. Drug Alcohol Depend 138:216–219

Hillmer AT, Esterlis I, Gallezot JD et al (2016a) Imaging of cerebral alpha4beta2* nicotinic acetylcholine receptors with (−)-[^{18}F]Flubatine PET: implementation of bolus plus constant infusion and sensitivity to acetylcholine in human brain. Neuroimage 141:71–80

Hillmer AT, Zheng MQ, Li S et al (2016b) PET imaging evaluation of [^{18}F]DBT-10, a novel radioligand specific to alpha7 nicotinic acetylcholine receptors, in nonhuman primates. Eur J Nucl Med Mol Imaging 43(3):537–547

Hillmer AT, Li S, Zheng MQ et al (2017) PET imaging of alpha7 nicotinic acetylcholine receptors: a comparative study of [^{18}F]ASEM and [^{18}F]DBT-10 in nonhuman primates, and further evaluation of [^{18}F]ASEM in humans. Eur J Nucl Med Mol Imaging 44(6):1042–1050

Hockley BG, Stewart MN, Sherman P et al (2013) (−)-[^{18}F]Flubatine: evaluation in rhesus monkeys and a report of the first fully automated radiosynthesis validated for clinical use. J Label Compd Radiopharm 56(12):595–599

Horti AG, Scheffel U, Koren AO et al (1998) 2-[^{18}F]Fluoro-A-85380, an in vivo tracer for the nicotinic acetylcholine receptors. Nucl Med Biol 25(7):599–603

Horti AG, Gao Y, Kuwabara H et al (2014) ^{18}F-ASEM, a radiolabeled antagonist for imaging the alpha7-nicotinic acetylcholine receptor with PET. J Nucl Med 55(4):672–677

Ishikawa M, Sakata M, Toyohara J et al (2011) Occupancy of alpha7 nicotinic acetylcholine receptors in the brain by tropisetron: a positron emission tomography study using [^{11}C]CHIBA-1001 in healthy human subjects. Clin Psychopharmacol Neurosci 9(3):111–116

Jacobsen JS, Wu CC, Redwine JM et al (2006) Early-onset behavioral and synaptic deficits in a mouse model of Alzheimer's disease. Proc Natl Acad Sci U S A 103(13):5161–5166

Kadir A, Almkvist O, Wall A, Langstrom B, Nordberg A (2006) PET imaging of cortical ^{11}C-nicotine binding correlates with the cognitive function of attention in Alzheimer's disease. Psychopharmacology (Berl) 188(4):509–520

Kendziorra K, Wolf H, Meyer PM et al (2011) Decreased cerebral alpha4beta2* nicotinic acetylcholine receptor availability in patients with mild cognitive impairment and Alzheimer's disease assessed with positron emission tomography. Eur J Nucl Med Mol Imaging 38(3):515–525

Koren AO, Horti AG, Mukhin AG et al (1998) 2-, 5-, and 6-Halo-3-(2(S)-azetidinylmethoxy)pyridines: synthesis, affinity for nicotinic acetylcholine receptors, and molecular modeling. J Med Chem 41(19):3690–3698

Logan J, Fowler JS, Volkow ND et al (1990) Graphical analysis of reversible radioligand binding from time-activity measurements applied to [*N*-^{11}C-methyl]-(−)-cocaine PET studies in human subjects. J Cereb Blood Flow Metab 10(5):740–747

Mamede M, Ishizu K, Ueda M et al (2004) Quantification of human nicotinic acetylcholine receptors with ^{123}I-5IA SPECT. J Nucl Med 45(9):1458–1470

Mamede M, Ishizu K, Ueda M et al (2007) Temporal change in human nicotinic acetylcholine receptor after smoking cessation: 5IA SPECT study. J Nucl Med 48(11):1829–1835

Mankoff DA (2007) A definition of molecular imaging. J Nucl Med 48(6):18N. 21N

Marks MJ, Smith KW, Collins AC (1998) Differential agonist inhibition identifies multiple epibatidine binding sites in mouse brain. J Pharmacol Exp Ther 285(1):377–386

Martin-Ruiz C, Court J, Lee M et al (2000) Nicotinic receptors in dementia of Alzheimer, Lewy body and vascular types. Acta Neurol Scand Suppl 176:34–41

Marutle A, Warpman U, Bogdanovic N, Nordberg A (1998) Regional distribution of subtypes of nicotinic receptors in human brain and effect of aging studied by (+/−)-[^{3}H]epibatidine. Brain Res 801(1–2):143–149

Matsuura Y, Ueda M, Higaki Y et al (2016) Noninvasive evaluation of nicotinic acetylcholine receptor availability in mouse brain using singlephoton emission computed tomography with [^{123}I]5IA. Nucl Med Biol 43(6):372–378

Meyer PM, Strecker K, Kendziorra K et al (2009) Reduced alpha4beta2*-nicotinic acetylcholine receptor binding and its relationship to mild cognitive and depressive symptoms in Parkinson disease. Arch Gen Psychiatry 66(8):866–877

Mitkovski S, Villemagne VL, Novakovic KE et al (2005) Simplified quantification of nicotinic receptors with 2[^{18}F]F-A-85380 PET. Nucl Med Biol 32(6):585–591

Mitsis EM, Reech KM, Bois F et al (2009) ^{123}I-5-IA-85380 SPECT imaging of nicotinic receptors in Alzheimer disease and mild cognitive impairment. J Nucl Med 50(9):1455–1463

Mukhin AG, Gundisch D, Horti AG et al (2000) 5-Iodo-A-85380, an alpha4beta2 subtype-selective ligand for nicotinic acetylcholine receptors. Mol Pharmacol 57(3):642–649

Mukhin AG, Kimes AS, Chefer SI et al (2008) Greater nicotinic acetylcholine receptor density in smokers than in nonsmokers: a PET study with 2-^{18}F-FA-85380. J Nucl Med 49(10):1628–1635

Musachio JL, Scheffel U, Finley PA et al (1998) 5-[I-125/123]lodo-3(2(S)-azetidinylmethoxy) pyridine, a radioiodinated analog of A-85380 for in vivo studies of central nicotinic acetylcholine receptors. Life Sci 62(22.): PL):351–357

Musachio JL, Villemagne VL, Scheffel UA et al (1999) Synthesis of an I-123 analog of A-85380 and preliminary SPECT imaging of nicotinic receptors in baboon. Nucl Med Biol 26(2):201–207

Muzic RF Jr, Berridge MS, Friedland RP, Zhu N, Nelson AD (1998) PET quantification of specific binding of carbon-11-nicotine in human brain. J Nucl Med 39(12):2048–2054

Nemecz A, Prevost MS, Menny A, Corringer PJ (2016) Emerging molecular mechanisms of signal transduction in pentameric ligand-gated ion channels. Neuron 90(3):452–470

Nickles RJ (1991) A shotgun approach to the chart of the nuclides. Radiotracer production with an 11 MeV proton cyclotron. Acta Radiol Suppl 376:69–71

Nickles RJ (2003) The production of a broader palette of PET tracers. J Labelled Comp Radiopharm 46(1):1–27

Nordberg A, Hartvig P, Lundqvist H, Antoni G, Ulin J, Langstrom B (1989) Uptake and regional distribution of (+)-(*R*)- and (−)-(*S*)-*N*-[methyl-^{11}C]-nicotine in the brains of rhesus monkey. An attempt to study nicotinic receptors in vivo. J Neural Transm Park Dis Dement Sect 1(3):195–205

Nordberg A, Lundqvist H, Hartvig P, Lilja A, Langstrom B (1995) Kinetic analysis of regional (*S*)(−)^{11}C-nicotine binding in normal and Alzheimer brains – in vivo assessment using positron emission tomography. Alzheimer Dis Assoc Disord 9(1):21–27

Nyback H, Halldin C, Ahlin A, Curvall M, Eriksson L (1994) PET studies of the uptake of (*S*)- and (*R*)-[^{11}C]nicotine in the human brain: difficulties in visualizing specific receptor binding in vivo. Psychopharmacology (Berl) 115(1–2):31–36

O'Brien JT, Colloby SJ, Pakrasi S et al (2007) Alpha4beta2 nicotinic receptor status in Alzheimer's disease using ^{123}I-5IA-85380 single-photonemission computed tomography. J Neurol Neurosurg Psychiatry 78(4):356–362

O'Brien JT, Colloby SJ, Pakrasi S et al (2008) Nicotinic alpha4beta2 receptor binding in dementia with Lewy bodies using ^{123}I-5IA-85380 SPECT demonstrates a link between occipital changes and visual hallucinations. Neuroimage 40(3):1056–1063

Oishi N, Hashikawa K, Yoshida H et al (2007) Quantification of nicotinic acetylcholine receptors in Parkinson's disease with ^{123}I-5IA SPECT. J Neurol Sci 256(1–2):52–60

Perry E, Ziabreva I, Perry R, Aarsland D, Ballard C (2005) Absence of cholinergic deficits in "pure" vascular dementia. Neurology 64(1):132–133

Picard F, Scheffer I (2005) Recently defined genetic epileptic syndromes. In: Roger J, Bureau M, Dravet C, Genton P, Tassinari CA, Wolf P (eds) Epileptic syndromes in infancy, childhood and adolescence. John Libbey Eurotext, Montrouge, pp 519–535

Picard F, Bruel D, Servent D et al (2006) Alteration of the in vivo nicotinic receptor density in ADNFLE patients: a PET study. Brain 129(Pt 8):2047–2060

Pietila K, Lahde T, Attila M, Ahtee L, Nordberg A (1998) Regulation of nicotinic receptors in the brain of mice withdrawn from chronic oral nicotine treatment. Naunyn Schmiedeberg's Arch Pharmacol 357(2):176–182

Pimlott SL, Piggott M, Owens J et al (2004) Nicotinic acetylcholine receptor distribution in Alzheimer's disease, dementia with Lewy bodies, Parkinson's disease, and vascular dementia: in vitro binding study using 5-[^{125}I]-A-85380. Neuropsychopharmacology 29(1):108–116

Provini F, Plazzi G, Tinuper P, Vandi S, Lugaresi E, Montagna P (1999) Nocturnal frontal lobe epilepsy. A clinical and polygraphic overview of 100 consecutive cases. Brain 122(Pt 6):1017–1031

Rinne JO, Myllykyla T, Lonnberg P, Marjamaki P (1991) A postmortem study of brain nicotinic receptors in Parkinson's and Alzheimer's disease. Brain Res 547(1):167–170

Robles N, Sabria J (2006) Ethanol consumption produces changes in behavior and on hippocampal alpha7 and alpha4beta2 nicotinic receptors. J Mol Neurosci 30(1–2):119–120

Rueter LE, Donnelly-Roberts DL, Curzon P, Briggs CA, Anderson DJ, Bitner RS (2006) A-85380: a pharmacological probe for the preclinical and clinical investigation of the alphabeta neuronal nicotinic acetylcholine receptor. CNS Drug Rev 12(2):100–112

Sabri O, Kendziorra K, Wolf H, Gertz HJ, Brust P (2008) Acetylcholine receptors in dementia and mild cognitive impairment. Eur J Nucl Med Mol Imaging 35(Suppl 1):S30–S45

Sabri O, Becker GA, Meyer PM et al (2015) First-in-human PET quantification study of cerebral alpha4beta2* nicotinic acetylcholine receptors using the novel specific radioligand (−)-[^{18}F] Flubatine. Neuroimage 118:199–208

Saji H, Magata Y, Yamada Y et al (1992) Synthesis of (*S*)-*N*-[methyl-^{11}C]nicotine and its regional distribution in the mouse brain: a potential tracer for visualization of brain nicotinic receptors by positron emission tomography. Chem Pharm Bull (Tokyo) 40(3):734–736

Saji H, Ogawa M, Ueda M et al (2002) Evaluation of radioiodinated 5-iodo-3-(2(S)-azetidinylmethoxy)pyridine as a ligand for SPECT investigations of brain nicotinic acetylcholine receptors. Ann Nucl Med 16(3):189–200

Saricicek A, Esterlis I, Maloney KH et al (2012) Persistent beta2*-nicotinic acetylcholinergic receptor dysfunction in major depressive disorder. Am J Psychiatry 169(8):851–859

Scheffel U, Horti AG, Koren AO et al (2000) 6-[^{18}F]Fluoro-A-85380: an in vivo tracer for the nicotinic acetylcholine receptor. Nucl Med Biol 27(1):51–56

Shimohama S, Taniguchi T, Fujiwara M, Kameyama M (1986) Changes in nicotinic and muscarinic cholinergic receptors in Alzheimer-type dementia. J Neurochem 46(1):288–293

Smits R, Fischer S, Hiller A et al (2014) Synthesis and biological evaluation of both enantiomers of [^{18}F]flubatine, promising radiotracers with fast kinetics for the imaging of alpha4beta2-nicotinic acetylcholine receptors. Bioorg Med Chem 22(2):804–812

Staley JK, Krishnan-Sarin S, Cosgrove KP et al (2006) Human tobacco smokers in early abstinence have higher levels of beta2* nicotinic acetylcholine receptors than nonsmokers. J Neurosci 26(34):8707–8714

Sullivan JP, Donnelly-Roberts D, Briggs CA et al (1996) A-85380 [3-(2(S)-azetidinylmethoxy) pyridine]: in vitro pharmacological properties of a novel, high affinity alpha 4 beta 2 nicotinic acetylcholine receptor ligand. Neuropharmacology 35(6):725–734

Terry AV Jr, Callahan PM, Hernandez CM (2015) Nicotinic ligands as multifunctional agents for the treatment of neuropsychiatric disorders. Biochem Pharmacol 97(4):388–398

Toda T, Noda Y, Ito G, Maeda M, Shimizu T (2011) Presenilin-2 mutation causes early amyloid accumulation and memory impairment in a transgenic mouse model of Alzheimer's disease. J Biomed Biotechnol 2011:617974

Toyohara J, Sakata M, Wu J et al (2009) Preclinical and the first clinical studies on [^{11}C] CHIBA-1001 for mapping alpha7 nicotinic receptors by positron emission tomography. Ann Nucl Med 23(3):301–309

Ueda M (2016) Development of radiolabeled molecular imaging probes for in vivo analysis of biological function. Yakugaku Zasshi 136(4):659–668

Ueda M, Iida Y, Mukai T et al (2004) 5-[^{123}I]Iodo-A-85380: assessment of pharmacological safety, radiation dosimetry and SPECT imaging of brain nicotinic receptors in healthy human subjects. Ann Nucl Med 18(4):337–344

Valette H, Bottlaender M, Dolle F et al (1999) Imaging central nicotinic acetylcholine receptors in baboons with [^{18}F]fluoro-A-85380. J Nucl Med 40(8):1374–1380

Valette H, Dolle F, Bottlaender M, Hinnen F, Marzin D (2002) Fluoro-A-85380 demonstrated no mutagenic properties in in vivo rat micronucleus and Ames tests. Nucl Med Biol 29(8):849–853

Wong DF, Kuwabara H, Pomper M et al (2014) Human brain imaging of alpha7 nAChR with [^{18}F]ASEM: a new PET radiotracer for neuropsychiatry and determination of drug occupancy. Mol Imaging Biol 16(5):730–738

Yates SL, Bencherif M, Fluhler EN, Lippiello PM (1995) Up-regulation of nicotinic acetylcholine receptors following chronic exposure of rats to mainstream cigarette smoke or alpha 4 beta 2 receptors to nicotine. Biochem Pharmacol 50(12):2001–2008

Chapter 3
A New Aspect of Cholinergic Transmission in the Central Nervous System

Ikunobu Muramatsu, Takayoshi Masuoka, Junsuke Uwada, Hatsumi Yoshiki, Takashi Yazama, Kung-Shing Lee, Kiyonao Sada, Matomo Nishio, Takaharu Ishibashi, and Takanobu Taniguchi

Abstract In the central nervous system, acetylcholine (ACh) is an important neurotransmitter related to higher brain functions and some neurodegenerative diseases. It is released from cholinergic nerve terminals and acts on presynaptic and postsynaptic ACh receptors (AChRs). Following release, ACh is rapidly hydrolyzed and the resultant choline is recycled as a substrate for new ACh synthesis. However, this classical concept of cholinergic transmission is currently reevaluated due to new evidence. In the cholinergic synapse, ACh may be itself taken up into postsynaptic neurons by a specific transport system and may act on AChRs at intracellular organelles (Golgi apparatus and mitochondria). Choline for ACh synthesis in cholinergic nerve terminals may be mainly supplied from choline at relevant concentration levels

I. Muramatsu (✉)
Department of Pharmacology, School of Medicine, Kanazawa Medical University, Uchinada, Ishikawa, Japan

Division of Genomic Science and Microbiology, School of Medicine, University of Fukui, Eiheiji, Fukui, Japan

Kimura Hospital, Awara, Fukui, Japan
e-mail: muramatu@u-fukui.ac.jp

T. Masuoka · M. Nishio · T. Ishibashi
Department of Pharmacology, School of Medicine, Kanazawa Medical University, Uchinada, Ishikawa, Japan

J. Uwada · T. Yazama · T. Taniguchi
Division of Cellular Signal Transduction, Department of Biochemistry, Asahikawa Medical University, Asahikawa, Hokkaido, Japan

H. Yoshiki · K. Sada
Division of Genomic Science and Microbiology, School of Medicine, University of Fukui, Eiheiji, Fukui, Japan

K.-S. Lee
Division of Genomic Science and Microbiology, School of Medicine, University of Fukui, Eiheiji, Fukui, Japan

Department of Surgery, Kaohsiung Medical University, Kaohsiung, Taiwan

A. Akaike et al. (eds.), *Nicotinic Acetylcholine Receptor Signaling in Neuroprotection*, https://doi.org/10.1007/978-981-10-8488-1_3

present in the extracellular space, rather than recycled from ACh-derived choline. Recent evidence has reopened the issue of classical cholinergic transmission and cognition, and may provide a novel approach to rational drug development for the treatment of neurodegenerative disorders such as Alzheimer's disease.

Keywords Cholinergic transmission · Intracellular acetylcholine receptors · Acetylcholine uptake · Acetylcholine esterase · Presynaptic muscarinic receptors

Abbreviations

ACh	Acetylcholine
AChE	Acetylcholine esterase
AChR	Acetylcholine receptor
AChT	Acetylcholine transporter
Ca^{2+}	Calcium
CHT1	High affinity-choline transporter 1
CNS	Central nervous system
DFP	Diisopropylfluorophosphate
ERK	Extracellular regulated kinase
HC-3	Hemicholinium-3
LTP	Long term-potentiation
mAChR	Muscarinic acetylcholine receptor
MAPK	Mitogen-activated protein kinase
nAChR	Nicotinic acetylcholine receptor
NMDAR	*N*-methyl-D-aspartate receptor
NMS	N-methyl-scopolamine
PIP_2	Phosphatidylinositol 4,5-bisphosphate
QNB	Quinuclidinyl benzilate
TEA	Tetraethylammonium

3.1 Introduction

In the central nervous system (CNS), acetylcholine (ACh) is one of the major neurotransmitters involved in higher brain functions, including cognitive processes such as learning and memory and extrapyramidal locomotor activity (Everitt and Robbins 1997; Terry and Buccafusco 2003; Mesulam 2004; Wess et al. 2007). In cholinergic transmission, released ACh acts on ACh receptors (AChRs) located on the presynaptic and/or postsynaptic plasma membranes. ACh is also rapidly hydrolyzed by ACh esterase (AChE), leading to the termination of synaptic neurotransmission. Then the resultant choline is transported back into the cholinergic nerve terminals by the high-affinity choline transporter 1 (CHT1), and is reutilized as a substrate for ACh synthesis (Parsons et al. 1993; Apparsundaram et al. 2000; Okuda et al. 2000; Sarter and Parikh 2005). However, this classical tenet of cholinergic transmission has recently been challenged by several new findings from recent studies. The first finding is with regard to the intracellular distribution and function of AChRs in postsynaptic neurons and neuroblastoma cells (Yamasaki et al. 2010: Uwada et al. 2011, 2014; Anisuzzaman et al. 2013; Muramatsu et al. 2015); the second is the incorporation of ACh itself into postsynaptic neurons (Muramatsu et al. 2016); and the third finding is that ACh-derived choline after hydrolysis may not be largely reused (Muramatsu et al. 2017). In this chapter, these findings were briefly summarized.

3.2 Intracellular Distribution of AChRs

It has been commonly accepted that most neurotransmitter receptors are located on the plasma membrane and transduce extracellular to intracellular signals. However, recent evidence suggests that several G-protein-coupled receptors including AChRs are located, and may also signal from, intracellular sites such as endosomes, Golgi apparatus, endoplasmic reticulum, mitochondria, and nuclear membranes (Boivin et al. 2008; Jong et al. 2009; Benard et al. 2012; den Boon et al. 2012; Uwada et al. 2011, 2014; Anisuzzaman et al. 2013).

3.2.1 Muscarinic AChRs

There are five subtypes of muscarinic AChRs (M1–M5 mAChRs), all of which are expressed in the CNS (Caulfield and Birdsall 1998; van Koppen and Kaiser 2003; Nathanson 2008). In general, the M1 subtype is the most abundant within the CNS, M2 and M4 subtypes are moderately expressed, and only low levels of M3 and M5 subtypes have been found (Volpicelli and Levery 2004). All of the mAChRs are generally located and function at the plasma membrane. However, recent studies have revealed that M1 mAChRs exist not only at the cell surface but also at intracellular membranes in the hippocampus and other telencephalon regions of rodents and humans and in neuroblastoma cells (Uwada et al. 2011; Anisuzzaman et al. 2013). Pharmacologically, the intracellular distribution of mAChRs is evaluated from the different binding densities of cell-permeable (hydrophobic) and cell-impermeable (hydrophilic) radioligands, [^{3}H]quinuclidinyl benzilate (QNB) and [^{3}H]N-methyl-scopolamine (NMS), respectively, in intact segments of brain tissue or whole neuronal cells to detect total (QNB binding) and cell surface (NMS binding) mAChRs (Muramatsu et al. 2005, 2015), and proportions of intracellular and surface M1 subtypes are estimated from the competing profiles of M1-selective ligands at the binding sites of both radioligands. Comparable amounts of surface and intracellular M1 mAChRs were identified under conditions where brain tissues or cultured neurons were not stimulated beforehand. Therefore, it is likely that approximately half the amount of M1 mAChR constitutively occurs at intracellular sites in the telencephalon and in neuroblastoma cells. Intracellular M1 mAChRs were immunohistochemically shown to localize at the Golgi apparatus, and a recent molecular biology study revealed that their intracellular localization requires the C-terminal tryptophan-based motif of M1 subtype, which does not exist in other subtypes (Uwada et al. 2014; Anisuzzaman et al. 2013). The abundant distribution of M1 mAChRs in the Golgi apparatus and endoplasmic reticulum of pyramidal neurons but not in astroglia was also demonstrated in immunoelectron microscopic studies (Yamasaki et al. 2010). A previous immunohistochemical study with a specific M1 antibody also reported intracellular detection in the cytoplasm of large and small dendrites and the dendritic spines of cerebral cortex neurons (Mrzljak et al. 1993).

M1 mAChRs cause phosphatidylinositol 4,5-bisphosphate (PIP_2) hydrolysis leading to calcium (Ca^{2+}) upregulation and activation of the mitogen-activated protein kinase (MAPK) pathway through the $G\alpha_{q/11}$ protein (van Koppen and Kaiser 2003; Morishima et al. 2013). In rat hippocampal and cortical neurons and neuroblastoma cells, the PIP_2-Ca^{2+} response is exclusively mediated by surface M1 mAChRs on a time scale of seconds. On the other hand, the extracellular signal-regulated kinase1/2 (ERK1/2) pathway is activated by intracellular M1 mAChRs on a slow time scale of minutes (Uwada et al. 2011; Anisuzzaman et al. 2013). These results indicate that M1 mAChRs at each site may be specifically activated and involved in distinct neuronal functions with different temporal courses (Fig. 3.1).

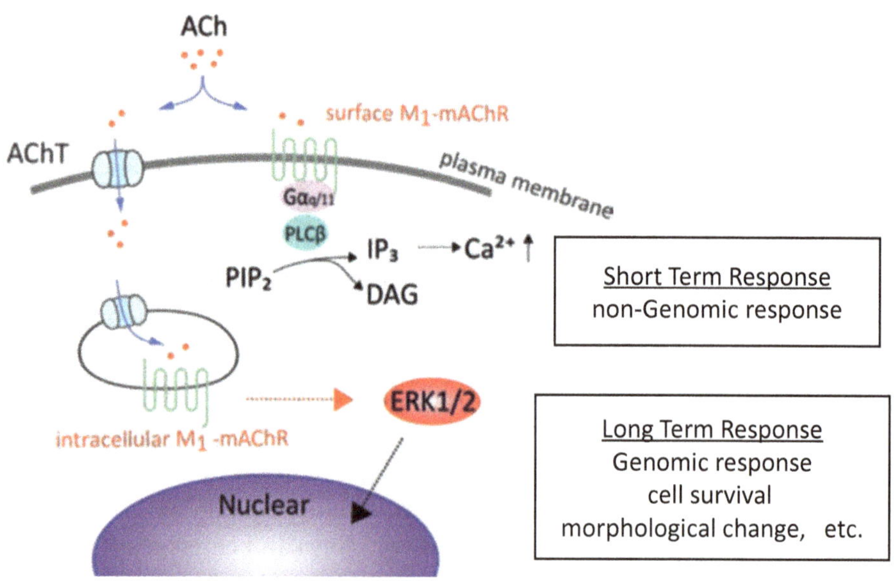

Fig. 3.1 Schematic representation of surface and intracellular M1 mAChRs in postsynaptic neurons, and their possible signal transduction pathways and physiological responses

As aforementioned, M1 mAChRs predominantly exist in the CNS and are involved in cognitive enhancement (Everitt and Robbins 1997; Kruse et al. 2014; Terry and Buccafusco 2003; Mesulam 2004; Wess et al. 2007). In the hippocampus, cholinergic activation induces a theta rhythm of neuronal activity and enhances or induces long-term potentiation (LTP) (Huerta and Lisman 1995; Williams and Kauer 1997; Fernandez de Sevilla et al. 2008), the primary experimental model for investigating the synaptic basis of learning and memory (Bliss and Collingridge 1993; Seol et al. 2007). M1 mAChR-knockout mice have severe deficits in working memory and memory consolidation, as well as impaired hippocampal LTP (Anagnostaras et al. 2003; Shinoe et al. 2005; Wess et al. 2007). M1-specific agonists have been shown to facilitate the induction of LTP and improve cognitive function in several animal models of amnesia (Caccamo et al. 2006; Langmead et al. 2008; Ma et al. 2009). Thus, the specific distribution of intracellular M1 mAChRs in the telencephalon may correlate with synaptic plasticity.

Our electrophysiological study with rat hippocampal slices revealed that cholinergic induction of a theta rhythm and cholinergic facilitation in the early part of *N*-methyl-d-aspartate receptor (NMDAR)-dependent LTP were mainly mediated by surface M1 mAChRs, whereas cholinergic facilitation in the late part of NMDAR-dependent LTP and the majority of non-NMDAR-dependent LTP were evoked by activation of intracellular M1 mAChRs (Anisuzzaman et al. 2013). The induction of LTP requires elevation of postsynaptic Ca^{2+} (Lynch et al. 1983) and activation of protein kinases (Soderling and Derkack 2000), whereas the maintenance of late-phase LTP depends on the MAPK/ERK cascade, gene transcription, protein synthesis, and posttranslational modification (Davi et al. 2000; Giovannini 2006; Nguyen et al. 1994; Frey et al. 1996; Bliss and Collingridge 1993; Routtenberg and Rekart 2005; Gold 2008). Taking these mechanisms into consideration, it is likely that cholinergic stimulation may primarily cause the selective enhancement of respective signaling processes in the early and late phases of LTP through M1 mAChRs located at two distinct sites, leading cholinergic facilitation (Fig. 3.2).

3.2.2 *Nicotinic AChRs*

The nicotinic AChRs (nAChRs) are widely expressed in the brain, where they maintain various neuronal functions including learning and memory (Terry and Buccafusco 2003; Dineley et al. 2015; Wu et al. 2016). They also control survival/death, proliferation/neurite outgrowth, and neurotransmitter release in neuronal cells (Akaike et al. 1994; Kihara et al. 2001; Shimohama et al. 1996; 2009; Rosa et al. 2006). The major nAChR subtypes in the CNS are heteromeric $\alpha4\beta2$, $\alpha3\beta2$, $\alpha7\beta2$ and homomeric $\alpha7$ assemblies, all of which have high permeability for Ca^{2+} as ionic channels and also transduce signals through the phosphatidylinositol 3-kinase (PI3K) signaling pathway (Kihara et al. 2001; Dajas-Bailador and Wonnacott 2004; also see other chapters in this book). To date, these responses have been mainly

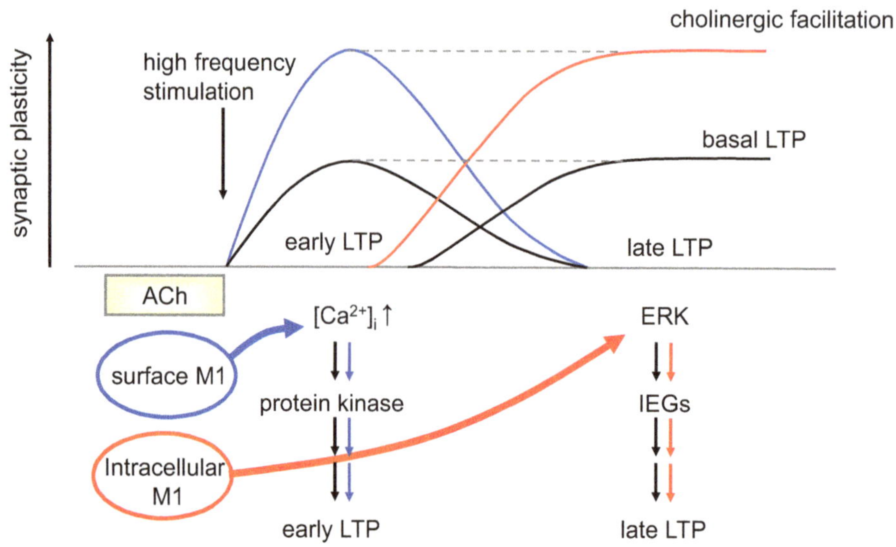

Fig. 3.2 Involvement of surface and intracellular M1 mAChRs in cholinergic facilitation of LTP in rat hippocampus. Note that early and late stages of basal LTP are represented to be primarily mediated by two distinct signal pathways, which are independently enhanced by surface and intracellular M1 mAChRs. Blue: surface M1 mAChR-mediated. Red: intracellular M1 mAChR-mediated. IEGs immediately early genes

discussed with special reference to nAChRs located on the plasma membrane; however, the intracellular distribution of nAChRs, especially in the mitochondria, was recently reported in immunochemical studies (Lykhmus et al. 2014; Gergalova et al. 2014). In brain mitochondria, α7β2 nAChRs mainly stimulate the PI3K/AKT pathway, and α3β2 and α4β2 nAChRs inhibit Src- and Ca^{2+}/calmodulin-dependent protein-kinase II pathways. Mitochondrial nAChRs and associated signaling pathways are associated with the induction of mitochondrial apoptosis (Lykhmus et al. 2014). However, more detailed analysis from different approaches is required in this issue.

3.3 Incorporation of ACh into Postsynaptic Neurons

To activate intracellular AChRs, the endogenous agonist ACh must cross the postsynaptic plasma and endosomal membranes. Because ACh is a hydrophilic molecule, the presence of a specific ACh transport system such as the ACh transporter (AChT) has been postulated (Muramatsu et al. 2016) (Fig. 3.1). Although detailed information on the AChT is lacking, incorporation of ACh into brain slices was reported more than four decades ago (Polak and Meeuws 1996; Liang and Quastel 1969; Katz et al. 1973; Kuhar and Simon 1974). More recently, previous evidence showing that [^{3}H]ACh is actively taken up into brain segments in time- and temperature-dependent manners was confirmed (Muramatsu et al. 2016, 2017). The uptake was clearly observed in the presence of irreversible but not reversible AChE inhibitors. [^{3}H]ACh uptake was high in the CNS but was negligible or minor in the peripheral tissues. The uptake was comparable among brain regions but was not related to the density of cholinergic innervation. Hemicholinium-3 (HC-3) and tetraethyammonium (TEA) inhibited [^{3}H]ACh uptake in a concentration-dependent manner. However, the uptake was little affected by the excitatory or inhibitory amino acid neurotransmitters glutamate and gamma-aminobutyric acid, respectively, biogenic amines, tetrodotoxin, and atropine. Therefore, it is likely that ACh uptake is facilitated by an intrinsic transport system (AChT), rather than a change in neuronal excitability and the involvement of amino acid neurotransmitters. Interestingly, [^{3}H]ACh uptake was potently suppressed by AChE inhibitors including drugs clinically used to treat the cognitive symptoms of Alzheimer's disease such as donepezil, galantamine and rivastigmine (Muramatsu et al. 2016). These results raise the interesting possibility that ACh concentrations released in the synapse may be regulated by both AChE and the postsynaptic uptake of ACh, which may be relevant to cholinergic therapy in Alzheimer's disease. As mentioned above, intracellular M1 mAChRs selectively activate ERK in hippocampal neurons and participate in the late stage of cholinergic facilitation of LTP. The intracellular M1-mediated responses both were inhibited by TEA and HC-3 at concentrations that inhibit ACh uptake. However, PIP_2 hydrolysis and the early phase of cholinergic facilitation of LTP, which were selectively caused by plasma membrane M1 AChRs, were not affected by TEA and HC-3 (Uwada and Masuoka unpublished observations). These pharmacological results further support the fact that cholinergic facilitation of LTP is caused independently by surface and intracellular M1 mAChRs through distinct signaling pathways (Figs. 3.1 and 3.2). These results also indicate that the ACh transport system serves as an intrinsic route for released ACh to access intracellular AChRs in postsynaptic neurons.

3.4 Regulation of Synaptic ACh Concentrations and the Choline-ACh Cycle

In the CNS, release of ACh from the cholinergic nerve terminals is negatively regulated through presynaptic mAChRs (Raiteri et al. 1989; Starke et al. 1989; Zhang et al. 2002; Alquicer et al. 2016). In vitro, this release is monitored with the superfusion technique, where ACh in synaptosomes (Raiteri and Raiteri 2000; Pittaluga 2016) and brain slices (Richardson and Szerb 1974; Zhang et al. 2002; Alquicer et al. 2016) has been synthesized/prelabeled in advance with [^{3}H]choline followed by superfusion. Figure 3.3a shows a representative result obtained from a superfusion experiment with rat striatal slices. Atropine dramatically increased [^{3}H]efflux evoked by electrical stimulation, indicating that blockade of presynaptic mAChRs suppressed autoinhibition of ACh release. Although the presynaptic mAChR

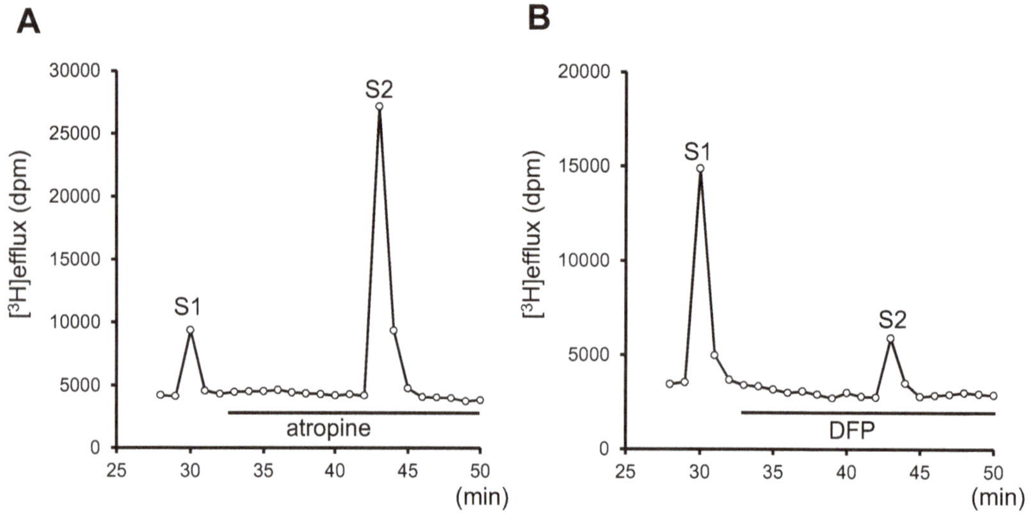

Fig. 3.3 Effects of atropine and diisopropyl phosphorofluoridate in [^{3}H]efflux in superfusion experiments. Rat striatal segments were incubated with 0.1 μM [^{3}H]choline for 30 min and then superfused. Electrical stimulation (3 Hz, for 30 s) was applied two times (S1 and S2). (**a**) 0.1 μM atropine. (**b**) 300 μM diisopropyl phosphorofluoridate (DFP). Ordinate: [^{3}H] count (dpm) in superfusate collected every minute. Abscissa: time after superfusion

subtypes that participate in autoregulation have been the subject of debate, it was recently concluded that the M2 subtype has dominant involvement and there is only minor participation of the M4 subtype (Dolezal and Tucek 1998; Fadel 2011; Zhang et al. 2002; Alquicer et al. 2016).

Released ACh is rapidly hydrolyzed by AChE. Compared with the peripheral tissues, AChE activity in the brain (except cerebellum) is extremely high, and esterase activity in the CNS is closely related to the density of cholinergic innervation (Muramatsu et al. 2016). The esterase activity in the rat striatum is more than five times higher than that in the cerebral cortex and hippocampus, whereas the lowest activity is in the cerebellum, on par with that of the heart and colon. Thus, concentrations of released ACh appear to be effectively regulated by AChE in the CNS.

Inhibition of AChE would be thought to elicit a dramatic increase in synaptic ACh concentration; however, the scenario is not so simple. As mentioned above, ACh release is negatively regulated by presynaptic autoreceptors. Thus, it is likely that AChE inhibitors suppress hydrolysis of released ACh, which in turn, enhances stimulation of presynaptic mAChRs. Figure 3.3b shows a representative result in rat striatal slices, where [^{3}H]efflux evoked by electrical stimulation (3 Hz, 30 s) was reduced after treatment with an irreversible AChE inhibitor (diisopropyl fluorophosphate [DFP]). This inhibitory effect of DFP was abolished by atropine (Muramatsu unpublished observations). These results strongly suggest that ACh release and synaptic concentrations of ACh are precisely controlled by the subtle balance between AChE activity and presynaptic autoinhibition.

In addition to presynaptic AChRs and AChE, the postsynaptic uptake of ACh itself also regulates synaptic ACh concentrations (Muramatsu et al. 2017). In Sect. 3.3, it was noted that ACh uptake is inhibited by TEA and HC-3. The concentration of both drugs that suppressed ACh uptake significantly increased the evoked [^{3}H] efflux by electrical stimulation in superfusion experiments. The effects of TEA or HC-3 were not related to inhibitory actions on presynaptic mAChRs or AChE activity, because the effects of both drugs were observed under conditions which mAChRs and AChE were completely inhibited. Therefore, it is possible that a portion of released ACh may be incorporated into postsynaptic neurons by AChT, participating in the regulation of synaptic ACh concentrations.

After hydrolysis by AChE, it has been classically proposed that ACh-derived choline is transported back into cholinergic nerve terminals and recycled for new ACh synthesis. In this process, choline uptake is mediated through CHT1, which shows high affinity for HC-3 (Ki = 0.001–0.01 μM) and choline (1–5 μM) (Guyenet et al. 1973; Haga and Noda 1973; Okuda et al. 2012). In most previous superfusion experiments, 10 μM HC-3 had been added into perfusion medium to suppress CHT1 activity. HC-3 at this concentration might act on presynaptic mAChRs in addition to inhibiting choline and ACh uptake. On the other hand, lower concentrations (0.1–1 μM) of HC-3, which selectively inhibit CHT1 but do not affect ACh uptake, failed to increase [^{3}H]efflux evoked by electrical stimulation in superfusion experiments (Muramatsu et al. 2017). These recent results suggest that the increase in [^{3}H] efflux by HC-3 is caused by an inhibition of ACh uptake but not choline uptake, implying that ACh-derived choline may not be significantly transported back into cholinergic terminals. Physiological concentrations of choline are relatively high (10–50 μM in plasma and 5–7 μM in cerebrospinal fluid) (Lockman and Allen 2002; Sweet et al. 2001), so that endogenous choline can be continuously supplied from extracellular spaces as a substrate for ACh synthesis. It is interesting to note that perturbations in brain choline homeostasis produce central cholinergic dysfunction (Koppen et al. 1993; Jenden et al. 1990; Sarter and Parikh 2005). These recent results were summarized in this review, and the modified cholinergic transmission mechanisms are proposed in Fig. 3.4.

3.5 Perspectives

Cholinergic transmission as well as adrenergic transmission is a prototype of neurotransmission, in which the transmitter is synthesized, stored and released from nerve terminals, and then acts on postsynaptic membrane receptors. Following release, the transmitter undergoes degradation and/or presynaptic reuptake, leading to termination of synaptic transmission. However, recent studies have revealed that the neurotransmission mechanisms may be more complex. In cholinergic transmission in the

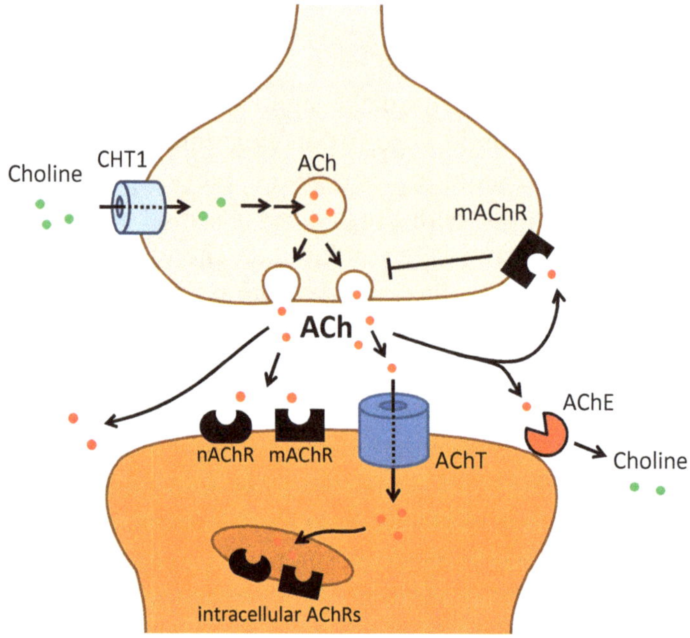

Fig. 3.4 A proposed model of cholinergic transmission in CNS. After release from cholinergic nerve terminals, ACh acts on plasma membrane and intracellular AChRs (mAChRs and/or nAChRs) in postsynaptic pyramidal neurons, in addition to presynaptic mAChRs. Thus, synaptic ACh concentrations are regulated by AChE hydrolysis, AChT-mediated postsynaptic uptake and presynaptic modulation of release itself. Choline for ACh synthesis may be largely supplied from endogenous choline present at relevant concentrations (>5 μM) in the extracellular space, rather than from ACh-degraded choline. Red circles: ACh. Green circles: choline

CNS, released ACh may act both the plasma membrane and intracellular receptors in postsynaptic neurons. ACh itself may be taken up into postsynaptic neurons and act on intracellular receptors. The proposed model (Fig. 3.4) has reopened the issue of classical cholinergic and other neurotransmission mechanisms, and may provide a significant impetus for the pharmacological therapy of neurodegenerative disorders such as Alzheimer's disease.

Acknowledgments We appreciate the kind support of the Life Science Research Laboratory, University of Fukui. This work was supported in part by a Grant-in-Aid for Scientific Research from the Japan Society of the Promotion of Sciences, and a grant from the Smoking Research Foundation of Japan.

Conflict of Interest The authors have no conflicts of interest to declare.

References

Akaike A, Tamura Y, Yokota T et al (1994) Nicotine-induced protection of cultured cortical neurons against N-methyl-D-aspartate receptor-mediated glutamate cytotoxicity. Brain Res 644:181–187

Alquicer G, Dolezal V, El-Fakahany EE (2016) Utilization of superfused cerebral slices in probing muscarinic receptor autoregulation of acetylcholine release. In: Myslivecek J, Jakubik J (eds) Muscarinic receptor: from structure to animal models, Neuromethods 107. Humana Press, New York, pp 221–233

Anagnostaras SG, Murphy GG, Hamilton SE et al (2003) Selective cognitive dysfunction in acetylcholine M1 muscarinic receptor mutant mice. Nat Neurosci 6:51–58

Anisuzzaman AMS, Uwada J, Masuoka T et al (2013) Novel contribution of cell surface and intracellular M1-muscarinic acetylcholine receptors to synaptic plasticity in hippocampus. J Neurochem 126:360–371

Apparsundaram S, Ferguson SM, George AL, Blakely RD (2000) Molecular cloning of a human, hemicholinium-3-sensitive choline transporter. Biochem Biophys Res Commun 276:862–867

Benard G, Massa F, Puemte N et al (2012) Mitochondrial CB_1 receptors regulate neuronal energy metabolism. Nat Neurosci 4:558–564

Bliss TV, Collingridge GL (1993) A synaptic model of memory: long-term potentiation in the hippocampus. Nature 361:31–39

Boivin B, Vaniotis G, Allen BG, Hebert TE (2008) G protein-coupled receptors in and on the cell nucleus: a new signaling paradigm? J Recept Signal Transduct Res 28:15–28

den Boon FS, Chameau P, Schaafsma-Zhao Q et al (2012) Excitability of prefrontal cortical pyramidal neurons id modulated y activation of intracellular type-2 cannabinoid receptors. Proc Natl Acad Sci U S A 109:3534–3539

Caccamo A, Oddo S, Billings LM et al (2006) M1 receptors play a central role in modulating AD-like pathology in transgenic mice. Neuron 49:671–682

Caulfield MP, Birdsall NJ (1998) International Union of Pharmacology. XVII. Classification of muscarinic acetylcholine receptors. Pharmacol Rev 50:279–290

Dajas-Bailador F, Wonnacott S (2004) Nicotinic acetylcholine receptors and the regulation of neuronal signaling. Trends Pharmacol Sci 25:317–324

Davi S, Vanhouute P, Pages C et al (2000) The MAPK/ERK cascade targets both Elk-1 and cAMP response element-binding protein to control long-term potentiation-dependent gene expression in the dentate gyrus in vivo. J Neurosci 20:4563–4572

Dineley KT, Pandya AA, Yakel JL (2015) Nicotinic ACh receptors as therapeutic targets in CNS disorders. Trends Pharmacol Sci 36:96–108

Dolezal V, Tucek S (1998) The effects of brucine and alcuronium on the inhibition of [^{3}H]acetylcholine release from rat striatum by muscarinic receptor agonists. Br J Pharmacol 124:1213–1218

Everitt BJ, Robbins TW (1997) Central cholinergic systems and cognition. Annu Rev Psychol 48:649–648

Fadel JR (2011) Regulation of cortical acetylcholine release: insights from in vivo microdialysis studies. Behav Brain Res 221:527–536

Fernandez de Sevilla D, Nunez A, Borde M et al (2008) Cholinergic-mediated IP3-receptor activation induces long-lasting synaptic enhancement in CA1 pyramidal neurons. J Neurosci 28:1469–1478

Frey U, Frey S, Schollmeier F et al (1996) Influence of actinomycin D, a RNA synthesis inhibitor, on long-term potentiation in rat hippocampal neurons in vivo and in vitro. J Physiol 490(Pt 3):703–711

Gergalova G, Lykhmus O, Komisarenko S et al (2014) α7 nicotinic acetylcholine receptors control cytochrome c release from isolated mitochondria through kinase-mediated pathways. Int J Biochem Cell Biol 49:26–31

Giovannini MG (2006) The role of the extracellular signal-regulated kinase pathway in memory encoding. Rev Neurosci 17:619–634

Gold PE (2008) Protein synthesis inhibition and memory: formation vs amnesia. Neurobiol Learn Mem 89:201–211

Guyenet P, Lefresne P, Rossier J et al (1973) Inhibition by hemicholinium-3 of [^{14}C]acetylcholine synthesis and [^{3}H]choline high-affinity uptake in rat striatal synaptosomes. Mol Pharmacol 9:630–639

Haga T, Noda H (1973) Choline uptake of rat brain synaptosomes. Biochim Biophys Acta 291:564–575

Huerta PT, Lisman JE (1995) Bidirectional synaptic plasticity induced by a single burst during cholinergic theta oscillation in CA1 in vitro. Neuron 15:1053–1063

Jenden DJ, Rice KM, Roch M et al (1990) Effects of nicotineamide on choline and acetylcholine levels. Adv Neurol 51:131–138

Jong YJ, Kumar V, O'Malley KL (2009) Intracellular metabotropic glutamate receptor 5 (mGluR5) activates signaling cascades activates signaling cascades distinct from cell surface counterparts. J Biol Chem 284:35827–35838

Katz HS, Salehmoghaddam S, Collier B (1973) The accumulation of radioactive acetylcholine by a sympathetic ganglion and by brain: failure to label endogenous stores. J Neurochem 20:569–579

Kihara T, Shimohama S, Sawada H et al (2001) α7 nicotinic receptor transduces signals to phosphatidylinositol 3-kinase to block a β-amyloid-induced neurotoxicity. J Boil Chem 276:13541–13546

van Koppen CJ, Kaiser B (2003) Regulation of muscarinic acetylcholine receptor signaling. Pharmacol Ther 98:197–220

Koppen A, Klein J, Huller T et al (1993) Synergistic effect of nicotineamide and choline administration on extracellular choline level in the brain. J Pharmacol Exp Ther 266:720–725

Kruse AC, Kobilka BL, Gautam D et al (2014) Muscarinic acetylcholine receptors: novel opportunities for drug development. Nat Rev Drug Discov 13:549–560

Kuhar MJ, Simon JR (1974) Acetylcholine uptake: lack of association with cholinergic neurons. J Neurochem 22:1135–1137

Langmead CJ, Watson J, Reavill C (2008) Muscarinic acetylcholine receptors as CNS drug targets. Pharmacol Ther 117:232–243

Liang CC, Quastel JH (1969) Effects of drugs on the uptake of acetylcholine in rat brain cortex slices. Biochem Pharmacol 18:1187–1194

Lockman PR, Allen DD (2002) The transport of choline. Drug Dev Ind Pharm 28:749–771

Lykhmus O, Gergalova G, Koval L et al (2014) Mitochondria express several nicotinic acetylcholine receptor subtypes to control various pathways of apoptosis induction. Int J Biochem Cell Biol 53:246–252

Lynch G, Larson J, Kelso S (1983) Intracellular injections of EGTA block induction of hippocampal long-term potentiation. Nature 305:719–721

Ma L, Seager MA, Wittmann M et al (2009) Selective activation of the M1 muscarinic acetylcholine receptor achieved by allosteric potentiation. Proc Natl Acad Sci U S A 106:15950–15955

Mesulam M (2004) The cholinergic lesion of Alzheimer's disease: pivotal factor or side show? Learn Mem 11:43–49

Morishima S, Anisuzzaman ASM, Uwada J et al (2013) Comparison of subcellular distribution and functions between exogenous and endogenous M1 muscarinic acetylcholine receptors. Life Sci 93:17–23

Mrzljak L, Levey AI, Goldman-Rakic P (1993) Association of m1 and m2 muscarinic receptor proteins with asymmetric synapses in the primate cerebral cortex: morphological evidence for cholinergic modulation of excitatory neurotransmission. Proc Natl Acad Sci U S A 90:5194–5198

Muramatsu I, Tanaka T, Suzuki F et al (2005) Quantifying receptor properties: the tissue segment binding method – a powerful tool for the pharmacome analysis of native receptors. J Pharmacol Sci 98:331–339

Muramatsu I, Yoshiki H, Sada K et al (2015) Binding method for detection of muscarinic receptor's natural environment. In: Myslivecek J, Jakubik J (eds) Muscarinic receptor: from structure to animal models, Neuromethods 107. Humana Press, New York, pp 69–81

Muramatsu I, Yoshiki H, Uwada J et al (2016) Pharmacological evidence of specific acetylcholine transport in rat cerebral cortex and other brain regions. J Neurochem 139:566–575

Muramatsu I, Uwada J, Masuoka T et al (2017) Regulation of synaptic acetylcholine concentrations by acetylcholine transport in rat striatal cholinergic transmission. J Neurochem 143:76–86

Nathanson NM (2008) Synthesis, trafficking, and localization of muscarinic acetylcholine receptors. Pharmacol Ther 119:33–43

Nguyen P, Abel T, Kandel ER (1994) Requirement of a critical period of transcription for induction of a late phase of LTP. Science 265:1104–1107

Okuda T, Haga T, Kanai Y et al (2000) Identification and characterization of the high-affinity choline transporter. Nat Neurosci 3:120–125

Okuda T, Osawa C, Yamada H et al (2012) Transmembrane topology and oligomeric structure of the high-affinity choline transporter. J Biol Chem 287:42826–42834

Parsons SM, Prior C, Marshall IG (1993) Acetylcholine transport, storage and release. In: Bradley RJ, Harris RA (eds) International review of neurobiology, vol 35. Academic, New York, pp 279–390

Pittaluga A (2016) Presynaptic release-regulating mGlu1 receptors in central nervous system. Front Pharmacol 7. doi:https://doi.org/10.3389/fphar.2016.00295

Polak RL, Meeuws MM (1996) The influence of atropine on the release and uptake of acetylcholine by the isolated cerebral cortex of the rat. Biochem Pharmacol 15:989–992

Raiteri L, Raiteri M (2000) Synaptosomes still viable after 25 years of superfusion. Neurochem Res 25:1265–1274

Raiteri M, Marchi M, Maura G, Bonanno G (1989) Presynaptic regulation of acetylcholine release in the CNS. Cell Biol Int Res 13:1109–1118

Richardson IW, Szerb JC (1974) The release of labelled acetylcholine and choline from cerebral cortical slices stimulated electrically. Br J Pharmacol 52:499–507

Rosa A, Egea J, Gandia L et al (2006) Neuroprotection by nicotine in hippocampal slices subjected to oxygen-glucose deprivation: involvement of alpha7 nAChR subtype. J Mol Neurosci 30:61–62

Routtenberg A, Rekart JL (2005) Post-translational protein modifications as the substrate for long-term memory. Trends Neurosci 28:12–19

Sarter M, Parikh V (2005) Choline transporters, cholinergic transmission and cognition. Nat Rev Neuosci 6:48–56

Seol GH, Ziburkus J, Huang S et al (2007) Neuromodulators control the polarity of spike-timing-dependent synaptic plasticity. Neuron 55:919–929

Shimohama S (2009) Nicotinic receptor-mediated neuroprotection in neurodegenerative disease models. Biol Pharm Bull 32:332–336

Shimohama S, Akaike A, Kimura J (1996) Nicotine-induced protection against glutamate cytotoxicity-nicotinic cholinergic receptor-mediated inhibition of nitric oxide formation. Ann N Y Acad Sci 777:356–361

Shinoe T, Matsui M, Takeko MM et al (2005) Modulation of synaptic plasticity of physiological activation of M1 muscarinic acetylcholine receptors in the mouse hippocampus. J Neurosci 25:11194–11200

Soderling TR, Derkack VA (2000) Postsynaptic protein phosphorylation and LTP. Trends Neurosci 23:75–80

Starke K, Gothert M, Kilbinger H (1989) Modulation of neurotransmitter release by presynaptic autoreceptors. Pharmacol Rev 69:864–989

Sweet DH, Miller DS, Pritchard JB (2001) Ventricular choline transport: a role for organic cation transporter 2 expressed in choroid plexus. J Biol Chem 276:41611–41619

Terry AV, Buccafusco JJ (2003) The cholinergic hypothesis of aged and Alzheimer's disease-related cognitive deficits: recent challenges and their implications for novel drug development. J Pharmacol Exp Ther 306:821–827

Uwada J, Anisuzzaman ASM, Nishimune A et al (2011) Intracellular distribution of functional M_1-muscarinic acetylcholine receptors in N1E-115 neuroblastoma cells. J Neurochem 118:958–967

Uwada J, Yoshiki H, Masuoka T et al (2014) Intracellular localization of M1 muscarinic acetylcholine receptor through clathrin-dependent constitutive internalization via a C-terminal tryptophan-based motif. J Cell Sci 127:3131–3140

Volpicelli LA, Levery AI (2004) Muscarinic acetylcholine receptor subtypes in cerebral cortex and hippocampus. Prog Brain Res 145:59–66

Wess J, Eglen RM, Gautam D (2007) Muscarinic acetylcholine receptors: mutant mice provide new insights for drug development. Nat Rev Drug Discov 6:21–733

Williams JH, Kauer JA (1997) Properties of carbachol-induced oscillatory activity in rat hippocampus. J Neurophysiol 78:2631–2640

Wu J, Liu Q, Tang P et al (2016) Heterometric α7β2 nicotinic acetylcholine receptors in the brain. Trends Pharmacol Sci 37:562–574

Yamasaki M, Matsui M, Watanabe M (2010) Preferential localization of muscarinic M1 receptor on dendritic shaft and spine of cortical pyramidal cells and its anatomical evidence for volume transmission. J Neurosci 30:4408–4418

Zhang W, Basile AS, Gomeza J et al (2002) Characterization of central inhibitory muscarinic autoreceptors by the use of muscarinic acetylcholine receptor knock-out mice. J Neurosci 22:1709–1717

Chapter 4
Nicotinic Acetylcholine Receptor Signaling: Roles in Neuroprotection

Toshiaki Kume and Yuki Takada-Takatori

Abstract Glutamate neurotoxicity is involved in various neurodegenerative disorders including brain ischemic stroke, trauma, and Alzheimer's and Parkinson's diseases. In addition to excitatory neuronal death, neuroinflammation accompanied by the activation of glial cells has been shown to be induced by these disorders. We previously reported the roles of nicotinic acetylcholine receptors (nAChRs) in the survival of central nervous system neurons during excitotoxic events and neuroinflammation. Nicotine and other nAChR agonists protected cortical neurons against glutamate neurotoxicity via α4- and α7-nAChRs in cultures of neurons obtained from the cerebral cortex of fetal rats. In addition, donepezil, a therapeutic acetylcholinesterase inhibitor currently being used for the treatment of Alzheimer's disease, protected neuronal cells from glutamate neurotoxicity. Moreover, nicotine and donepezil induced the upregulation of nAChRs. Thus, we propose that nicotine as well as donepezil prevents glutamate neurotoxicity through A4- and α7-nAChRs and the phosphatidylinositol 3-kinase (PI3K)/Akt pathway. In addition to the beneficial effect on neuronal cells, we have reported the responses of astrocytes to bradykinin, an inflammatory mediator, and the effect of nAChR stimulation on these responses using cultured cortical astrocytes. Bradykinin induced a transient increase of intracellular calcium concentration ($[Ca^{2+}]_i$) in cultured astrocytes. Both nicotine and donepezil reduced this bradykinin-induced $[Ca^{2+}]_i$ increase. This reduction was inhibited not only by mecamylamine, an nAChR antagonist, but also by PI3K and Akt inhibitors. These results suggest that nAChR stimulation suppresses the inflammatory response induced by bradykinin via the PI3K-Akt pathway in astrocytes.

T. Kume (✉)
Department of Pharmacology, Graduate School of Pharmaceutical Sciences, Kyoto University, Kyoto, Japan

Department of Applied Pharmacology, Graduate School of Medicine and Pharmaceutical Sciences, University of Toyama, Toyama, Japan
e-mail: tkume@pharm.kyoto-u.ac.jp

Y. Takada-Takatori
Department of Pharmacology, Faculty of Pharmaceutical Sciences, Doshisha Women's College, Kyoto, Japan

A. Akaike et al. (eds.), *Nicotinic Acetylcholine Receptor Signaling in Neuroprotection*, https://doi.org/10.1007/978-981-10-8488-1_4

Keywords Nicotine · Donepezil · Neuroprotection · Astrocyte · Nicotinic acetylcholine receptor · Neuroinflammation

4.1 Introduction

Nicotinic acetylcholine receptors (nAChRs) are distributed across various organs, such as the central nervous system (CNS), and are involved in changing cell functions and controlling cell survival via several intracellular signal transduction mechanisms. Many endogenous compounds such as glutamate are known to trigger neuronal death via apoptosis in degenerative diseases of the CNS (Bresnick 1989; Choi et al. 1987). To date, we have elucidated that excitatory neurotoxicity triggered by excitative glutamate can be inhibited by various endogenous factors. In research using cultured rat embryonic cortical neurons, nicotine was shown to exert neuroprotective effects against glutamate neurotoxicity via neuronal nAChRs (Akaike et al. 1994; Kaneko et al. 1997; Shimohama et al. 1998). These studies raised awareness of this issue among many researchers, and numerous groups subsequently reported that nAChR agonists inhibit acute glutamate-induced neuronal death.

Alzheimer's disease (AD) is a common type of dementia. Its pathological characteristics include the formation of senile plaques primarily consisting of amyloid-β (Aβ) proteins, neurofibrillary tangles, and neurologic deficit; thus, AD has aspects of neurodegenerative disease (Whitehouse et al. 1982; Perry et al. 1995). Various disorders related to cholinergic nerves have also been found in the postmortem brain of AD patients, such as atrophy of the nucleus of origin of cholinergic nerves, reduction of acetylcholinergic nerves that project to the cortex from the Meynert nucleus, reduced activity of acetylcholine transferase activity in the cortex, and reduced expression of ACh and nAChRs (Bartus et al. 1982; Coyle et al. 1983). Since the cholinergic nervous system is involved in the functions of cognition and learning, attempts have been made to relieve symptoms by supplementing ACh, which led to the emergence of treatment drugs that act as acetylcholinesterase (AChE) inhibitors, such as donepezil. In addition to the neuronal injury, inflammation in the brain is involved in the pathogenesis of AD (Heppner et al. 2015; Heneka et al. 2015; Rogers 2008; Lee et al. 2010). In inflammatory conditions, it is reported that glial cells, such as astrocytes and microglia, are abnormally activated (Morris et al. 2013; Lee et al. 1995). This abnormal activation of glial cells contributes to the pathogenesis of various neurodegenerative disorders (Heppner et al. 2015; Heneka et al. 2015; Rogers 2008; Lee et al. 2010; Yan et al. 2014). Astrocytes are the most abundant cells in the CNS and play important roles in the maintenance of neuronal activity through the release of neurotrophic factors, the maintenance of ion gradients such as extracellular K^+, and the construction of the blood–brain barrier (Giaume et al. 2010). However, a recent study revealed that, in various pathological conditions, astrocytes were abnormally activated and could be deleterious to adjacent neurons through the release of various inflammatory cytokines (Allan and Rothwell 2001).

Therefore, inhibition of the abnormal activation of astrocytes is considered to be a therapeutic strategy for several CNS diseases involving inflammation.

As a therapeutic drug of AD, donepezil is an effective AChE inhibitor for slowing the progression of cognitive function disorders. In addition to AChE inhibitory activity, several other mechanisms have been noted for their possible relationships to the therapeutic effects of these drugs. AD is a neurodegenerative disease, and some of the therapeutic effects of donepezil may be attributable to its neuroprotective action; however, the assessment of its protective action and analysis of its mechanism of action have not been fully investigated, and much has yet to be clarified. In addition to the effect of donepezil on neurons, another group reported that donepezil inhibited the production of inflammatory cytokines induced by the treatment of Aβ oligomer in cultured microglia (Kim et al. 2014). However, the effect of donepezil on the function of astrocytes has not been elucidated.

This chapter summarizes the effects of nAChR stimulation using nicotine and nAChR ligands, including donepezil, on excitatory neuronal death in rat cultured neurons and neuroinflammation in astrocytes.

4.2 Neuroprotective Effect via Nicotine Receptors

On the basis of the above findings, we have focused on the neuroprotective action of donepezil and found that it exerts its protective effect against glutamate neurotoxicity, as determined through research seeking to reveal its mechanism of action. At the same time, we found that donepezil did not exhibit a protective effect when neurons were treated simultaneously with glutamate and that it expressed its protective action in a manner dependent on the duration and concentration of the pretreatment. This strongly suggests that donepezil exerts its protective effect by a mechanism of action other than AChE inhibition (Takada et al. 2003).

Thus, we continued our analysis with the objective of elucidating the mechanism of the neuroprotective effect of donepezil against glutamate neurotoxicity. It has been shown that nicotine exerted a protective effect against glutamate neurotoxicity via nAChR in the primary culture of cortical neurons by pretreatment (Akaike et al. 1994). Since donepezil exerted a neuroprotective effect in a manner dependent on the duration of the pretreatment, we examined the possible involvement of acetylcholine receptors in the protective action of donepezil. Upon treatment with glutamate after treatment for 24 h with the nAChR antagonist mecamylamine and donepezil, we found that mecamylamine treatment significantly prevented the protective effect of AChE inhibitors. Upon pretreatment with the muscarine acetylcholine receptor antagonist scopolamine and donepezil, there was no impact on the protective effect of donepezil. These results suggested that the protective effect of donepezil against glutamate neurotoxicity involves nAChRs.

Next, we examined nAChR subtypes which are involved in the protective action of donepezil. The brain-expressed primary subtypes among the currently known 12 nAChR subtypes are α4- and α7-nAChR. First, when we verified the expression of primary component subunits of α4- and α7-nAChR in the primary culture of rat embryonic cortical neurons used in our laboratory, we detected nAChR mRNA and proteins of α4 and α7 subunits, which are the subunits composing α7-nAChR. We also used dihydro-β-erythroidine (DHβE) and methyllycaconitine (MLA), which are α4- nAChR and α7-nAChR-specific antagonists, to examine the involvement of neuronal nAChR subtypes in the neuroprotective action of donepezil. We applied glutamate treatment after treatment with donepezil and DHβE or MLA for 24 h and found that the protective action of donepezil was significantly inhibited. The above results showed that the protective action of donepezil against glutamate neurotoxicity involved nAChRs (Takada et al. 2003).

4.3 Mechanisms of Neuroprotective Effects by Stimulating Nicotinic Receptors

Nicotine exerts a neuroprotective effect against neuronal apoptosis via α7-nAChR. The phosphatidylinositol 3-kinase (PI3K)/Akt signal pathway has been reported to be involved in this protective mechanism (Kihara et al. 2001; Shaw et al. 2002). In addition to the protective effect of nicotine against glutamate neurotoxicity reportedly being inhibited by various kinase inhibitors through the PI3K pathway, the phosphorylation of Akt by nicotine treatment and the increase in the expression of Bcl-2, an anti-apoptotic protein, have also been reported. Since donepezil exerts its protective effect through α7-nAChR, we considered the possibility of the involvement of the PI3K-Akt signal pathway in this protective action and investigated specific inhibitors of kinases that form the PI3K signal pathway. Janus-activated kinase 2 (JAK2), a non-receptor tyrosine kinase, and Fyn activate PI3K in conjunction with α7-nAChR, so we examined the involvements of AG490 and PP2, inhibitors of JAK2 and Fyn. After pretreating cerebral cortical cells with either AG 490 or PP2 along with donepezil 24 h ahead of time, the application of glutamate significantly inhibited the protective action of donepezil. Next, to clarify the involvement of PI3K, we examined the effect of the PI3K inhibitor LY294002 on donepezil and found the protective effect of donepezil to be significantly inhibited. After that, we examined whether the MAPK pathway might be involved by observing the effect of the MAPK inhibitor PD98059 on donepezil; we found that the protective effect of donepezil was unaffected. The results of using these different kinase inhibitors suggested that the protective effect of donepezil is expressed through the PI3K signal pathway.

To further examine the role of donepezil in the PI3K signal transmission pathway, we observed the phosphorylation of Akt and the change in the amount of Bcl-2 expression in cerebral cortical cells treated with donepezil. Akt is known to be recruited by active PI3K in the vicinity of cell membranes, activated through phosphorylation, which in turn activates proteins and caspases of the Bcl-2 family of apoptotic control factors to regulate apoptosis. Using western blotting to observe

Akt phosphorylation in cerebral cortical neurons treated for 1 h with donepezil, we found a marked increase of phosphorylated Akt in the neurons treated with donepezil. Likewise, in assessing change in the amount of Bcl-2 expression in cerebral cortical cells treated for 24 h with donepezil, an increase of Bcl-2 expression could be seen from the donepezil treatment. By integrating these results, the protective effect of donepezil against glutamate neurotoxicity is thought to be linked to the activation of PI3K by α7-nAChR via JAK2 and Fyn and, by virtue of activating p-Akt, to be expressed through initiation of an apoptosis control program involving an increase in Bcl-2 expression (Takada-Takatori et al. 2006).

4.4 Mechanism of the Nicotinic Acetylcholine Receptor Upregulation upon Long-Term Nicotine Stimulation

Unlike other receptors, the amount of protein increases in nAChR and its function is accelerated—that is, upregulation is provoked—as a result of long-term exposure to nicotine and other agonists. However, much remains unknown about the details of this mechanism. Thus, further research has been performed on the signals related to nAChR upregulation and increased sensitivity of the neuroprotective action in order to elucidate the mechanism that promotes the survival of neurons associated with nAChR and to understand the changes in cellular and receptor functions that are caused by long-term stimulation of nAChR, which has a neuroprotective effect. It is assumed that long-term nicotine stimulus is subjected to complex regulation by the desensitization of nAChR. Therefore, the study described below investigated this mechanism using donepezil, as an nAChR activator, which is currently indicated for long-term clinical use.

When we observed the amounts of nAChR expression in primary cortical neuron cultures as a result of long-term treatment with donepezil using western blot analysis, the expression level of α7-nAChR protein was increased. In addition, when we observed the immunohistochemical changes in the amount of nAChR expression as a result of long-term treatment with donepezil, we observed that the number of α7-nAChR-expressing cells increased in the cell membrane, which is important for the exertion of nAChR function. These results suggest that long-term stimulation of nAChR not only increases the amount of α7-nAChR that is expressed as a protein but also promotes a shift of that expression to the cell membrane, which is thought to be responsible for the function of α7-nAChR.

Next, to investigate the effect that increased expression of α7-nAChR has on the function of nAChR, we investigated the involvement of nicotine in increased intracellular concentrations of calcium ($[Ca^{2+}]_i$). Temporary increases in $[Ca^{2+}]_i$ as a result of nicotine treatment increased even further as a result of nicotine stimulation in cells that were treated with donepezil for 4 days. This indicates that long-term treatment with donepezil enhanced the response to nicotine stimulation immediately after administration and induced upregulation (Kume et al. 2005).

Since it is clear that nAChR upregulation occurs as a result of long-term stimulation of nAChR receptors in cortical neuron cultures, we continued our investigation of the mechanism behind this effect. To investigate the involvement of nAChR stimulation and its downstream signal, we simultaneously carried out both long-term donepezil treatment and treatment with MLA, which is an α7-nAChR antagonist. The results indicated that the increases in the amount of nAChR proteins caused by long-term donepezil treatment were suppressed by simultaneous treatment with MLA. Therefore, we simultaneously carried out both long-term donepezil treatment and treatment with either LY294002, which is a PI3K inhibitor, or the MAPKK inhibitor PD98059 and found that simultaneous treatment with either LY294002 or PD98059 suppressed increases in the amount of nAChR proteins. These results indicate that the nAChR and the PI3K and MAPK signal pathways are involved in nAChR upregulation caused by long-term donepezil treatment. Next, to elucidate the mechanism of action of the promotion of nAChR function caused by long-term donepezil treatment, we investigated the involvement of the actions of nAChR antagonist, PI3K inhibitor, and MAPKK inhibitor on the increases in $[Ca^{2+}]_i$ that are caused by nicotine. We carried out simultaneous long-term treatment with donepezil and treatment with the α7-nAChR antagonist MLA. This resulted in the suppression of further increases in $[Ca^{2+}]_i$ as a result of nicotine. We then carried out simultaneous long-term treatment with donepezil and either the PI3K inhibitor LY294002 or the MAPKK inhibitor PD98059. This also resulted in the suppression of further increases in $[Ca^{2+}]_i$ as a result of nicotine. These results suggest that nAChR as well as the PI3K and MAPK pathways are involved in the promotion of nAChR function in cell membranes, such as seen when $[Ca^{2+}]_i$ increases as a result of long-term treatment with donepezil (Takada-Takatori et al. 2008a).

4.5 Mechanism of Increased Sensitivity in the Neuronal Protective Effect of Nicotine That Accompanies Receptor Upregulation Caused by Long-Term Stimulation of Nicotine Receptors

Next, to investigate whether the increased sensitivity to the neuronal protective effect results from nAChR causing upregulation, we conducted long-term treatment with donepezil and investigated its effect on donepezil against glutamate neurotoxicity during a state of increased nAChR function. The concentrations of donepezil that are sufficiently low that they do not lead to expression of the normal protective action (1 nM) in the treatment of neurons that have been subjected to long-term treatment with donepezil resulted in the marked suppression of glutamate neurotoxicity. This indicates that the protective effect that is induced by long-term treatment with donepezil is dependent on both the treatment duration and the concentration. Therefore, to elucidate the mechanism of neuroprotection that occurs under the conditions of long-term treatment, we investigated the effect of simultaneous long-term treatment with donepezil, nAChR antagonist, and either PI3K or MAPK pathway inhibitor on increased sensitivity to the neuroprotective action of donepezil. First, when we examined simultaneous long-term treatment with donepezil and treatment with the α7-nAChR antagonist MLA, we observed that the neuroprotective action caused by low concentrations of donepezil administered after long-term treatment with donepezil was suppressed by the simultaneous treatment with MLA. Next, when we examined simultaneous long-term treatment with donepezil and treatment with either the PI3K inhibitor LY294002 or the MAPKK inhibitor PD98059, we found that both had the same suppressive effect. Finally, to elucidate the mechanism by which the survival signal is enhanced by the phosphorylation of Akt in the downstream PI3K pathway, we observed the phosphorylation of Akt in cortical neurons with long-term donepezil treatment and pretreatment using western blotting. The results indicated that, although the amount of phosphorylated Akt in neurons with long-term donepezil treatment and pretreatment increased markedly, when we carried out treatment with nAChR inhibitor and PI3K inhibitor simultaneously with donepezil pretreatment, increases in the amount of phosphorylated Akt were suppressed. These results indicate that when receptors are in a state of upregulation as a result of long-term nAChR stimulation, the promotive function of nAChR in cell membranes increases sensitivity to the neuroprotective effect of donepezil, which in turn indicates that the nAChR and either the PI3K or the MAPK signal pathways are involved in that action. When nAChR is in an upregulated state, the survival signal via the nAChR, PI3K-Akt, and MAPK pathways is more efficiently transmitted, and thus, we assume that this is why even lower concentrations of donepezil exerted the protective effect (Takada-Takatori et al. 2008b).

The mechanism of the neuroprotective effect of donepezil via nAChR that we assume is at work as a result of the above results is shown in Fig. 4.1. We hypothesize the following: As a result of the stimulation of α4- and α7-nAChR, donepezil exerts its neuroprotective effect via the PI3K-Akt signal pathway. Long-term nAChR stimulation induces the upregulation of nAChR in cell membranes, and the resulting promotion of nAChR function causes increased sensitivity to the neuroprotective effect (Takada-Takatori et al. 2009).

4.6 Effect of the Stimulation of Nicotinic Acetylcholine Receptor in Astrocytes on Inflammatory Response in the Brain

Not only direct nAChR receptor stimulation on neuronal cells but also an indirect effect through glial cells is considered to mediate the neuroprotective effect. Therefore, we investigated the effect of nAChR stimulation on the inflammatory responses of astrocytes, which play a crucial role in brain inflammation. As an inflammatory mediator in the brain, bradykinin is produced in the early stage of inflammation and induces the expression of several inflammatory genes (Lin et al.

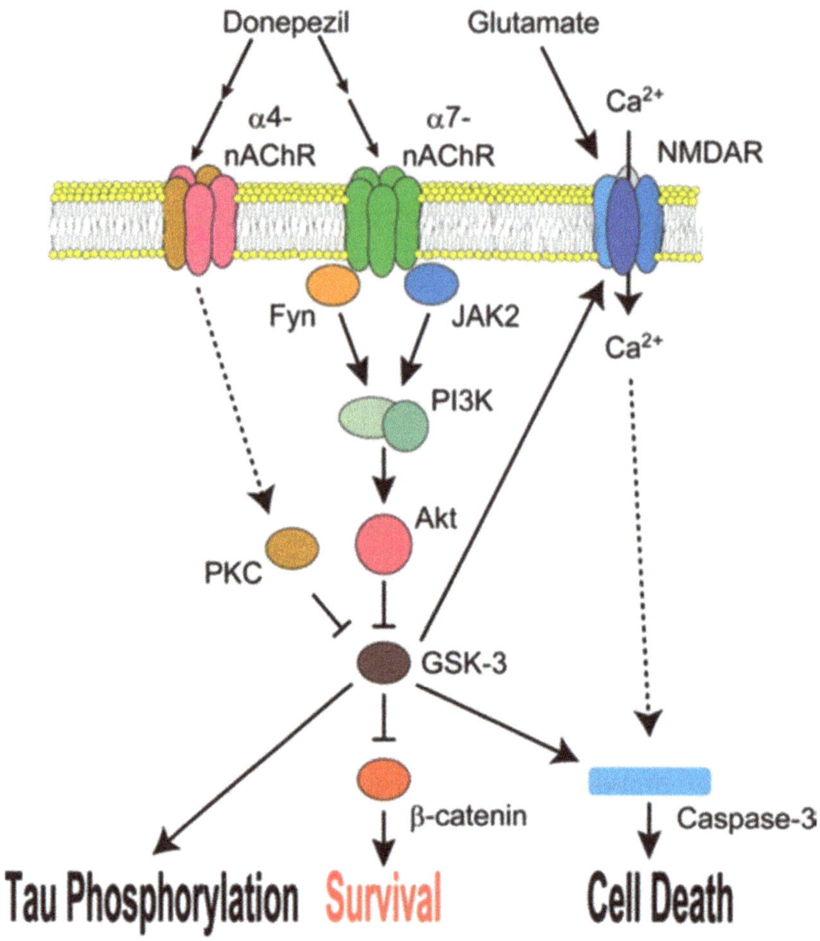

Fig. 4.1 The mechanism of the neuroprotective effects of donepezil via nicotinic acetylcholine receptors

2012; Hsieh et al. 2007; Schwaninger et al. 1999). In particular, bradykinin induces a variety of responses, such as a transient increase of intracellular calcium concentration ($[Ca^{2+}]_i$) (Akita and Okada 2011), the expression of matrix metalloprotease-9 (Lin et al. 2012) and cyclooxygenase-2 (COX-2) (Hsieh et al. 2007), and the release of interleukin-6 (IL-6) (Schwaninger et al. 1999) and glutamate (Liu et al. 2009) in astrocytes. In addition, it was previously reported that the cleavage of high-molecular-weight kininogen, the precursor of bradykinin, was increased in the cerebrospinal fluid of AD patients (Iores-Marçal et al. 2006; Bergamaschini et al. 1998) and that bradykinin receptor antagonists ameliorated the cognitive deficits in AD model mice (Bicca et al. 2015; Prediger et al. 2008; Lacoste et al. 2013). Accordingly, it can be speculated that inflammation induced by bradykinin in astrocytes is involved in the pathogenesis of AD. On the basis of these findings, to elucidate the effect of nAChR stimulation using nicotine and donepezil on the function in astrocytes, we investigated the responses of astrocytes to bradykinin and the effects of donepezil on these responses using cultured cortical astrocytes.

We first examined the effect of bradykinin on $[Ca^{2+}]_i$ in cultured cortical astrocytes. Bradykinin induced a transient increase in $[Ca^{2+}]_i$ in a concentration-dependent manner. Next, we verified the gene expression of B_1 and B_2 receptors in cultured cortical astrocytes. Both B_1 and B_2 receptors were expressed in our cultured astrocytes. We investigated the involvement of B_1 and B_2 receptors in the increase in $[Ca^{2+}]_i$ induced by bradykinin using subtype-specific antagonists. Des-Arg9-[Leu8]-bradykinin, an antagonist of B_1 receptors, did not affect the increase in $[Ca^{2+}]_i$ induced by bradykinin, but HOE140, an antagonist of B_2 receptors, almost completely inhibited the Ca^{2+} response induced by bradykinin. We further determined whether the $[Ca^{2+}]_i$ increase induced by bradykinin was due to Ca^{2+} influx from the extracellular space or Ca^{2+} release from the intracellular Ca^{2+} store. Bradykinin-induced $[Ca^{2+}]_i$ increase did not change upon excluding extracellular Ca^{2+}. In contrast, depletion of Ca^{2+} stored in the endoplasmic reticulum (ER) by treating cells with thapsigargin, a blocker of Ca^{2+}-ATPase on the ER, significantly reduced the Ca^{2+} response. These results suggest that bradykinin-induced $[Ca^{2+}]_i$ response is attributable not to Ca^{2+} influx from the extracellular space but to Ca^{2+} release from the ER. Next, we examined the effect of nicotine and donepezil on the increase in $[Ca^{2+}]_i$ induced by bradykinin. Simultaneous treatment of nicotine and donepezil did not affect the increase of $[Ca^{2+}]_i$. However, 24 h pretreatment of these drugs significantly reduced the Ca^{2+} response in a concentration-dependent manner, while these drugs did not affect the cell morphology and cell proliferation in astrocytes. These results suggest that nicotinic receptor stimulation suppressed the increase of $[Ca^{2+}]_i$ induced by bradykinin and that pretreatment is required for this inhibitory effect.

We attempted to elucidate the mechanism of the inhibitory effect of nicotinic receptor stimulation on the increase of $[Ca^{2+}]_i$ induced by bradykinin. We previously reported that donepezil exerted a neuroprotective effect on glutamate neurotoxicity via nAChRs in cultured cortical neurons (Takada-Takatori et al. 2006). Thus, we herein investigated the involvement of nAChRs in this effect of donepezil using nAChR antagonists. When cortical astrocytes were treated with a nAChR antagonist, mecamylamine, for 24 h before Ca^{2+} imaging, the inhibitory effect of donepezil was significantly antagonized. Previous studies reported that the most abundant nAChR subtypes in the brain are the α7- and α4- nAChRs (Paterson and Nordberg 2000) and that both of the receptor subtypes were also expressed in astrocytes (Oikawa et al. 2005). Thus, we examined the effects of MLA, an α7- nAChR antagonist, and DHβE, an α4- nAChR antagonist, on the inhibition by donepezil of the $[Ca^{2+}]_i$ increase induced by bradykinin. When cortical astrocytes were pretreated with either MLA or DHβE for 24 h, the inhibitory effect of donepezil did not change. However, the effect of donepezil was significantly suppressed by treating cortical astrocytes with both MLA and DHβE for 24 h prior to bradykinin. These results suggested that both α7- and α4- nAChRs were involved in the inhibitory effect of donepezil on the increase of $[Ca^{2+}]_i$ induced by bradykinin.

Previous studies demonstrated that JAK2 was activated in the downstream signaling of nAChRs (Razani-Boroujerdi et al. 2007; Marrero and Bencherif 2009). Therefore, we used AG490, a JAK2 inhibitor, to investigate the involvement of

JAK2 in the inhibitory effect of donepezil. Treatment with AG490 significantly suppressed the inhibitory effect of donepezil on the increase in $[Ca^{2+}]_i$ induced by bradykinin.

We previously reported that the stimulation of nAChRs activated PI3K and that the phosphorylation and activation of Akt downstream of PI3K were induced (Kihara et al. 2001). Thus, we examined the involvement of the PI3K-Akt pathway in the inhibitory effect of donepezil on the Ca^{2+} response induced by bradykinin. LY294002, a PI3K inhibitor, and Akt inhibitor significantly suppressed the effect of donepezil. In addition, we investigated the effect of donepezil on the phosphorylation state of Akt in cultured cortical astrocytes. The phosphorylation level of Akt was significantly elevated by treating cells with donepezil for 6 h.

Taking the obtained findings together, nAChR stimulation using donepezil induced the activation of the PI3K-Akt pathway in both cultured astrocytes and cultured neurons. However, there are some differences between astrocytes and neurons with respect to the signaling pathway mediated by nAChRs. For example, we previously showed that Akt phosphorylation was induced 1 h after the treatment of donepezil in cultured neurons, although donepezil induced Akt phosphorylation 6 h after the treatment in cultured astrocytes. Moreover, treatment of MLA or DHβE alone did not inhibit the effect of donepezil, and the combination of MLA and DHβE significantly reduced this effect. Thus, further studies are needed to elucidate the differences of the time course of Akt phosphorylation and the involvement of nAChR subtypes between neurons and astrocytes. Here we demonstrated that the Akt inhibitor suppressed the effect of donepezil on the increase in $[Ca^{2+}]_i$ induced by bradykinin. Other researchers reported that, as the downstream signaling of the PI3K-Akt pathway, the activated Akt induced the phosphorylation of inositol trisphosphate (IP_3) receptors and lowered the function of IP_3 receptors (Khan et al. 2006; Szado et al. 2008). Taken together, these findings suggest that the phosphorylation and hypofunction of IP_3 receptors by Akt could be involved in the effect of donepezil.

A previous study showed that bradykinin induced the production of intracellular reactive oxygen species (ROS) after the $[Ca^{2+}]_i$ increase in cultured astrocytes (Akita and Okada 2011). To elucidate the effect of donepezil on ROS production, we examined ROS production induced by bradykinin using a fluorescent ROS indicator, H_2DCF-DA. Bradykinin induced ROS production in a time-dependent manner. Donepezil significantly inhibited the increase of intracellular ROS level induced by bradykinin. Previous studies reported that an increase in intracellular ROS level activated transcription factors, such as nuclear factor-kappa B (NF-κB) and activator protein 1, and this activation led to inflammatory responses in astrocytes (Yang et al. 2012; Park et al. 2004). In fact, bradykinin induced the expression of IL-6 and COX-2 downstream of ROS production and activation of NF-κB in cultured astrocytes (Hsieh et al. 2007; Schwaninger et al. 1999). We here demonstrated that donepezil inhibited ROS production induced by bradykinin. Taking these results and reports into account, we suggest that nAChR stimulation using donepezil decreases the inflammatory response induced by bradykinin by regulating the increase of intracellular ROS level.

4.7 Conclusion and Future Prospects

It was previously reported that nAChR is involved in AD and many neurodegenerative diseases. We investigated the involvement of nAChRs in the neuroprotective action that is induced through the use of AD drugs and found that PI3K-Akt and other intracellular information transmission systems play an important role in the neuroprotective effect and nAChR upregulation. In addition, we found that nAChR stimulation exerted an inhibitory effect on the $[Ca^{2+}]_i$ increase induced by bradykinin via the PI3K-Akt pathway and also inhibited the increase of the ROS level in cultured cortical astrocytes. The cholinergic hypothesis was first proposed in the 1970s, but interesting new discoveries relating to the mechanism of action of AD drugs based on this hypothesis continue to be made. Research into the molecular mechanism that targets the signals that are related to nAChR, which is still only slightly understood, should make major contributions to the development of new drugs for neurodegenerative disorders including AD.

Acknowledgment This study was supported in part by JSPS KAKENHI Grant Numbers JP24590111 and JP24390139 to Toshiaki Kume, and JP25860069 and JP17K08323 to Yuki Takada-Takatori. It was also supported in part by a grant from the Smoking Research Foundation and the Naito Foundation of Japan.

References

Akaike A, Tamura Y, Yokota T et al (1994) Nicotine-induced protection of cultured cortical neurons against *N*-methyl-D-aspartate receptor-mediated glutamate cytotoxicity. Brain Res 644:181–187

Akita T, Okada Y (2011) Regulation of bradykinin-induced activation of volume-sensitive outwardly rectifying anion channels by Ca^{2+} nanodomains in mouse astrocytes. J Physiol 589:3909–3927

Allan SM, Rothwell NJ (2001) Cytokines and acute neurodegeneration. Nat Rev Neurosci 2:734–744

Bartus RT, Dean RL 3rd, Beer B et al (1982) The cholinergic hypothesis of geriatric memory dysfunction. Science 217:408–414

Bergamaschini L, Parnetti L, Pareyson D et al (1998) Activation of the contact system in cerebrospinal fluid of patients with Alzheimer disease. Alzheimer Dis Assoc Disord 12:102–108

Bicca MA, Costa R, Loch-Neckel G et al (2015) B2 receptor blockage prevents Aβ-induced cognitive impairment by neuroinflammation inhibition. Behav Brain Res 278:482–491

Bresnick GH (1989) Excitotoxins: a possible new mechanism for the pathogenesis of ischemic retinal damage. Arch Ophthalmol 107:339–341

Choi DW, Maulucci-Gedde M, Kriegstein AJ (1987) Glutamate neurotoxicity in cortical cell culture. J Neurosci 7:357–368

Coyle JT, Price DL, DeLong MR et al (1983) Alzheimer's disease: a disorder of cortical cholinergic innervation. Science 219:1184–1190

Giaume C, Koulakoff A, Roux L et al (2010) Astroglial networks: a step further in neuroglial and gliovascular interactions. Nat Rev Neurosci 11:87–99

Heneka MT, Carson MJ, El Khoury J et al (2015) Neuroinflammation in Alzheimer's disease. Lancet Neurol 14:388–405

Heppner FL, Ransohoff RM, Becher B (2015) Immune attack: the role of inflammation in Alzheimer disease. Nat Rev Neurosci 16:358–372
Hsieh HL, Wang HH, Wu CY et al (2007) BK-induced COX-2 expression via PKC-δ-dependent activation of p42/p44 MAPK and NF-κB in astrocytes. Cell Signal 19:330–340
Iores-Marçal LM, Viel TA, Buck HS et al (2006) Bradykinin release and inactivation in brain of rats submitted to an experimental model of Alzheimer's disease. Peptides 27:3363–3369
Kaneko S, Maeda T, Kume T et al (1997) Nicotine protects cultured cortical neurons against glutamate-induced cytotoxicity via α7 neuronal receptors and neuronal CNS receptors. Brain Res 765:135–140
Khan MT, Wagner L 2nd, Yule DI et al (2006) Akt kinase phosphorylation of inositol 1,4,5-trisphosphate receptors. J Biol Chem 281:3731–3737
Kihara T, Shimohama S, Sawada H et al (2001) α7 nicotinic receptor transduces signals to phosphatidylinositol 3-kinase to block A β-amyloid-induced neurotoxicity. J Biol Chem 276:13541–13546
Kim HG, Moon M, Choi JG et al (2014) Donepezil inhibits the amyloid-β oligomer-induced microglial activation in vitro and in vivo. Neurotoxicology 40:23–32
Kume T, Sugimoto M, Takada Y et al (2005) Up-regulation of nicotinic acetylcholine receptors by central-type acetylcholinesterase inhibitors in rat cortical neurons. Eur J Pharmacol 527:77–85
Lacoste B, Tong XK, Lahjouji K et al (2013) Cognitive and cerebrovascular improvements following kinin B1 receptor blockade in Alzheimer's disease mice. J Neuroinflammation 4:10–57
Lee SC, Dickson DW, Brosnan CF (1995) Interleukin-1, nitric oxide and reactive astrocytes. Brain Behav Immun 9:345–354
Lee YJ, Han SB, Nam SY, Oh KW et al (2010) Inflammation and Alzheimer's disease. Arch Pharm Res 33:1539–1556
Lin CC, Hsieh HL, Shih RH et al (2012) NADPH oxidase 2-derived reactive oxygen species signal contributes to bradykinin-induced matrix metalloproteinase-9 expression and cell migration in brain astrocytes. Cell Commun Signal 10:35
Liu HT, Akita T, Shimizu T et al (2009) Bradykinin-induced astrocyte-neuron signaling: glutamate release is mediated by ROS-activated volume-sensitive outwardly rectifying anion channels. J Physiol 587:2197–2209
Marrero MB, Bencherif M (2009) Convergence of α7 nicotinic acetylcholine receptor-activated pathways for anti-apoptosis and anti-inflammation: central role for JAK2 activation of STAT3 and NF-κB. Brain Res 1256:1–7
Morris GP, Clark IA, Zinn R et al (2013) Microglia: a new frontier for synaptic plasticity, learning and memory, and neurodegenerative disease research. Neurobiol Learn Mem 105:40–53
Oikawa H, Nakamichi N, Kambe Y et al (2005) An increase in intracellular free calcium ions by nicotinic acetylcholine receptors in a single cultured rat cortical astrocyte. J Neurosci Res 79:535–544
Park J, Choi K, Jeong E et al (2004) Reactive oxygen species mediate chloroquine-induced expression of chemokines by human astroglial cells. Glia 47:9–20
Paterson D, Nordberg A (2000) Neuronal nicotinic receptors in the human brain. Prog Neurobiol 61:75–111
Perry EK, Morris CM, Court JA et al (1995) Alteration in nicotine binding sites in Parkinson's disease, Lewy body dementia and Alzheimer's disease: possible index of early neuropathology. Neuroscience 64:385–395
Prediger RD, Medeiros R, Pandolfo P et al (2008) Genetic deletion or antagonism of kinin B(1) and B(2) receptors improves cognitive deficits in a mouse model of Alzheimer's disease. Neuroscience 151:631–643
Razani-Boroujerdi S, Boyd RT, Dávila-García MI et al (2007) T cells express α7-nicotinic acetylcholine receptor subunits that require a functional TCR and leukocyte-specific protein tyrosine kinase for nicotine-induced Ca2+ response. J Immunol 179:2889–2998
Rogers J (2008) The inflammatory response in Alzheimer's disease. J Periodontol 79:1535–1543
Schwaninger M, Sallmann S, Petersen N et al (1999) Bradykinin induces interleukin-6 expression in astrocytes through activation of nuclear factor- κB. J Neurochem 73:1461–1466

Shaw S, Bencherif M, Marrero MB et al (2002) Janus kinase 2, an early target of α7 nicotinic acetylcholine receptor-mediated neuroprotection against Aβ-(1-42) amyloid. J Biol Chem 277:44920–44924

Shimohama S, Greenwald DL, Shafron DH et al (1998) Nicotinic α7 receptors protect against glutamate neurotoxicity and neuronal ischemic damage. Brain Res 779:359–363

Szado T, Vanderheyden V, Parys JB et al (2008) Phosphorylation of inositol 1,4,5-trisphosphate receptors by protein kinase B/Akt inhibits Ca^{2+} release and apoptosis. Proc Natl Acad Sci U S A 105:2427–2432

Takada Y, Yonezawa A, Kume T et al (2003) Nicotinic acetylcholine receptor-mediated neuroprotection by donepezil against glutamate neurotoxicity in rat cortical neurons. J Pharmacol Exp Ther 306:772–777

Takada-Takatori Y, Kume T, Sugimoto M et al (2006) Acetylcholinesterase inhibitors used in treatment of Alzheimer's disease prevent glutamate neurotoxicity via nicotinic acetylcholine receptors and phosphatidylinositol 3-kinase cascade. Neuropharmacology 51:474–486

Takada-Takatori Y, Kume T, Ohgi Y et al (2008a) Mechanisms of α7-nicotinic receptor up-regulation and sensitization to donepezil-induced by chronic donepezil treatment. Eur J Pharmacol 590:150–156

Takada-Takatori Y, Kume T, Ohgi Y et al (2008b) Mechanism of neuroprotection by donepezil pretreatment in rat cortical neurons chronically treated with donepezil. J Neurosci Res. 2008 86:3575–3583

Takada-Takatori Y, Kume T, Izumi Y (2009) Roles of nicotinic receptors in acetylcholinesterase inhibitor-induced neuroprotection and nicotinic receptor up-regulation. Biol Pharm Bull 32:318–324

Whitehouse PJ, Price DL, Struble RG et al (1982) Alzheimer's disease and senile dementia: loss of neurons in the basal forebrain. Science 215:1237–1239

Yan J, Fu Q, Cheng L et al (2014) Inflammatory response in Parkinson's disease (review). Mol Med Rep 10:2223–2233

Yang CM, Lin CC, Lee IT et al (2012) Japanese encephalitis virus induces matrix metalloproteinase-9 expression via a ROS/c-Src/PDGFR/PI3K-Akt/MAPKs-dependent AP-1 pathway in rat brain astrocytes. J Neuroinflammation 18:9–12

Chapter 5
Regulation by Nicotinic Acetylcholine Receptors of Microglial Glutamate Transporters: Role of Microglia in Neuroprotection

Norimitsu Morioka, Kazue Hisaoka-Nakashima, and Yoshihiro Nakata

Abstract Accumulated evidence shows that activation of microglia is associated with a change in morphology, from ramified to globular, which also represents a transition to M1 microglia. M1 microglia contribute to the induction and development of various neuroinflammatory disorders, including stroke, spinal cord injury, multiple sclerosis, Parkinson's disease, Alzheimer's disease psychiatric disorders, neuropathic pain and epilepsy. Thus, inhibition of microglial activation would be crucial in treating neurological disorders. Recent studies suggest a number of attractive molecular targets for blocking microglial activation. Among them, the nicotinic ACh receptor (nAChR), which especially contains the α7 subunit, contributes to the regulation of microglial activity through the inhibition of the synthesis of proinflammatory molecules. In addition, the glutamate transporter GLAST expressed in microglia is upregulated by α7 nAChR stimulation, which is mediated through both inositol triphosphate-Ca^{2+}/calmodulin-dependent protein kinase II and fibroblast growth factor-2 pathways. It is possible, then, that activation of microglial α7 nAChR could be neuroprotective through inhibition of the production of proinflammatory molecules and enhancement of glutamate clearance from the synapse. This chapter will give an overview of the role of the α7 nAChR in microglial functioning and its potential as a therapeutic target for neurological disorders.

Keywords Microglia · α7 nicotinic ACh receptor · Glutamate transporter · GLAST · Ca^{2+} · Calmodulin-dependent protein kinase II · Fibroblast growth factor-2

N. Morioka (✉) · K. Hisaoka-Nakashima · Y. Nakata
Department of Pharmacology, Hiroshima University Graduate School of Biomedical & Health Sciences, Hiroshima, Japan
e-mail: mnori@hiroshima-u.ac.jp

A. Akaike et al. (eds.), *Nicotinic Acetylcholine Receptor Signaling in Neuroprotection*, https://doi.org/10.1007/978-981-10-8488-1_5

5.1 Microglia

Neuroinflammation is involved in the induction of various neurodegenerative and neuropsychiatric disorders including stroke, spinal cord injury, multiple sclerosis, Parkinson's disease, Alzheimer's disease, depressive disorders, schizophrenia, neuropathic pain and epilepsy (Blank and Prinz 2013; Frank-Cannon et al. 2009; Yrjänheikki et al. 1998). Neuroinflammation is mainly mediated by CNS glial cells such as microglia and astrocytes. Microglia, originally derived from the reticuloendothelial system, have a pivotal role as the main effector cells of the immune system (Kettenmann and Verkhratsky 2008). Although present in all region of the CNS, microglia are not uniformly distributed, representing between 0.5 and 16.6% of all cells in human and mouse brain (Lawson et al. 1990; Mittelbronn et al. 2001). Microglia act as a type of macrophage in peripheral tissues. Microglia are highly ramified, with long processes and small cell bodies, under the normal physiological state (Kettenmann et al. 2011). The recent emergence of live cell imaging technology reveals that microglia have highly motile processes that continuously survey the surrounding environment (Nimmerjahn et al. 2005; Davalos et al. 2005). This state represents the "resting" phenotype, which is involved in maintaining homeostasis (Kettenmann et al. 2011). Therefore, changes in microglial activity and functionality are indicative of pathological conditions.

5.2 Neuroinflammatory and Neuroprotective Roles of Microglia

It is widely known that activation of microglia, in response to illness, infection and injury, lead to morphological changes, from the highly ramified configuration to a globular, amoeboid shape (Kitamura et al. 1978; Stence et al. 2001; Thomas 1992). Activated microglia demonstrate increased proliferation, migration to the site of injury, scavenging of exogenous substances, cellular debris and pathogens, and production of proinflammatory molecules, including cytokines, chemokines, prostaglandins, nitric oxide and reactive oxygen species (Suzuki et al. 2004; Hide et al. 2000; Koizumi et al. 2007; Stence et al. 2001; Nolte et al. 1996; Morioka et al. 2013; Garrido-Gil et al. 2013; Fernandes et al. 2014). Cells that exhibit this phenotype are identified as "M1 microglia" (Kigerl et al. 2009). In fact, it has been demonstrated that hyper- or chronic activation of microglia could lead to the initiation of neurodegenerative disorders (Moehle and West 2015; Henkel et al. 2009). In addition, treatment with the microglial inhibitor minocycline, a tetracycline antibiotic, reduces inflammation in animal models of neurodegeneration (Wu et al. 2002; Hou et al. 2016).

At the same time, microglia also contribute to tissue recovery. Microglia produce anti-inflammatory and neuroprotective molecules, such as brain-derived neurotrophic factor (BDNF), glial cell-derived neurotrophic factor (GDNF), transforming growth factor-β (TGF-β), tumor necrosis factor (TNF), interleukin-4 (IL-4) and interleukin-10 (IL-10) (Suzuki et al. 2004; Lai and Todd 2008; Polazzi and Monti 2010; Amantea et al. 2015). Microglia showing anti-inflammatory and neuroprotective properties are called "M2 microglia". Stimulation of microglia with IL-4 and interleukin-13 (IL-13), which are secreted by Th2 lymphocytes (Freilich et al. 2013), induces the M2 phenotype. M2 microglia express markers such as heparin-binding lectin, cysteine-rich protein FIZZ-1 and arginase-1 (Freilich et al. 2013). Transient middle cerebral artery occlusion induces brain tissue infraction and cell apoptosis. The number of apoptotic cells in infarcted tissue in transgenic mice in which microglia were selectively ablated was significantly more than that of wild-type mice (Lalancette-Hébert et al. 2007). Microglial phenotype is altered depending on environmental conditions—thus, microglial functioning show apparently opposing properties, either pro-inflammatory or anti-inflammatory (Ponomarev et al. 2007). Previous findings also indicate that blockade of microglial activity alone may not be sufficient as a treatment for neuroinflammatory disorders, so further elucidating changes in microglial phenotypes and properties under specific pathological conditions is crucial. Although there are a number of studies on the role of M1 microglia in proinflammatory responses and their involvement in neurological disorders, their roles in neuroprotection and their function in neuroinflammatory and neurodegenerative diseases have yet to be fully elaborated. In this vein, more research is necessary on identifying the neuroprotective molecules released by microglia under pathological conditions.

5.3 Nicotinic Acetylcholine Receptors and Microglia

Nicotinic acetylcholine receptors (nAChRs) are ligand-gated ion channels, consisting of hetero- or homo-pentameric subunits. These receptors have important roles in neurobiological processes such as memory, learning, locomotion, attention and anxiety (Dajas-Bailador and Wonnacott 2004; Dani and Bertrand 2007; Zoli et al. 2015). In the mammalian brain, 12 genes each encode a subunit, and nine different nAChR subunits have been identified (α2-α10 and β2-β4) (Dani and Bertrand 2007). The homomeric α7 nAChR is one of the most abundantly expressed and widely distributed subtype in the brain (Gotti and Clementi 2004; Sargent 1993). The α7 nAChR is expressed not only in neurons, but also in non-neuronal cells such as astrocytes, microglia, oligodendrocyte precursor cells and brain endothelial cells (Liu et al. 2015; Kihara et al. 2001; Suzuki et al. 2006; Hawkins et al. 2005; Rogers et al. 2001). Human microglia express the α3, α5, α7 and β4 subunits (Rock et al. 2008), whereas the α7 nAChR is the only functional nAChR subtype in rat cortical microglia (Morioka et al. 2014). The rat cortical microglia, then, makes an ideal system to study the neurobiological role of the α7 nAChR.

The α7 nAChR appears to have a critical role in neuroprotection. Peripheral macrophages express α7 nAChR, which regulate the systemic response to inflammation

(Wang et al. 2003). Microglial α7 nAChR could be responsible for modulating the response to inflammation in the mouse brain. Prevention of lipopolysaccharide (LPS)-induced TNF release from murine microglia is mediated through activation of the α7 nAChR (Shytle et al. 2004). Activation of microglial α7 nAChR suppresses the production of a number of proinflammatory molecules (Suzuki et al. 2006; Giunta et al. 2004; De Simone et al. 2005; Rock et al. 2008; Zhang et al. 2017). Furthermore, stimulation of the α7 nAChR suppresses the production of reactive oxygen species (ROS) in microglia stimulated with fibrillar β-amyloid peptide (Moon et al. 2008), in addition, treatment of cultured microglia with galantamine, a nAChR allosteric ligand, induces phagocytosis of β-amyloid in an α7 nAChR-dependent manner (Takata et al. 2010), suggesting a potential role of the α7 nAChR in the pathophysiology of Alzheimer's disease. Stimulation of the α7 nAChR also increases expression of anti-inflammatory and neuroprotective molecules such as TGF-β1, IL-4, IL-10 and heme oxygenase-1 (De Simone et al. 2005; Parada et al. 2013; Rock et al. 2008; Zhang et al. 2017). Treatment of a microglial cell line BV2 with an α7 nAChR agonist increases autophagy, an anti-inflammatory response (Shao et al. 2017). Furthermore, treatment with nicotine inhibits LPS-induced H^+ currents through α7 nAChR (Noda and Kobayashi 2017). It is known that H^+ channel-mediated currents are required for NAPDH oxidase-dependent ROS generation in brain microglia, a key step in the neuroinflammatory pathway (Wu et al. 2012). While it is currently unknown whether the stimulation of α7 nAChR induces the switching of microglial phenotype from M1 to M2, studies clearly indicate the importance of microglia-expressed α7 nAChR in reducing neuroinflammation, and suggest that microglial α7 nAChR could be utilized as a therapeutic target for the treatment of neuropathological disorders (Table 5.1).

5.4 Glutamate Transporters and Microglia

Glutamate is not only one of the major excitatory neurotransmitters mediating memory, learning and acute pain perception, but is excitotoxic at high concentrations in the synapse. Therefore, the regulation of synaptic glutamate concentration, to prevent the overstimulation of post-synaptic neurons, is important in preventing excitotoxicity, and is mainly conducted through Na^+/K^+-dependent glutamate transporters located in glial cells and neurons (Robinson and Dowd 1997). Thus far, five glutamate transporters have been cloned and pharmacologically characterized: excitatory amino acid transporter (EAAT) 1 (glutamate/aspartate transporter; GLAST) and EAAT2 (glutamate transporter 1; GLT-1), which are mainly expressed in glial cells, and EAAT3 (excitatory amino acid carrier 1; EAAC1), EAAT4 and EAAT5, which are mainly expressed in neurons (Arriza et al. 1997; Fairman et al. 1995; Kanai and Hediger 1992; Pines et al. 1992). In general, astrocytic GLAST and GLT-1 are important for maintaining low concentration of glutamate (Shibata et al. 1997), and astrocytic glutamate uptake at synapses account for about 90% of total clearance under physiological conditions (Tanaka et al. 1997).

Table 5.1 Effect of α7 nAChR stimulation on microglial function

Authors	Species	Cell types	Agonists	Actions
Shytle et al. (2004)	Mouse	Primary culture	ACh, nicotine	Inhibition of LPS-induced TNF expression
Giunta et al. (2004)	Mouse	Primary culture	Nicotine+galantamine	Inhibition of gp120+IFN-γ-induced TNF expression, NO production, and ERK phosphorylation
Noda and Kobayashi (2017)	Mouse	Primary culture	Nicotine	Inhibition of LPS-induced proton current
De Simone et al. (2005)	Rat	Primary culture	Nicotine	Inhibition of LPS-induced TNF, NO, and IL-10 expression increase of LPS-induced PGE2; no effect on IL-1β expression
Suzuki et al. (2006)	Rat	Primary culture	Nicotine	Inhibition of LPS-induced TNF production, increased ATP-induced TNF production
Moon et al. (2008)	Rat	Primary culture	Nicotine	Inhibition of Aβ-induced ROS production
Takata et al. (2010)	Rat	Primary culture	Nicotine, galantamine	Enhancement of Aβ clearance
Parada et al. (2013)	Rat	Organotypic hippocampal cultures	PNU282987	Induction of heme oxygenase-1 expression
Rock et al. (2008)	Human	Primary culture	Nicotine	Increased TGF-β1, IL-4, CX3CL1, CCR2, CXCR6 expression, inhibition of IL-8, IL-10, TNF, CCL2, CXCR4 expression
Zhang et al. (2017)	Mouse	BV2	ACh	Inhibition of LPS-induced IL-1β and IL-6 expression, p38 phosphorylation increased IL-4, and IL-10 expression rescue of LPS-suppressed JAK/STAT3 phosphorylation, and PI3K/Akt phosphorylation
Shao et al. (2017)	Mouse	BV2	PNU282987	Increased autophagy

Microglia express functional glutamate transporters, which are involved in regulating glutamate homeostasis in synapses (Morioka et al. 2008). It has been shown that activated microglia express GLAST and GLT-1 both in vivo and in vitro (Noda et al. 1999). Microglial glutamate uptake at synapses is about 10% of that of astrocytes under physiological conditions (Persson et al. 2005; Shaked et al. 2005). Under excitotoxic conditions induced by high concentrations of glutamate, however, activity and expression of microglial glutamate transporters are enhanced by excluding excess glutamate. For example, GLT-1 expression is increased in activated microglia following nerve injury (López-Redondo et al. 2000). Furthermore, stimulation of cultured microglia with LPS increases GLT-1 expression and glutamate transport capacity (Persson et al. 2005). A clinical study demonstrated that microglial glutamate transporters are involved in the control of neuronal damage in traumatic brain injury. Upregulation of GLAST expression in microglia is observed in brain white matter 1 week after ischemia (Beschorner et al. 2007). In addition, the expression of glutamate transporters (GLAST, GLT-1 and EAAC1) is observed in microglia/macrophages within the infract region at 7 and 28 days after ischemia (Arranz et al. 2010). Thus, these observations indicate that microglial glutamate transporters could be crucial in reducing glutamate-mediated excitotoxicity. Although astrocytes generally have a crucial role in clearing glutamate from the synapses, the activity of glutamate transport in astrocytes is in fact downregulated under pathological conditions (Fine et al. 1996; Xin et al. 2009). Therefore, microglial glutamate transporters, which are upregulated under pathological conditions, serve as a back-up to astrocytic glutamate uptake (López-Redondo et al. 2000; Xin et al. 2009). However, microglial glutamate transporter function and the functional relationship between α7 nAChR and glutamate transporters in microglia, have yet to be elaborated.

5.5 Nicotinic Acetylcholine Receptor and Glutamate Transporters

A number of studies have described significant interactions between nAChR and monoamine transporters, which comprise of noradrenaline, dopamine and serotonin transporters. For example, treatment with nicotine induced increased expression and functioning of these transporters in frontal cortical neurons and other cell types (Danielson et al. 2011; Itoh et al. 2010; Awtry and Werling 2003; Middleton et al. 2004). By contrast, few studies have demonstrated a positive functional interaction between the nAChR and glutamate transporters. Basal glutamate uptake in cultured glial cells derived from rat pups prenatally exposed to nicotine is higher than normal (Lim and Kim 2001). Furthermore, increased activity of astrocytic glutamate transporters (GLAST and GLT-1) is observed following neuronal nAChR stimulation, which increases synaptic levels of glutamate (Poitry-Yamate et al. 2002). Chronic treatment of Xenopus oocytes overexpressing EAAC1 with nicotine reduces EAAC1 activity (Yoon et al. 2014). Stimulation of cultured cerebellar astrocytes with nicotine modulates glutamate uptake, which is probably mediated through either a cAMP-independent or cAMP-dependent mechanism (Lim and Kim 2003).

5.6 Alpha7 Nicotinic Acetylcholine Receptors and Microglial Glutamate Transporters

Although nicotine modulates activity and expression of glutamate transporters in the CNS, the actual nAChR subtype involved and the intracellular signal cascade mediating the transporter's response to nAChR stimulation are not clear. Furthermore, a potential role of α7 nAChR modulating microglial glutamate transporters has yet to be elaborated. A recent study showed that activation of the microglial α7 nAChR system is crucial in the regulation of glutamate transporters (Morioka et al. 2014, 2015). Cultured rat cortical microglia mainly express GLAST and not GLT-1, as shown by RT-PCR and pharmacological analysis using selective inhibitors for GLAST and GLT-1. Treatment with nicotine increases GLAST mRNA expression and glutamate transport activity and the effect of nicotine is blocked by pretreatment with a selective α7 nAChR antagonist, indicating that α7 nAChR mediates nicotine-induced GLAST expression. Understanding the role of the α7 subtype, this is the only nAChR subtype expressed in the cortical microglia.

The concentration of nicotine needed to induce GLAST expression is relatively high (300–1000 μM) compared to concentrations utilized in other in vitro assays. It is possible that, compared to α7 nAChR expressed in other cell types, cortical microglial α7 nAChR has unique properties. Microglial α7 nAChR demonstrates a different pattern of electrical current compared with that demonstrated by neurons, in which stimulation of cortical microglia with nicotine does not evoke current, although ATP treatment evokes current (Suzuki et al. 2006). Furthermore, the α7 nAChR has two isoforms with different pharmacological properties: a low and a high affinity nicotinic binding site (Severance et al. 2004). In fact, high concentrations of nicotine (>1000 μM) is used to stimulate microglia/macrophage α7 nAChR (Takata et al. 2010; Sun et al. 2013). Thus, in the case of microglial α7 nAChR, high concentrations of nicotine may be needed to activate microglia. Further investigation is necessary to elucidate precise pharmacological and functional properties of α7 nAChR.

Various intracellular signal molecules are involved following stimulation of α7 nAChR in vitro (Kihara et al. 2001; Arredondo et al. 2006; Maouche et al. 2013). In rat cortical microglia, stimulation of the α7 nAChR induced a rapid and transient increase in the concentration of cytosolic Ca^{2+} through the activation of phospholipase C (PLC) and the release of Ca^{2+} from inositol triphosphate (IP_3)-sensitive intracellular stores, but not through the influx of extracellular Ca^{2+} (Suzuki et al. 2006). Increased cytosolic Ca^{2+} concentration through an IP_3 receptor-dependent mechanism is one of the key events underlying nicotine-α7 nAChR-mediated GLAST expression, block of the IP_3 receptor, but not removal of extracellular Ca^{2+}, inhibits nicotine's effect. Likewise, Mashimo et al. previously demonstrated that an IP_3 receptor signaling cascade is crucial in the regulation of GLAST expression in Bergmann glial cells, which are a type of astrocyte found in the cerebellum (Mashimo et al. 2010).

A number of studies have indicated that several signaling molecules are activated following increased cytosolic Ca^{2+} concentration in microglia (Takata et al. 2010; Suzuki et al. 2006; Hide et al. 2000). The calmodulin-Ca^{2+}/calmodulin-dependent protein kinase II (CaMKII) pathway is activated following an α7 nAChR-mediated Ca^{2+} influx, eventually leading to microglia phagocytosis of amyloid β (Takata et al. 2010). CaMKII activation is crucial since inhibiting CaMKII blocks nicotine-induced GLAST expression and glutamate transport in cortical microglia. Others have confirmed that CaMKII activity has an important role in glutamate uptake in cortical astrocytes induced through other pharmacological stimuli (Smith and Navratilova 1999). By contrast, other signal molecules, including protein kinase A, protein kinase C, phosphatidylinositol 3-kinase, janus-activated kinase, Src tyrosine kinase and extracellular signal-regulated protein kinase, do not appear to have a major role in nicotine-mediated GLAST expression in microglia.

Increased cytosolic Ca^{2+} concentration is observed within 1–2 min following nicotine treatment (Suzuki et al. 2006). Thus, it is speculated that CaMKII is rapidly activated in parallel with increased intracellular Ca^{2+}. However, upregulation of GLAST mRNA expression is observed only after 18 h of nicotine treatment. Therefore, this delay between increased cytosolic Ca^{2+} concentration and GLAST expression suggests the induction of intermediary molecules which could have a role in GLAST expression. In fact, the protein synthesis inhibitor cycloheximide blocks nicotine-induced GLAST mRNA expression, indicating the presence of a protein intermediary between increased Ca^{2+} concentration and GLAST expression.

Stimulation of nAChRs contributes to the production of several molecules such as cytokines, chemokines, and neurotrophic factors (Hawkins et al. 2015; Maggio et al. 1998; Son and Winzer-Serhan 2009; Takarada et al. 2012). These substances in turn could enhance clearance of glutamate from the synapse by increasing GLAST expression. A number of studies have demonstrated that growth factors, including epidermal growth factor (EGF), fibroblast growth factor (FGF), insulin-like growth factor-1 (IGF-1) and TGF-β1, modulate GLAST expression in astrocytes (Figiel et al. 2003; Lee et al. 2009; Suzuki et al. 2001). In addition, treatment of cultured microglia with nicotine increases FGF-2 mRNA, but not EGF, IGF-1 and TGF-β1 mRNAs, via the stimulation of the α7 nAChR. FGF-2 protein is also increased after treatment with nicotine. Thus, these findings indicate that FGF-2 could be the crucial intermediary between α7 nAChR and GLAST upregulation.

In fact, treatment of cultured microglia with recombinant FGF-2 increases expression of GLAST and increases glutamate transport. In addition, pretreatment with a selective inhibitor of FGF receptor (FGFR) tyrosine kinase blocks the stimulatory effect of nicotine on GLAST expression and glutamate transport. The FGFR has four subtypes (FGFR1-FGFR4). Cultured cortical microglia express FGFR1 mRNA, but not FGFR2 mRNA, FGFR3 mRNA, and FGFR4 mRNA. In neurons, FGF2 exerts neuroprotection by activating FGFR1, thereby decreasing glutamate-induced damage of hippocampal neurons through the production of GDNF (Lenhard et al. 2002). Thus, the microglial α7 nAChR-FGF-2-FGFR1 pathway elicited by nicotine could be neuroprotective through the enhancement of glutamate clearance

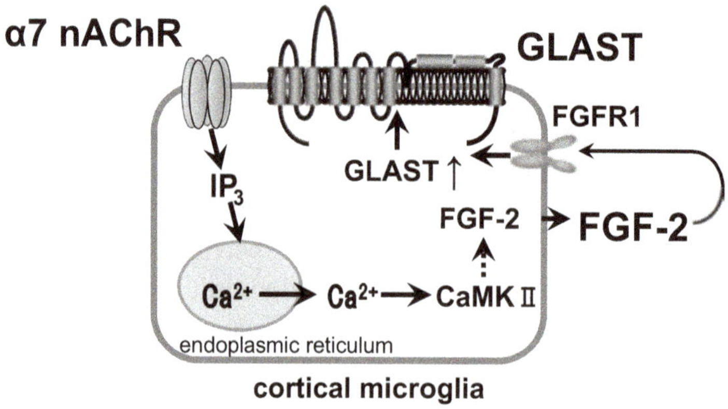

Fig. 5.1 Schematic representation of nicotine-α7 nAChR mediating GLAST expression in microglia. Long-term treatment (more than 18 h) of microglia with nicotine (300–1000 μM) upregulates the expression of GLAST (mRNA and protein) through the stimulation of the α7 nAChR. The stimulation of α7 nAChR increases transient Ca^{2+} concentration through phospholipase C and inositol triphosphate (IP_3)-dependent pathways, and subsequent activation of Ca^{2+}/calmodulin-dependent protein kinase II (CaMKII). The treatment of microglia with nicotine induces expression of fibroblast growth factor-2 (FGF-2) mRNA and protein. FGF-2 produced stimulates FGFR1 expressed in microglia in an autocrine and paracrine manner, and increases both GLAST expression and glutamate transport. Thus, clearance of synaptic glutamate is achieved via activation of a nicotine-α7 nAChR system, through regulation of GLAST expression and glutamate transport in microglia through IP_3-Ca^{2+}- CaMKII and FGF-2 pathways

by GLAST upregulation. FGF-2 has a neuroprotective role in preclinical animal models of neuroinflammation and neurodegenerative disorders. FGF-2 secreted from injured neurons could lead to microglia transformation and neuroprotective activities such as migration and phagocytosis (Noda et al. 2014). Enhancing brain FGF-2 expression restores hippocampal functioning in a preclinical model of Alzheimer's disease (Kiyota et al. 2011).

Although further investigation is needed to elaborate the relationship between transformed M2 microglia and neuroprotection, the findings so far indicate that the nicotine-α7 nAChR system modulates microglial GLAST function and regulates the clearance of synaptic glutamate (Fig. 5.1).

5.7 Drug Development Targeting α7 nAChR for Neurological Disorders

Targeting the α7 nAChR is a potential strategy to treat neurological disorders which currently have no effective treatments. In fact, a selective α7 nAChR agonist reduces 6-hydroxydopamine-induced dopaminergic neuronal damage in a rat model of Parkinson's disease (Suzuki et al. 2013; Bordia et al. 2015). Furthermore, the α7 nAChR is a potential target for the treatment of cognitive dysfunction associated with Alzheimer's disease. Systemic treatment with selective α7 nAChR agonists, either PHA-543613 or galantamine, improves cognitive dysfunction in β-amyloid-treated mice (Sadigh-Eteghad et al. 2015). In addition, the α7 nAChR may be involved in regulating nociceptive transduction, as α7 nAChR agonists ameliorate experimental painful peripheral neuropathies (Di Cesare Mannelli et al. 2014; Freitas et al. 2013). Studies uncovering the relationship between α7 nAChR and microglial function in particular suggest the possibility that α7 nAChR expressed by microglia are a novel therapeutic target for the treatment of neurological disorders. For example, stimulation of the α7 nAChR enhances microglial β-amyloid clearance (Takata et al. 2010). Direct activation of microglial α7 nAChR is neuroprotective, through upregulation of heme oxtgenase-1, against oxygen and glucose deprivation in organotrophic hippocampal culture (Parada et al. 2013). Recent findings also demonstrate that stimulation of α7 nAChR enhances GLAST expression and glutamate transport in microglia, suggesting that enhancing glutamate reuptake at the synapse is crucial in maintaining normal functioning of the glutamatergic system. Furthermore, it is also possible that downregulation of the α7 nAChR itself is associated with the induction of neurological disorders. Thus, direct stimulation of α7 nAChR or gene therapy to enhance α7 nAChR expression, especially in microglia, could be useful for treatment of various neurological disorders.

5.8 Conclusions

Hyperactivation of microglia, especially transitioning to the M1 phenotype, contributes to the induction of neuropathology in the CNS, suggesting that targeting M1 microglia could be an appropriate treatment for neurological disorders. Although mechanisms regulating the switching of microglial phenotypes have yet to be fully elaborated, inducing the transitioning of microglia from the M1 phenotype to the M2 phenotype could be an alternate therapeutic approach. As described above, the α7 nAChR contributes to the regulation of a number of microglial functions, especially in the reduction of neuroinflammatory responses and the clearance of potentially excitotoxic levels of synaptic glutamate. Therefore, further understanding of the molecular and cellular mechanisms underlying α7 nAChR expressed in microglia could aid in the development of therapeutic strategies for neuroinflammatory and neurodegenerative diseases, which in general, are lacking in effective treatments.

Acknowledgement This work was supported in part by grants from Smoking Research Foundation. We also thank Dr. Aldric T. Hama for his careful editing of the manuscript.

References

Amantea D, Micieli G, Tassorelli C, Cuartero MI, Ballesteros I, Certo M, Moro MA, Lizasoain I, Bagetta G (2015) Rational modulation of the innate immune system for neuroprotection in ischemic stroke. Front Neurosci 9:147. https://doi.org/10.3389/fnins.2015.00147

Arranz AM, Gottlieb M, Pérez-Cerdá F, Matute C (2010) Increased expression of glutamate transporters in subcortical white matter after transient focal cerebral ischemia. Neurobiol Dis 37(1):156–165. https://doi.org/10.1016/j.nbd.2009.09.019

Arredondo J, Chernyavsky AI, Jolkovsky DL, Pinkerton KE, Grando SA (2006) Receptor-mediated tobacco toxicity: cooperation of the Ras/Raf-1/MEK1/ERK and JAK-2/STAT-3 pathways downstream of alpha7 nicotinic receptor in oral keratinocytes. FASEB J 20(12):2093–2101. https://doi.org/10.1096/fj.06-6191com

Arriza JL, Eliasof S, Kavanaugh MP, Amara SG (1997) Excitatory amino acid transporter 5, a retinal glutamate transporter coupled to a chloride conductance. Proc Natl Acad Sci U S A 94(8):4155–4160

Awtry TL, Werling LL (2003) Acute and chronic effects of nicotine on serotonin uptake in prefrontal cortex and hippocampus of rats. Synapse 50(3):206–211. https://doi.org/10.1002/syn.10259

Beschorner R, Simon P, Schauer N, Mittelbronn M, Schluesener HJ, Trautmann K, Dietz K, Meyermann R (2007) Reactive astrocytes and activated microglial cells express EAAT1, but not EAAT2, reflecting a neuroprotective potential following ischaemia. Histopathology 50(7):897–910. https://doi.org/10.1111/j.1365-2559.2007.02703.x

Blank T, Prinz M (2013) Microglia as modulators of cognition and neuropsychiatric disorders. Glia 61(1):62–70. https://doi.org/10.1002/glia.22372

Bordia T, McGregor M, Papke RL, Decker MW, McIntosh JM, Quik M (2015) The α7 nicotinic receptor agonist ABT-107 protects against nigrostriatal damage in rats with unilateral 6-hydroxydopamine lesions. Exp Neurol 263:277–284. https://doi.org/10.1016/j.expneurol.2014.09.015

Dajas-Bailador F, Wonnacott S (2004) Nicotinic acetylcholine receptors and the regulation of neuronal signalling. Trends Pharmacol Sci 25(6):317–324. https://doi.org/10.1016/j.tips.2004.04.006

Dani JA, Bertrand D (2007) Nicotinic acetylcholine receptors and nicotinic cholinergic mechanisms of the central nervous system. Annu Rev Pharmacol Toxicol 47:699–729. https://doi.org/10.1146/annurev.pharmtox.47.120505.105214

Danielson K, Truman P, Kivell BM (2011) The effects of nicotine and cigarette smoke on the monoamine transporters. Synapse 65(9):866–879. https://doi.org/10.1002/syn.20914

Davalos D, Grutzendler J, Yang G, Kim JV, Zuo Y, Jung S, Littman DR, Dustin ML, Gan WB (2005) ATP mediates rapid microglial response to local brain injury in vivo. Nat Neurosci 8(6):752–758. https://doi.org/10.1038/nn1472

De Simone R, Ajmone-Cat MA, Carnevale D, Minghetti L (2005) Activation of alpha7 nicotinic acetylcholine receptor by nicotine selectively up-regulates cyclooxygenase-2 and prostaglandin E2 in rat microglial cultures. J Neuroinflammation 2(1):4. https://doi.org/10.1186/1742-2094-2-4

Di Cesare Mannelli L, Pacini A, Matera C, Zanardelli M, Mello T, De Amici M, Dallanoce C, Ghelardini C (2014) Involvement of α7 nAChR subtype in rat oxaliplatin-induced neuropathy: effects of selective activation. Neuropharmacology 79:37–48. https://doi.org/10.1016/j.neuropharm.2013.10.034

Fairman WA, Vandenberg RJ, Arriza JL, Kavanaugh MP, Amara SG (1995) An excitatory amino-acid transporter with properties of a ligand-gated chloride channel. Nature 375(6532):599–603. https://doi.org/10.1038/375599a0

Fernandes A, Miller-Fleming L, Pais TF (2014) Microglia and inflammation: conspiracy, controversy or control? Cell Mol Life Sci 71(20):3969–3985. https://doi.org/10.1007/s00018-014-1670-8

Figiel M, Maucher T, Rozyczka J, Bayatti N, Engele J (2003) Regulation of glial glutamate transporter expression by growth factors. Exp Neurol 183(1):124–135

Fine SM, Angel RA, Perry SW, Epstein LG, Rothstein JD, Dewhurst S, Gelbard HA (1996) Tumor necrosis factor alpha inhibits glutamate uptake by primary human astrocytes. Implications for pathogenesis of HIV-1 dementia. J Biol Chem 271(26):15303–15306

Frank-Cannon TC, Alto LT, McAlpine FE, Tansey MG (2009) Does neuroinflammation fan the flame in neurodegenerative diseases? Mol Neurodegener 4:47. https://doi.org/10.1186/1750-1326-4-47

Freilich RW, Woodbury ME, Ikezu T (2013) Integrated expression profiles of mRNA and miRNA in polarized primary murine microglia. PLoS One 8(11):e79416. https://doi.org/10.1371/journal.pone.0079416

Freitas K, Ghosh S, Ivy Carroll F, Lichtman AH, Imad Damaj M (2013) Effects of α7 positive allosteric modulators in murine inflammatory and chronic neuropathic pain models. Neuropharmacology 65:156–164. https://doi.org/10.1016/j.neuropharm.2012.08.022

Garrido-Gil P, Rodriguez-Pallares J, Dominguez-Meijide A, Guerra MJ, Labandeira-Garcia JL (2013) Brain angiotensin regulates iron homeostasis in dopaminergic neurons and microglial cells. Exp Neurol 250:384–396. https://doi.org/10.1016/j.expneurol.2013.10.013

Giunta B, Ehrhart J, Townsend K, Sun N, Vendrame M, Shytle D, Tan J, Fernandez F (2004) Galantamine and nicotine have a synergistic effect on inhibition of microglial activation induced by HIV-1 gp120. Brain Res Bull 64(2):165–170. https://doi.org/10.1016/j.brainresbull.2004.06.008

Gotti C, Clementi F (2004) Neuronal nicotinic receptors: from structure to pathology. Prog Neurobiol 74(6):363–396. https://doi.org/10.1016/j.pneurobio.2004.09.006

Hawkins BT, Egleton RD, Davis TP (2005) Modulation of cerebral microvascular permeability by endothelial nicotinic acetylcholine receptors. Am J Physiol Heart Circ Physiol 289(1):H212–H219. https://doi.org/10.1152/ajpheart.01210.2004

Hawkins JL, Denson JE, Miley DR, Durham PL (2015) Nicotine stimulates expression of proteins implicated in peripheral and central sensitization. Neuroscience 290C:115–125. https://doi.org/10.1016/j.neuroscience.2015.01.034

Henkel JS, Beers DR, Zhao W, Appel SH (2009) Microglia in ALS: the good, the bad, and the resting. J NeuroImmune Pharmacol 4(4):389–398. https://doi.org/10.1007/s11481-009-9171-5

Hide I, Tanaka M, Inoue A, Nakajima K, Kohsaka S, Inoue K, Nakata Y (2000) Extracellular ATP triggers tumor necrosis factor-alpha release from rat microglia. J Neurochem 75(3):965–972

Hou Y, Xie G, Liu X, Li G, Jia C, Xu J, Wang B (2016) Minocycline protects against lipopolysaccharide-induced cognitive impairment in mice. Psychopharmacology (Berl) 233(5):905–916. https://doi.org/10.1007/s00213-015-4169-6

Itoh H, Toyohira Y, Ueno S, Saeki S, Zhang H, Furuno Y, Takahashi K, Tsutsui M, Hachisuka K, Yanagihara N (2010) Upregulation of norepinephrine transporter function by prolonged exposure to nicotine in cultured bovine adrenal medullary cells. Naunyn Schmiedeberg's Arch Pharmacol 382(3):235–243. https://doi.org/10.1007/s00210-010-0540-7

Kanai Y, Hediger MA (1992) Primary structure and functional characterization of a high-affinity glutamate transporter. Nature 360(6403):467–471. https://doi.org/10.1038/360467a0

Kettenmann H, Verkhratsky A (2008) Neuroglia: the 150 years after. Trends Neurosci 31(12):653–659. https://doi.org/10.1016/j.tins.2008.09.003

Kettenmann H, Hanisch UK, Noda M, Verkhratsky A (2011) Physiology of microglia. Physiol Rev 91(2):461–553. https://doi.org/10.1152/physrev.00011.2010

Kigerl KA, Gensel JC, Ankeny DP, Alexander JK, Donnelly DJ, Popovich PG (2009) Identification of two distinct macrophage subsets with divergent effects causing either neurotoxicity or regeneration in the injured mouse spinal cord. J Neurosci 29(43):13435–13444. https://doi.org/10.1523/JNEUROSCI.3257-09.2009

Kihara T, Shimohama S, Sawada H, Honda K, Nakamizo T, Shibasaki H, Kume T, Akaike A (2001) alpha 7 nicotinic receptor transduces signals to phosphatidylinositol 3-kinase to block A beta-amyloid-induced neurotoxicity. J Biol Chem 276(17):13541–13546. https://doi.org/10.1074/jbc.M008035200

Kitamura T, Tsuchihashi Y, Fujita S (1978) Initial response of silver-impregnated "resting microglia" to stab wounding in rabbit hippocampus. Acta Neuropathol 44(1):31–39

Kiyota T, Ingraham KL, Jacobsen MT, Xiong H, Ikezu T (2011) FGF2 gene transfer restores hippocampal functions in mouse models of Alzheimer's disease and has therapeutic implications for neurocognitive disorders. Proc Natl Acad Sci U S A 108(49):E1339–E1348. https://doi.org/10.1073/pnas.1102349108

Koizumi S, Shigemoto-Mogami Y, Nasu-Tada K, Shinozaki Y, Ohsawa K, Tsuda M, Joshi BV, Jacobson KA, Kohsaka S, Inoue K (2007) UDP acting at P2Y6 receptors is a mediator of microglial phagocytosis. Nature 446(7139):1091–1095. nature05704 [pii] 391038/nature05704

Lai AY, Todd KG (2008) Differential regulation of trophic and proinflammatory microglial effectors is dependent on severity of neuronal injury. Glia 56(3):259–270. https://doi.org/10.1002/glia.20610

Lalancette-Hébert M, Gowing G, Simard A, Weng YC, Kriz J (2007) Selective ablation of proliferating microglial cells exacerbates ischemic injury in the brain. J Neurosci 27(10):2596–2605. https://doi.org/10.1523/JNEUROSCI.5360-06.2007

Lawson LJ, Perry VH, Dri P, Gordon S (1990) Heterogeneity in the distribution and morphology of microglia in the normal adult mouse brain. Neuroscience 39(1):151–170

Lee ES, Sidoryk M, Jiang H, Yin Z, Aschner M (2009) Estrogen and tamoxifen reverse manganese-induced glutamate transporter impairment in astrocytes. J Neurochem 110(2):530–544. https://doi.org/10.1111/j.1471-4159.2009.06105.x

Lenhard T, Schober A, Suter-Crazzolara C, Unsicker K (2002) Fibroblast growth factor-2 requires glial-cell-line-derived neurotrophic factor for exerting its neuroprotective actions on glutamate-lesioned hippocampal neurons. Mol Cell Neurosci 20(2):181–197

Lim DK, Kim HS (2001) Changes in the glutamate release and uptake of cerebellar cells in perinatally nicotine-exposed rat pups. Neurochem Res 26(10):1119–1125

Lim DK, Kim HS (2003) Opposite modulation of glutamate uptake by nicotine in cultured astrocytes with/without cAMP treatment. Eur J Pharmacol 476(3):179–184

Liu Y, Zeng X, Hui Y, Zhu C, Wu J, Taylor DH, Ji J, Fan W, Huang Z, Hu J (2015) Activation of α7 nicotinic acetylcholine receptors protects astrocytes against oxidative stress-induced apoptosis: implications for Parkinson's disease. Neuropharmacology 91:87–96. https://doi.org/10.1016/j.neuropharm.2014.11.028

López-Redondo F, Nakajima K, Honda S, Kohsaka S (2000) Glutamate transporter GLT-1 is highly expressed in activated microglia following facial nerve axotomy. Brain Res Mol Brain Res 76(2):429–435

Maggio R, Riva M, Vaglini F, Fornai F, Molteni R, Armogida M, Racagni G, Corsini GU (1998) Nicotine prevents experimental parkinsonism in rodents and induces striatal increase of neurotrophic factors. J Neurochem 71(6):2439–2446

Maouche K, Medjber K, Zahm JM, Delavoie F, Terryn C, Coraux C, Pons S, Cloëz-Tayarani I, Maskos U, Birembaut P, Tournier JM (2013) Contribution of α7 nicotinic receptor to airway epithelium dysfunction under nicotine exposure. Proc Natl Acad Sci U S A 110(10):4099–4104. https://doi.org/10.1073/pnas.1216939110

Mashimo M, Okubo Y, Yamazawa T, Yamasaki M, Watanabe M, Murayama T, Iino M (2010) Inositol 1,4,5-trisphosphate signaling maintains the activity of glutamate uptake in Bergmann glia. Eur J Neurosci 32(10):1668–1677. https://doi.org/10.1111/j.1460-9568.2010.07452.x

Middleton LS, Cass WA, Dwoskin LP (2004) Nicotinic receptor modulation of dopamine transporter function in rat striatum and medial prefrontal cortex. J Pharmacol Exp Ther 308(1):367–377. https://doi.org/10.1124/jpet.103.055335

Mittelbronn M, Dietz K, Schluesener HJ, Meyermann R (2001) Local distribution of microglia in the normal adult human central nervous system differs by up to one order of magnitude. Acta Neuropathol 101(3):249–255

Moehle MS, West AB (2015) M1 and M2 immune activation in Parkinson's disease: foe and ally? Neuroscience 302:59–73. https://doi.org/10.1016/j.neuroscience.2014.11.018

Moon JH, Kim SY, Lee HG, Kim SU, Lee YB (2008) Activation of nicotinic acetylcholine receptor prevents the production of reactive oxygen species in fibrillar beta amyloid peptide (1-42)-stimulated microglia. Exp Mol Med 40(1):11–18. https://doi.org/10.3858/emm.2008.40.1.11

Morioka N, Abdin MJ, Kitayama T, Morita K, Nakata Y, Dohi T (2008) P2X(7) receptor stimulation in primary cultures of rat spinal microglia induces downregulation of the activity for glutamate transport. Glia 56(5):528–538. https://doi.org/10.1002/glia.20634

Morioka N, Tokuhara M, Harano S, Nakamura Y, Hisaoka-Nakashima K, Nakata Y (2013) The activation of P2Y6 receptor in cultured spinal microglia induces the production of CCL2 through the MAP kinases-NF-κB pathway. Neuropharmacology 75C:116–125. https://doi.org/10.1016/j.neuropharm.2013.07.017

Morioka N, Tokuhara M, Nakamura Y, Idenoshita Y, Harano S, Zhang FF, Hisaoka-Nakashima K, Nakata Y (2014) Primary cultures of rat cortical microglia treated with nicotine increases in the expression of excitatory amino acid transporter 1 (GLAST) via the activation of the α7 nicotinic acetylcholine receptor. Neuroscience 258:374–384. https://doi.org/10.1016/j.neuroscience.2013.11.044

Morioka N, Harano S, Tokuhara M, Idenoshita Y, Zhang FF, Hisaoka-Nakashima K, Nakata Y (2015) Stimulation of α7 nicotinic acetylcholine receptor regulates glutamate transporter GLAST via basic fibroblast growth factor production in cultured cortical microglia. Brain Res 1625:111–120. https://doi.org/10.1016/j.brainres.2015.08.029

Nimmerjahn A, Kirchhoff F, Helmchen F (2005) Resting microglial cells are highly dynamic surveillants of brain parenchyma in vivo. Science 308(5726):1314–1318. https://doi.org/10.1126/science.1110647

Noda M, Kobayashi AI (2017) Nicotine inhibits activation of microglial proton currents via interactions with α7 acetylcholine receptors. J Physiol Sci 67(1):235–245. https://doi.org/10.1007/s12576-016-0460-5

Noda M, Nakanishi H, Akaike N (1999) Glutamate release from microglia via glutamate transporter is enhanced by amyloid-beta peptide. Neuroscience 92(4):1465–1474

Noda M, Takii K, Parajuli B, Kawanokuchi J, Sonobe Y, Takeuchi H, Mizuno T, Suzumura A (2014) FGF-2 released from degenerating neurons exerts microglial-induced neuroprotection via FGFR3-ERK signaling pathway. J Neuroinflammation 11:76. https://doi.org/10.1186/1742-2094-11-76

Nolte C, Möller T, Walter T, Kettenmann H (1996) Complement 5a controls motility of murine microglial cells in vitro via activation of an inhibitory G-protein and the rearrangement of the actin cytoskeleton. Neuroscience 73(4):1091–1107

Parada E, Egea J, Buendia I, Negredo P, Cunha AC, Cardoso S, Soares MP, López MG (2013) The microglial α7-acetylcholine nicotinic receptor is a key element in promoting neuroprotection by inducing heme oxygenase-1 via nuclear factor erythroid-2-related factor 2. Antioxid Redox Signal 19(11):1135–1148. https://doi.org/10.1089/ars.2012.4671

Persson M, Brantefjord M, Hansson E, Rönnbäck L (2005) Lipopolysaccharide increases microglial GLT-1 expression and glutamate uptake capacity in vitro by a mechanism dependent on TNF-alpha. Glia 51(2):111–120. https://doi.org/10.1002/glia.20191

Pines G, Danbolt NC, Bjørås M, Zhang Y, Bendahan A, Eide L, Koepsell H, Storm-Mathisen J, Seeberg E, Kanner BI (1992) Cloning and expression of a rat brain L-glutamate transporter. Nature 360(6403):464–467. https://doi.org/10.1038/360464a0

Poitry-Yamate CL, Vutskits L, Rauen T (2002) Neuronal-induced and glutamate-dependent activation of glial glutamate transporter function. J Neurochem 82(4):987–997

Polazzi E, Monti B (2010) Microglia and neuroprotection: from in vitro studies to therapeutic applications. Prog Neurobiol 92(3):293–315. https://doi.org/10.1016/j.pneurobio.2010.06.009

Ponomarev ED, Maresz K, Tan Y, Dittel BN (2007) CNS-derived interleukin-4 is essential for the regulation of autoimmune inflammation and induces a state of alternative activation in microglial cells. J Neurosci 27(40):10714–10721. https://doi.org/10.1523/JNEUROSCI.1922-07.2007

Robinson MB, Dowd LA (1997) Heterogeneity and functional properties of subtypes of sodium-dependent glutamate transporters in the mammalian central nervous system. Adv Pharmacol 37:69–115

Rock RB, Gekker G, Aravalli RN, Hu S, Sheng WS, Peterson PK (2008) Potentiation of HIV-1 expression in microglial cells by nicotine: involvement of transforming growth factor-beta 1. J NeuroImmune Pharmacol 3(3):143–149. https://doi.org/10.1007/s11481-007-9098-7

Rogers SW, Gregori NZ, Carlson N, Gahring LC, Noble M (2001) Neuronal nicotinic acetylcholine receptor expression by O2A/oligodendrocyte progenitor cells. Glia 33(4):306–313

Sadigh-Eteghad S, Talebi M, Mahmoudi J, Babri S, Shanehbandi D (2015) Selective activation of α7 nicotinic acetylcholine receptor by PHA-543613 improves Aβ25-35-mediated cognitive deficits in mice. Neuroscience 298:81–93. https://doi.org/10.1016/j.neuroscience.2015.04.017

Sargent PB (1993) The diversity of neuronal nicotinic acetylcholine receptors. Annu Rev Neurosci 16:403–443. https://doi.org/10.1146/annurev.ne.16.030193.002155

Severance EG, Zhang H, Cruz Y, Pakhlevaniants S, Hadley SH, Amin J, Wecker L, Reed C, Cuevas J (2004) The alpha7 nicotinic acetylcholine receptor subunit exists in two isoforms that contribute to functional ligand-gated ion channels. Mol Pharmacol 66(3):420–429. https://doi.org/10.1124/mol.104.000059

Shaked I, Tchoresh D, Gersner R, Meiri G, Mordechai S, Xiao X, Hart RP, Schwartz M (2005) Protective autoimmunity: interferon-gamma enables microglia to remove glutamate without evoking inflammatory mediators. J Neurochem 92(5):997–1009. https://doi.org/10.1111/j.1471-4159.2004.02954.x

Shao BZ, Ke P, Xu ZQ, Wei W, Cheng MH, Han BZ, Chen XW, Su DF, Liu C (2017) Autophagy plays an important role in anti-inflammatory mechanisms stimulated by Alpha7 nicotinic acetylcholine receptor. Front Immunol 8:553. https://doi.org/10.3389/fimmu.2017.00553

Shibata T, Yamada K, Watanabe M, Ikenaka K, Wada K, Tanaka K, Inoue Y (1997) Glutamate transporter GLAST is expressed in the radial glia-astrocyte lineage of developing mouse spinal cord. J Neurosci 17(23):9212–9219

Shytle RD, Mori T, Townsend K, Vendrame M, Sun N, Zeng J, Ehrhart J, Silver AA, Sanberg PR, Tan J (2004) Cholinergic modulation of microglial activation by alpha 7 nicotinic receptors. J Neurochem 89(2):337–343. https://doi.org/10.1046/j.1471-4159.2004.02347.x

Smith TL, Navratilova E (1999) Increased calcium/calmodulin protein kinase activity in astrocytes chronically exposed to ethanol: influences on glutamate transport. Neurosci Lett 269(3):145–148

Son JH, Winzer-Serhan UH (2009) Chronic neonatal nicotine exposure increases mRNA expression of neurotrophic factors in the postnatal rat hippocampus. Brain Res 1278:1–14. https://doi.org/10.1016/j.brainres.2009.04.046

Stence N, Waite M, Dailey ME (2001) Dynamics of microglial activation: a confocal time-lapse analysis in hippocampal slices. Glia 33(3):256–266

Sun Y, Li Q, Gui H, Xu DP, Yang YL, Su DF, Liu X (2013) MicroRNA-124 mediates the cholinergic anti-inflammatory action through inhibiting the production of pro-inflammatory cytokines. Cell Res 23(11):1270–1283. https://doi.org/10.1038/cr.2013.116

Suzuki K, Ikegaya Y, Matsuura S, Kanai Y, Endou H, Matsuki N (2001) Transient upregulation of the glial glutamate transporter GLAST in response to fibroblast growth factor, insulin-like growth factor and epidermal growth factor in cultured astrocytes. J Cell Sci 114(Pt 20):3717–3725

Suzuki T, Hide I, Ido K, Kohsaka S, Inoue K, Nakata Y (2004) Production and release of neuroprotective tumor necrosis factor by P2X7 receptor-activated microglia. J Neurosci 24(1):1–7. 24/1/1 [pii] 10.1523/JNEUROSCI.3792-03.2004

Suzuki T, Hide I, Matsubara A, Hama C, Harada K, Miyano K, Andrä M, Matsubayashi H, Sakai N, Kohsaka S, Inoue K, Nakata Y (2006) Microglial alpha7 nicotinic acetylcholine receptors drive a phospholipase C/IP3 pathway and modulate the cell activation toward a neuroprotective role. J Neurosci Res 83(8):1461–1470. https://doi.org/10.1002/jnr.20850

Suzuki S, Kawamata J, Matsushita T, Matsumura A, Hisahara S, Takata K, Kitamura Y, Kem W, Shimohama S (2013) 3-[(2,4-Dimethoxy)benzylidene]-anabaseine dihydrochloride protects against 6-hydroxydopamine-induced parkinsonian neurodegeneration through α7 nicotinic acetylcholine receptor stimulation in rats. J Neurosci Res 91(3):462–471. https://doi.org/10.1002/jnr.23160

Takarada T, Nakamichi N, Kawagoe H, Ogura M, Fukumori R, Nakazato R, Fujikawa K, Kou M, Yoneda Y (2012) Possible neuroprotective property of nicotinic acetylcholine receptors in association with predominant upregulation of glial cell line-derived neurotrophic factor in astrocytes. J Neurosci Res 90(11):2074–2085. https://doi.org/10.1002/jnr.23101

Takata K, Kitamura Y, Saeki M, Terada M, Kagitani S, Kitamura R, Fujikawa Y, Maelicke A, Tomimoto H, Taniguchi T, Shimohama S (2010) Galantamine-induced amyloid-{beta} clearance mediated via stimulation of microglial nicotinic acetylcholine receptors. J Biol Chem 285(51):40180–40191. https://doi.org/10.1074/jbc.M110.142356

Tanaka K, Watase K, Manabe T, Yamada K, Watanabe M, Takahashi K, Iwama H, Nishikawa T, Ichihara N, Kikuchi T, Okuyama S, Kawashima N, Hori S, Takimoto M, Wada K (1997) Epilepsy and exacerbation of brain injury in mice lacking the glutamate transporter GLT-1. Science 276(5319):1699–1702

Thomas WE (1992) Brain macrophages: evaluation of microglia and their functions. Brain Res Brain Res Rev 17(1):61–74

Wang H, Yu M, Ochani M, Amella CA, Tanovic M, Susarla S, Li JH, Yang H, Ulloa L, Al-Abed Y, Czura CJ, Tracey KJ (2003) Nicotinic acetylcholine receptor alpha7 subunit is an essential regulator of inflammation. Nature 421(6921):384–388. https://doi.org/10.1038/nature01339

Wu DC, Jackson-Lewis V, Vila M, Tieu K, Teismann P, Vadseth C, Choi DK, Ischiropoulos H, Przedborski S (2002) Blockade of microglial activation is neuroprotective in the 1-methyl-4-phenyl-1,2,3,6-tetrahydropyridine mouse model of Parkinson disease. J Neurosci 22(5):1763–1771

Wu LJ, Wu G, Akhavan Sharif MR, Baker A, Jia Y, Fahey FH, Luo HR, Feener EP, Clapham DE (2012) The voltage-gated proton channel Hv1 enhances brain damage from ischemic stroke. Nat Neurosci 15(4):565–573. https://doi.org/10.1038/nn.3059

Xin WJ, Weng HR, Dougherty PM (2009) Plasticity in expression of the glutamate transporters GLT-1 and GLAST in spinal dorsal horn glial cells following partial sciatic nerve ligation. Mol Pain 5:15. https://doi.org/10.1186/1744-8069-5-15

Yoon HJ, Lim YJ, Zuo Z, Hur W, Do SH (2014) Nicotine decreases the activity of glutamate transporter type 3. Toxicol Lett 225(1):147–152. https://doi.org/10.1016/j.toxlet.2013.12.002

Yrjänheikki J, Keinänen R, Pellikka M, Hökfelt T, Koistinaho J (1998) Tetracyclines inhibit microglial activation and are neuroprotective in global brain ischemia. Proc Natl Acad Sci U S A 95(26):15769–15774

Zhang Q, Lu Y, Bian H, Guo L, Zhu H (2017) Activation of the α7 nicotinic receptor promotes lipopolysaccharide-induced conversion of M1 microglia to M2. Am J Transl Res 9(3):971–985

Zoli M, Pistillo F, Gotti C (2015) Diversity of native nicotinic receptor subtypes in mammalian brain. Neuropharmacology 96(Pt B):302–311. https://doi.org/10.1016/j.neuropharm.2014.11.003

Chapter 6
Shati/Nat8l and *N*-acetylaspartate (NAA) Have Important Roles in Regulating Nicotinic Acetylcholine Receptors in Neuronal and Psychiatric Diseases in Animal Models and Humans

Atsumi Nitta, Hiroshi Noike, Kazuyuki Sumi, Hajime Miyanishi, Takuya Tanaka, Kazuya Takaoka, Miyuki Nagakura, Noriyuki Iegaki, Jin-ichiro Kaji, Yoshiaki Miyamoto, Shin-Ichi Muramatsu, and Kyosuke Uno

Abstract Shati/Nat8l was originally isolated as a methamphetamine-related-molecule from the nucleus accumbens of mice. Since then, Shati/Nat8l has been characterized as an *N*-acetyltransferase-8-like protein (Nat8l) that catalyzes *N*-acetylaspartate (NAA) synthesis from aspartate and acetyl-coenzyme A. It has been shown that elevated NAA levels detected by proton magnetic resonance spectroscopy (^{1}H-MRS) brain imaging indicates increased neuronal activity. Our group produced Shati/Nat8l knock out mice (Shati/Nat8l KO mice), which exhibit hyper locomotion, anxiety behaviors, and social dysfunction. These mice have a high sensitivity to methamphetamine, as evidenced by their results in assessments of locomotor activity and conditioned place preference, as well as their elevated dopamine levels. We used an adeno-associated virus (AAV) vector containing *Shati/Nat8l* (AAV-*Shati/Nat8l*) to overexpress the protein in different brain regions such as the striatum and the nucleus accumbens, in order to investigate their involvement in methamphetamine-induced behavioral and pharmacological changes. We showed that overexpression of accumbal Shati/Nat8l attenuates methamphetamine-induced behaviors.

A. Nitta (✉) · H. Noike · K. Sumi · H. Miyanishi · T. Tanaka · K. Takaoka · M. Nagakura
N. Iegaki · J. Kaji · Y. Miyamoto · K. Uno
Department of Pharmaceutical Therapy and Neuropharmacology, Faculty of Pharmaceutical Sciences, Graduate School of Medicine and Pharmaceutical Sciences, University of Toyama, Toyama, Japan
e-mail: nitta@pha.u-toyama.ac.jp

S.-I. Muramatsu
Division of Neurology, Department of Medicine, Jichi Medical University, Tochigi, Japan

Center for Gene & Cell Therapy, Institute of Medical Science, The University of Tokyo, Tokyo, Japan

A. Akaike et al. (eds.), *Nicotinic Acetylcholine Receptor Signaling in Neuroprotection*, https://doi.org/10.1007/978-981-10-8488-1_6

Recent clinical studies have revealed further novel roles of Shati/Nat8l in psychiatric and neuronal diseases. We are just beginning to appreciate the various actions of this intriguing, recently discovered molecule in the central nervous system.

Keywords Shati/Nat8l · Methamphetamine · Addiction · Depression · Alzheimer's disease · ATP

6.1 Introduction

Shati is a molecule originally isolated from the nucleus accumbens of mice that had received repeated administration of methamphetamine (Niwa et al. 2007, 2008). Shati was later identified as an *N*-acetyltransferase-8-like protein (Nat8l) and was found to catalyze *N*-acetylaspartate (NAA) synthesis from aspartate and acetyl-coenzyme A (Ariyannur et al. 2010) (Fig. 6.1). We renamed the novel molecule from Shati to Shati/Nat8l following this finding. NAA is present at high concentrations in the central nervous system and is combined with glutamate and converted into *N*-acetylaspartylglutamate (NAAG) by NAAG synthetase (NAAGS) (Becker et al. 2010). NAAG is widely distributed in the brains of mammals (Neale et al. 2000) and acts as a highly selective neurotransmitter for group II metabotropic glutamate receptor 3 (mGluR3) (Neale et al. 2011). Following the release of NAAG into the synaptic cleft, NAAG binds mGluR3 and is metabolized to NAA and glutamate by glutamate carboxypeptidase II (GCPII) (Bzdega et al. 1997; Fig. 6.1). A postmortem study showed that the levels of NAA and NAAG are significantly lower in the brains of subjects with major depressive disorder, schizophrenia and bipolar disorder (Reynolds and Reynolds 2011). In patients with pre-Alzheimer's disease, NAA levels are significantly reduced in the cingulate gyrus. A clinical study using magnetic resonance spectroscopy (MRS) showed that NAA was significantly increased in adult patients with autism spectrum disorder when compared with a control group (Aoki et al. 2012). Together, these observations suggest that the NAA synthetase, Shati/Nat8l, may play important roles in psychiatric, neurodegenerative, and neurodevelopmental disorders.

Furthermore, treatment of a neuroblastoma-derived cell line with a physiological level of NAA resulted in apoptosis of cancerous cells and enhanced neuronal differentiation (Mazzoccoli et al. 2016). NAA is of unique clinical significance and hence is exploited in MRS. Treatment of an SH-SY5Y neuroblastoma-derived cell line with sub-cytotoxic physiological concentrations of NAA has been shown to inhibits cell growth (Mazzoccoli et al. 2016). This effect is partly due to enhanced apoptosis, which is indicated by a decrease in the anti-apoptotic factors survivin and Bcl-xL, and partly due to the arrest of the cell-cycle progression, linked to enhanced expression of the cyclin-inhibitors p53, p21Cip1/Waf1, and p27Kip1 (Mazzoccoli et al. 2016). NAA-pre-treated SH-SY5Y cells were more sensitive to the cytotoxic effect of the chemotherapeutic drugs cisplatin and 5-fluorouracil (Mazzoccoli et al. 2016).

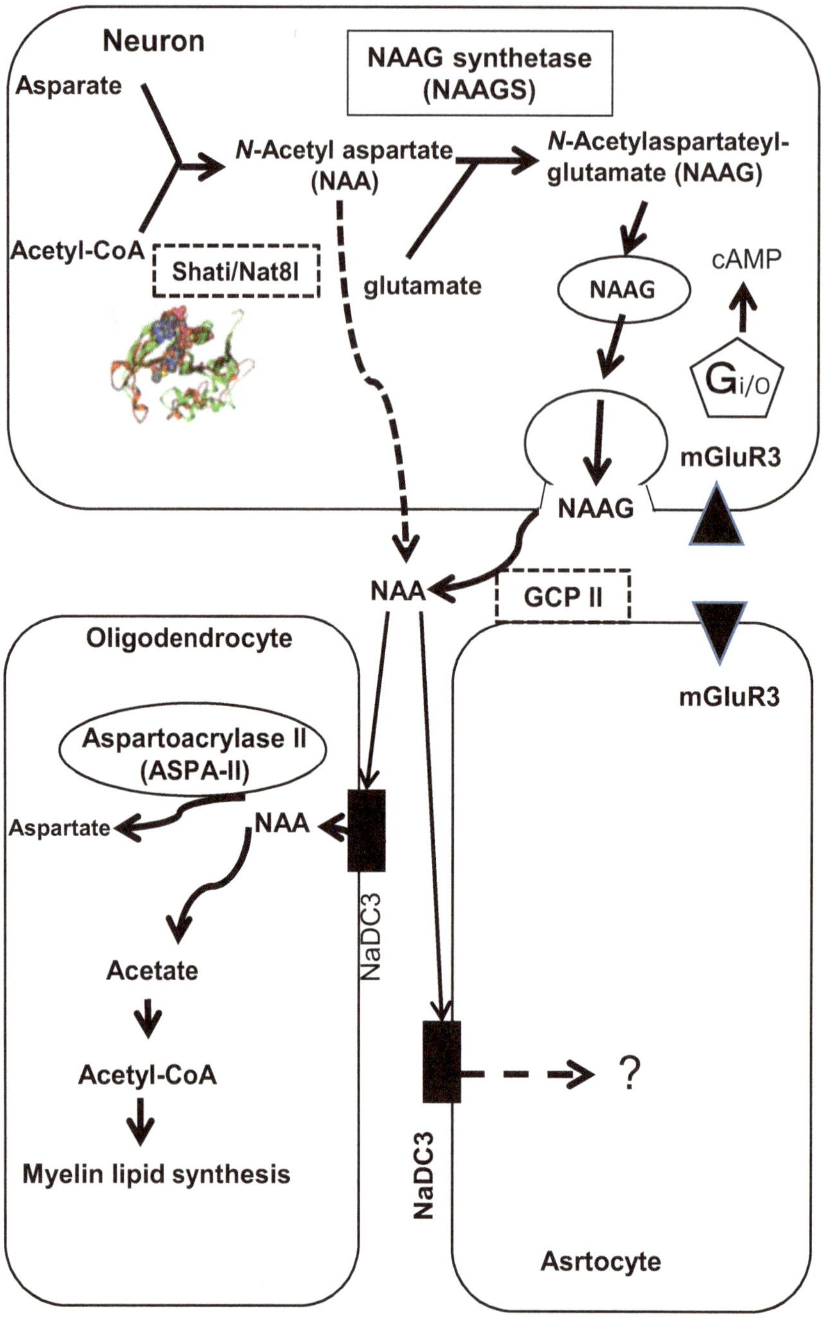

Fig. 6.1 Schematic overview of Shati/Nat8l function. *Shati/Nat8l* catalyzes the *N*-acetylation of aspartate, forming *N*-acetylaspartate (NAA). The condensation of NAA and glutamate is catalyzed by *N*-acetylaspartylglutamate (NAAG) synthetase (NAAGS). NAAG is released from nerve terminals most likely via synaptic vesicles. The transporter responsible for the translocation of NAAG into synaptic vesicles is unknown. Released NAAG can be degraded by glutamate carboxypeptidase II (GCP-II), membrane-bound enzymes mainly expressed by astrocytes, liberating NAA and glutamate (Moffett et al. 2007). NAAG may also bind to metabotropic glutamate receptor 3 (mGluR3) on presynaptic membranes and astrocytes. mGluR3 is coupled to a G_i protein and negatively coupled to adenylyl cyclase (Conn and Pin 1997). The NAA transporter, sodium-dependent dicarboxylate (NaDC3), is expressed by astrocytes and oligodendrocytes (Huang et al. 2000). In oligodendrocytes, NAA can be degraded by aspartoacylase II (ASPA-II, liberating aspartate and acetate (Moffett et al. 2007). The released acetate may be used for lipid synthesis by myelinating oligodendrocytes (Burri et al. 1991; Namboodiri et al. 2006). To what extent NAA is taken up by astrocytes *in vivo* or its metabolic fate in these cells is unclear

In this review, we will introduce the various functions of Shati/Nat8l and NAA in psychiatric behaviors, especially addictive behaviors, and summarize their roles in neuronal and psychiatric diseases.

6.2 Shati/Nat8l and Drug Reward

6.2.1 Function of Accumbal Shati/Nat8l in Nicotinic Effects

We previously reported that overexpression of Shati/Nat8l in the nucleus accumbens (NAc) of mice depressed the pharmacological effects of methamphetamine, especially addiction-related behaviors, hyperactivity, and place preference. In an in vivo microdialysis experiment, the extracellular dopamine (DA) level was increased by 200–300% of the base line by peripheral methamphetamine injection. In the NAc of these mice, NAA and NAAG levels were significantly reduced (Miyamoto et al. 2014). The mGluR3 antagonist, LY341495, cancelled the Shati-Nat8l-indeuced reduction of hyperlocomotion and conditioned place preference after methamphetamine treatment. Furthermore, LY341495 also cancelled the Shati/Nat8l-associated increase in extracellular DA levels in the NAc of methamphetamine-treated mice. These results indicate that the overexpression of Shati/Nat8l in the NAc suppresses the increase in dopamine release caused by methamphetamine *via* mGluR3 (Miyamoto et al. 2014).

We also investigated the effects of Shati/Nat8l on nicotine preference using a three-bottle paradigm. Experiments were performed as follows: I. Both NAc-Mock and NAc-Shati/Nat8l overexpressing mice were habituated to an experimental chamber which contained three water bottles on days 1–3. II. The tap water in all three bottles was changed to 2% saccharin to habituate animals to saccharin on days 4–6. III. The contents of all three bottles were replaced with a mixture of 75 μg/mL and 2% saccharin on days 8–14 (Fig. 6.2). During the subsequent test phase, three bottles containing either 0 μg/mL nicotine +2% saccharin, 75 μg/mL nicotine +2% saccharin or 150 μg/mL nicotine +2% saccharin, were presented to each mouse, and the total intake of nicotine was measured in each mouse on days 15–21 (Fig. 6.2). The daily amounts of nicotine intake are shown in Fig. 6.3a. On the first day of the test phase, an average of 300 μg of nicotine was consumed by both groups. In the NAc-Mock mice, the amount of nicotine consumed increased each day during days 15–17 (Fig. 6.3a). In contrast, the Shati/Nat8l mice showed a lower intake of nicotine enriched solution during this period (Fig. 6.3a). These results suggest that overexpression of Shati/Nat8l in NAc lowers nicotine intake and preference. The 2% of saccharin were essential for the experimental protocol, since nicotine also has aversive effects due to its bitter taste. While overexpression of Shati/Nat8l in NAc lowered nicotine preference during days 16–17 (Fig. 6.3a), total intake (water and nicotine solution) was not changed (Fig. 6.3c, d).

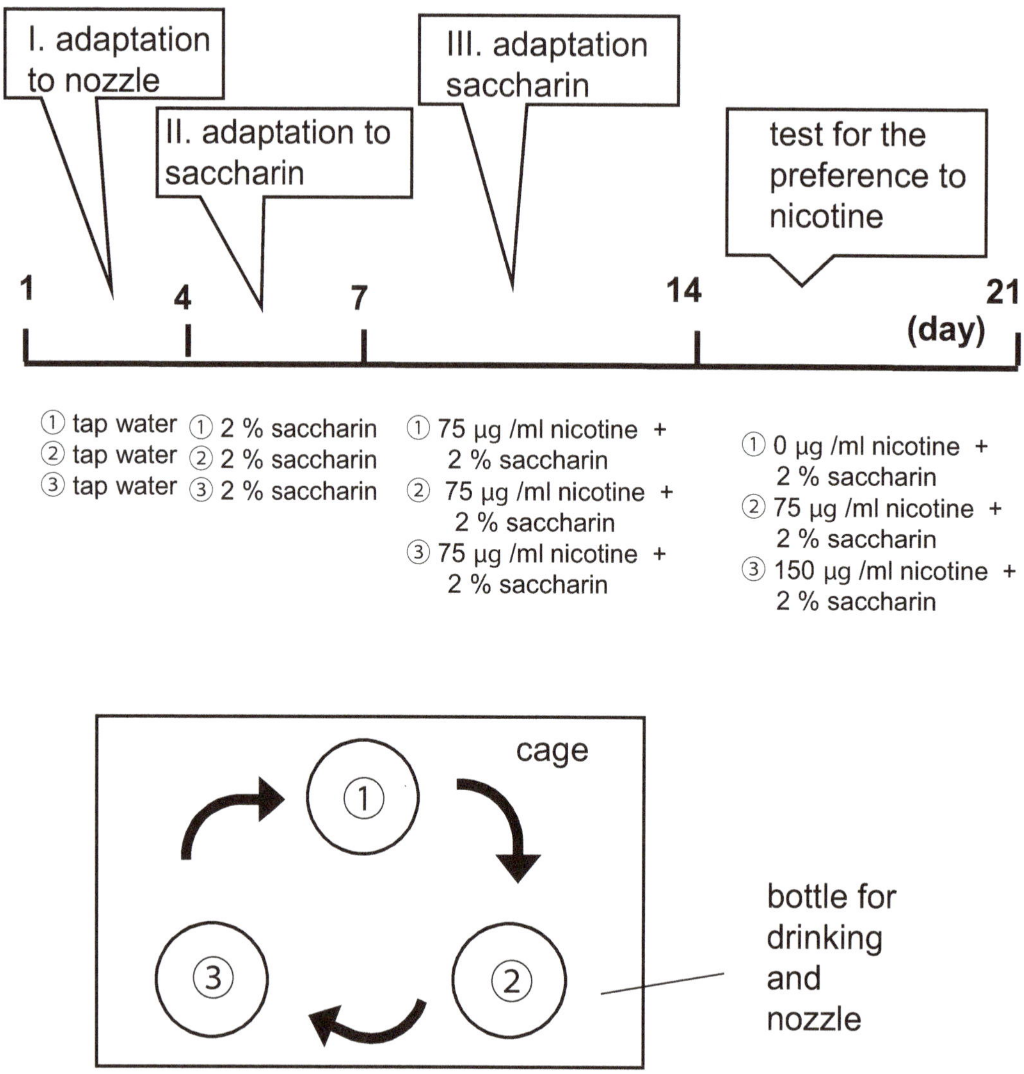

Fig. 6.2 Procedure for the three bottle test to evaluate nicotine preference. I. Both NAc-Mock and NAc-Shati/Nat8l mice were habituated to an experimental chamber which contained three water bottles on days 1–3. II. The tap water in all three bottles was changed to 2% saccharin to habituate animals to saccharin on days 4–6. III. The contents of all three bottles were replaced with a mixture of 75 µg/mL nicotine and 2% saccharin on days 8–14. During the test phase, three bottles containing either 0 µg/ mL nicotine +2% saccharin, 75 µg/mL + 2% saccharin or 150 µg/mL + 2% saccharin were presented to each mouse, and the total intake of nicotine was measured in each mouse on days 15–21

Next, we performed in vivo microdialysis experiments to measure the amount of extracellular DA induced by nicotine in the system (Fig. 6.4a). Basal levels of extracellular DA in the NAc of Shati/Nat8l-overexpressing mice were significantly lower than those of NAc-Mock mice (Fig. 6.4b). In the NAc-Mock mice group, the extracellular DA level was significantly increased 60–120 min after nicotine injection, up to a level of approximately 170% of that of the saline injection. Nicotine-injected NAc-Shati/Nat8l mice showed low levels of extracellular DA at the 60–120 min time point similar to saline-injected groups (Fig. 6.5). Furthermore, the suppressive

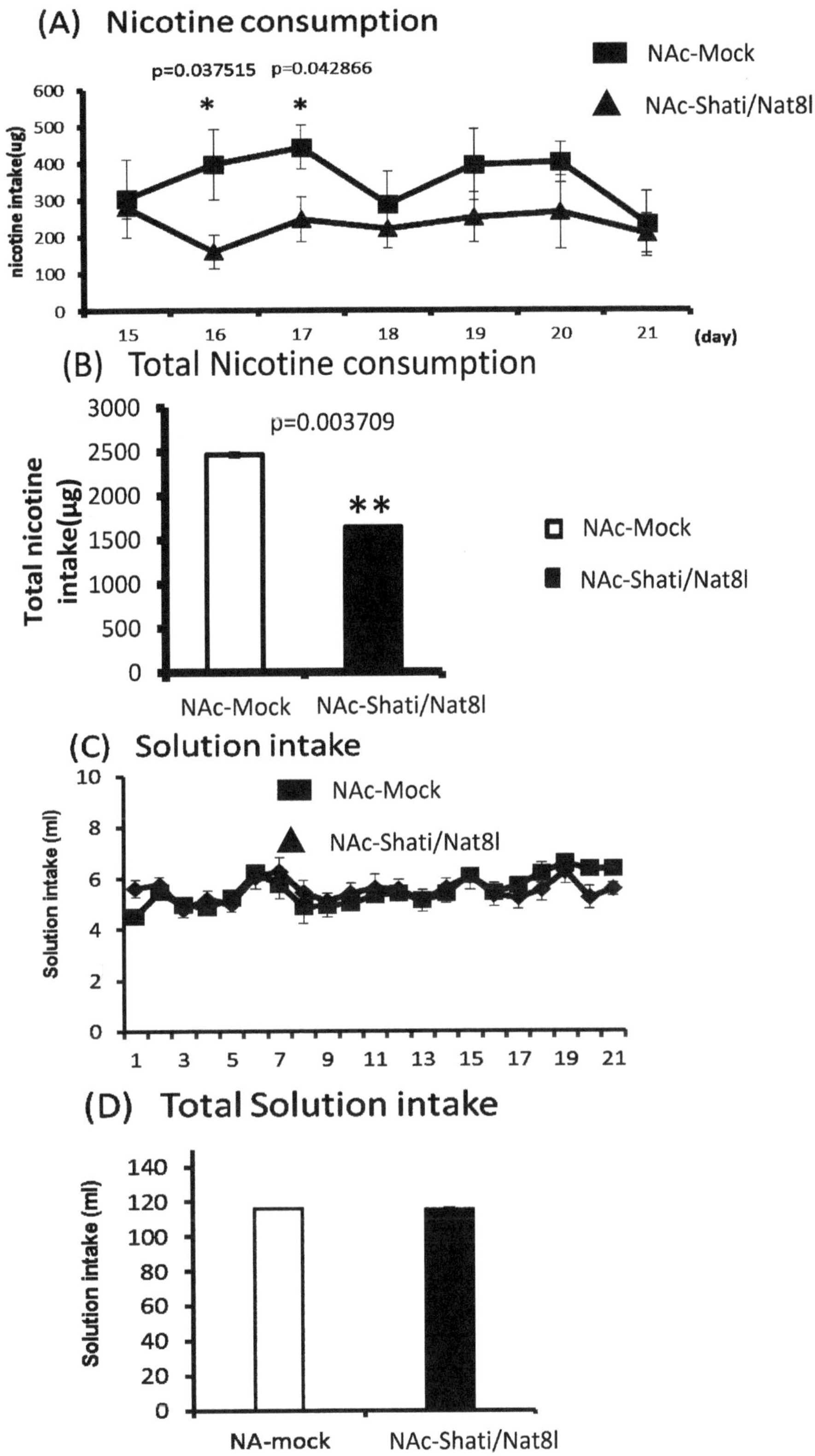

Fig. 6.3 Effects on nicotine preference of overexpression of Shati/Nat8l in NAc of mice. (**a**) Daily nicotine consumption in the test phase from days 15–21. (**b**) Total nicotine consumption during the test phase. (**c**) Daily solution intake in the test phase. (**d**) Total solution intake during the test phase

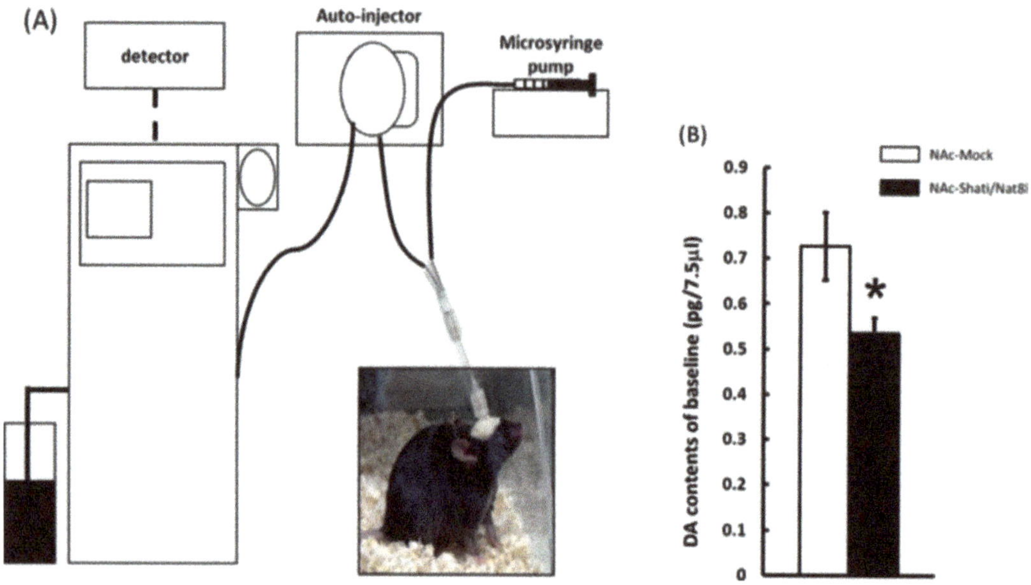

Fig. 6.4 Apparatus for in vivo microdialysis and quantification of basal DA levels. (**a**) Apparatus for in vivo microdialysis to measure dopamine (DA). (**b**) Effects of Shati/Nat8l overexpression in the basal levels of extracellular DA. Each column represents the mean ± S.E.M. n = 10, *P < 0.05 vs. NAc-Mock, Student's t-test)

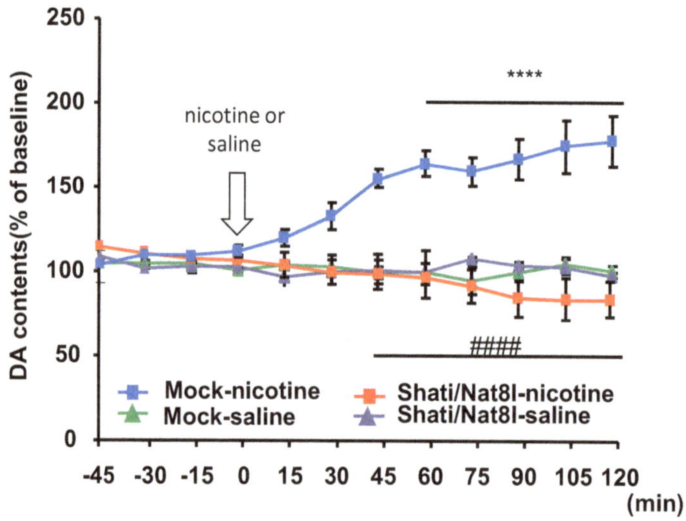

Fig. 6.5 Effect of Shati/Nat8l overexpression on nicotine (NIC)-induced dopamine (DA) release in the NAc. At 0 min, NAc-Shati/Nat8l and NAc-Mock mice were injected with either nicotine (0.4 mg/kg as free base) or saline (sal) subcutaneously. Each value represents the mean ± S.E.M. (n = 5, ****P < 0.001 vs. Mock-sal group, #P < 0.05 vs. Mock-NIC group, two- way repeated measure ANOVA with Bonferroni's post hoc test)

effects of Shati/Nat8l on nicotine-induced DA elevation were partially reversed by LY341495, an mGluR2/3 antagonist (Fig. 6.6). These results indicate that the function of Shati/Nat8l to suppress the effect of nicotine-induced extracellular DA in the NAc is partially dependent on mGluR3. These results are similar to those showing

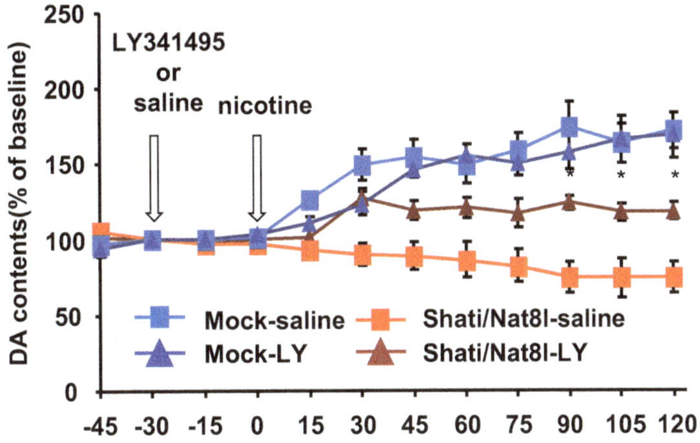

Fig. 6.6 The suppressant effect of Shati/Nat8l overexpression on nicotine-induced dopamine (DA) elevation was partially blocked by the mGluR2/3 antagonist, LY341495. At −30 min, NAc-Shati/Nat8l and NAc-Mock mice were injected with the mGluR2/3 antagonist, LY341495 (LY, 0.1 mg/kg, *i.p.*). Mice were injected with nicotine (NIC) (0.4 mg/kg, s.c.) 30 min after LY341495 injection. Each value represents the mean ± SEM. (n = 5, *P < 0.05 vs. Shati/Nat8l-Saline group, two-way repeated measures ANOVA with Bonferroni post hoc test)

the action of Shati/Nat8l against the pharmacological effects of methamphetamine. One difference is the complete or partial contribution of mGluR3 in methamphetamine and nicotine use, respectively. Both nicotine and methamphetamine regulate the DA reward system in the brain. Methamphetamine directly alters dopamine uptake and release, while nicotine first binds to the nicotinic acetylcholine receptor (nAChR) and, following signal transduction contributes to the potentiation of DA release. The suppressive effects of Shati/Nat8l on the DA release might happen downstream of the mGluR3 pathway. Further studies are required to discern whether there is a mechanistic crossover between the pharmacological actions of nicotine and methamphetamine. We attempted to investigate *Shati/Nat8l* mRNA changes in the NAc, the hippocampus and the frontal cortex, related to reward pathways following single or repeated treatments with nicotine. Unfortunately, we could not reproduce the results of the mRNA measurements, potentially because the levels of Shati/Nat8l or NAAG do not change based on the activation of nAChR. In relation to Shati/Nat8l production, methamphetamine and nicotine most likely act through different pathways.

Taken together, our results show that Shati/Nat8l in the NAc has a protective effect against the deleterious physiological changes associated with nicotine or methamphetamine administration.

6.2.2 *Striatal Shati/Nat8l and the Reward System*

We produced Shati/Nat8l transgenic mice (*Shati/Nat8l*-Tg) to investigate global overexpression in the brain. A targeting vector was used to produce the *Shati/Nat8l*-Tg mice, which ubiquitously expressed his-tagged *Shati/Nat8l* gene. A transgene

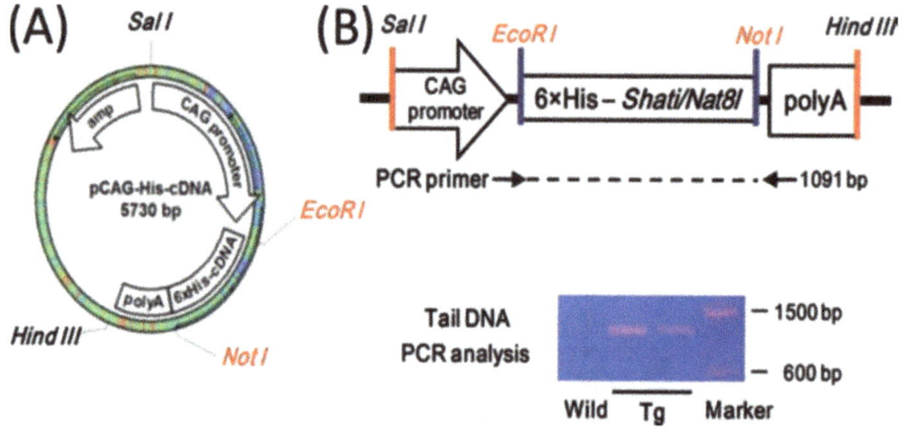

Fig. 6.7 Genetic scheme of *Shati/Nat8l*-Tg mice. (**a**) Targeting vector used to produce *Shati/Nat8l*-Tg mice. Transgenic mice ubiquitously expressing the His-tagged *Shati/Nat8l* gene were produced by Unitech (Chiba, Japan). Briefly, the transgene cassette including the CAG promoter followed by the his-*Shati/Nat8l* sequence was obtained from the CAG promoter his-*Shati/Nat8l* expression plasmid. The transgene cassette was microinjected into fertilized eggs from C57BL/6J females mated with males. (**b**) Genotyping results of *Shati/Nat8l*-Tg mice using a wild type mouse

cassette including the CAG promoter followed by the his-*Shati/Nat8l* sequence was obtained from a CAG promoter the his-*Shati/Nat8l* expression plasmid (Fig. 6.7a). The transgene cassette was microinjected into fertilized eggs from C57BL/6 J females mated with males. Genotyping confirmation of *Shati/Nat8l*-Tg mice using a wild type mouse as a control is shown in Fig. 6.7b. *Shati/Nat8l* mRNA levels were measured by quantitative real-time reverse transcriptase (RT)-PCR in the brain and are presented relative to the expression of the housekeeping gene, 36B4. *Shati/Nat8l* mRNA was highly expressed in the whole brain of 8-week-old transgenic mice (Fig. 6.8). However, *Shati/Nat8l* mRNA levels were increased in relation to wild type expression in the striatum only, not in other brain regions, such as the olfactory bulb, the prefrontal cortex or the NAc (Fig. 6.9). These *Shati/Nat8l*-Tg mice were therefore used for striatal Shati/Nat8l-overexpression mice. The mice showed no differences in basal locomotor activity compared to wild-type mice when observed in a novel environment (Fig. 6.10). These mice also performed a Y maze task as well as novel object recognition tests, to assess their learning abilities (Fig. 6.11). In the Y maze task, neither the number of total entries nor spontaneous alternation behaviors were different between *Shati/Nat8l*-Tg and wild type mice (Fig. 6.12). In the novel recognition test, both time and trial exploratory preference (in %) were similar between wild type and *Shati/Nat8l*-Tg mice (Fig. 6.12). Next, anxiety-like emotional behaviors in *Shati/Nat8l*-Tg mice were investigated using the light/dark box test, and no difference in the time spent on the light side was observed between *Shati/Nat8l*-Tg mice and wild type mice (Fig. 6.13). Results from both the light/dark box and elevated plus maze tests indicated no effect of increased levels of striatal Shati/Nat8l on anxiety-like behaviors. We also investigated the social abilities of the *Shati/Nat8l*-Tg mice. The experimental schedule of the three-chamber social interaction test is shown in Fig. 6.13a. In trial 1, the test mouse was placed in the

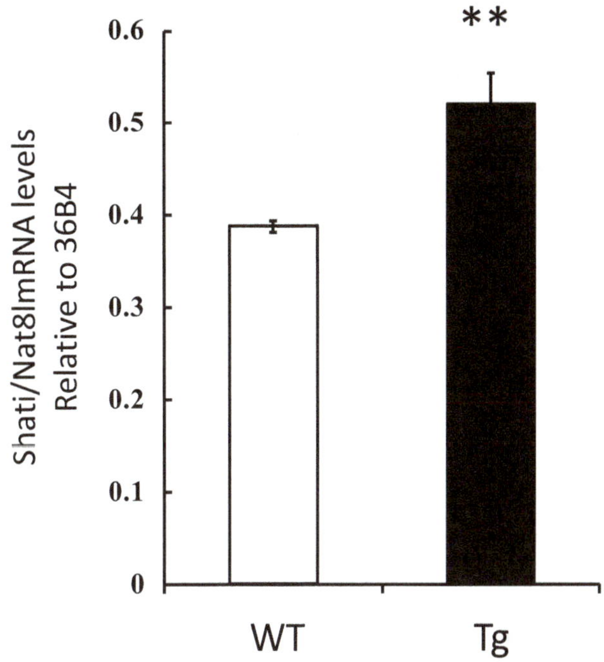

Fig. 6.8 Expression of *Shati/Nat8l* mRNA in the whole brain of *Shati/Nat8l*-Tg mice. *Shati/Nat8l* mRNA levels were measured by quantitative real-time RT-PCR in the brain and are presented as relative to the expression of the housekeeping gene, 36B4. Values are mean ± SEM (n = 5 mice/group, $^{**}P < 0.01$ vs. wild type group, Student's t-test)

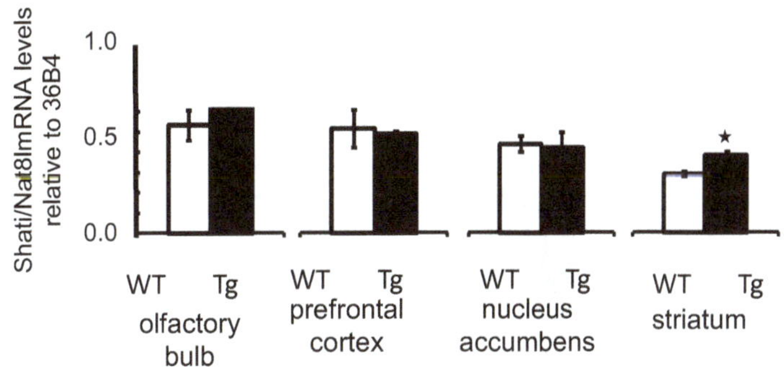

Fig. 6.9 Expression of *Shati/Nat8l* mRNA in various brain regions of *Shati/Nat8l*-Tg mice. *Shati/Nat8l* mRNA levels were measured by quantitative real-time RT-PCR in the brain and are presented as relative to 36B4. Values are mean ± SEM (n = 3 mice/group, $^{*}P < 0.05$ vs. wild type group, Student's t-test)

center of the chamber, while the other side of the chamber remained empty and no wire cage was placed. Both *Shati/Nat8l*-Tg and wild type mice were more interested in the novel object (Fig. 6.13b, left). In trial 2, another novel object was placed in the wire cage on one side, and an unfamiliar mouse (C57BL/6J) was placed in a wire cage on the opposite side. The *Shati/Nat8l*-Tg mice and wild type mice showed a similar level of interest in the unfamiliar mouse (Fig. 6.13b, right). In a prepulse inhibition (PPI) test, auditory startle response (Fig. 6.14a) and sensory motor control function (Fig. 6.14b) were not changed in *Shati/Nat8l*-Tg mice. Furthermore, in forced swimming and tail suspension tests, the immobility times of *Shati/Nat8l*-Tg mice were the same as those found for wild type mice (Figs. 6.15 and 6.16). These

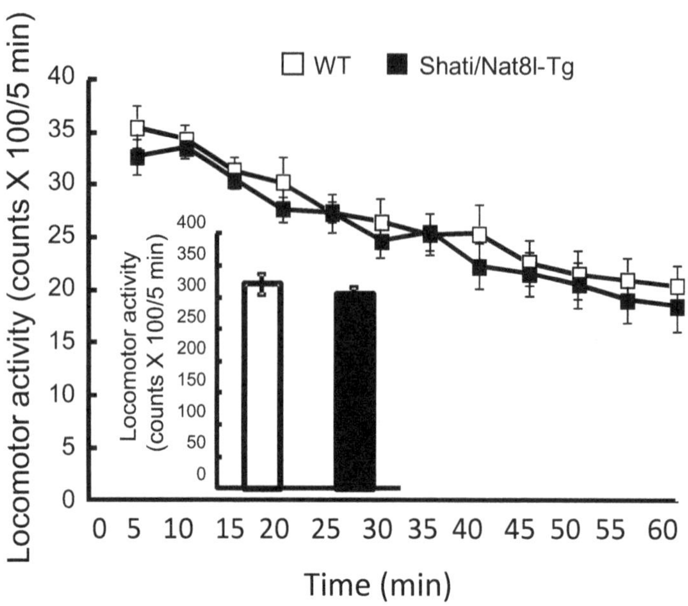

Fig. 6.10 Locomotor activity in *Shati/Nat8l*-Tg mice. No difference in basal locomotor activity was observed in a novel environment between *Shati/Nat8l*-Tg mice and wild type mice. Values are mean ± SEM (n = 10 or 14 mice/group)

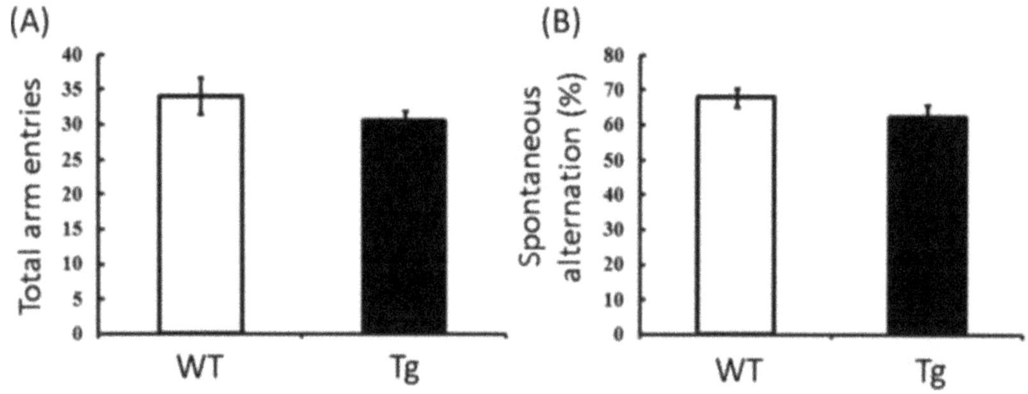

Fig. 6.11 Spontaneous alternation behavior in *Shati/Nat8l*-Tg mice. There was no difference in (**a**) total arm entries or (**b**) spontaneous alternation behavior in the Y-maze test observed between *Shati/Nat8l*-Tg mice and wild type mice. Values are mean ± SEM (n = 10 or 14 mice/group)

results indicate *Shati/Nat8l*-Tg mice do not demonstrate schizophrenia or depression-like behaviors.

Shati/Nat8l-Tg mice were not stable for the overexpression of Shati/Nat8l in the striatum, depending on their generation. In general, mouse lines generated with transgenes are often not stable, since transecting genes is a process that does not happen naturally. Therefore, to measure the effect of increased striatal Shati/Nat8l on the reward system, we injected an EGFP-tagged AAV containing *Shati/Nat8l* into the striatum of mice (Str-Shati/Nat8l) and confirmed localized overexpression by *in situ* hybridization and EGFP immunohistochemistry in the dorsal striatum

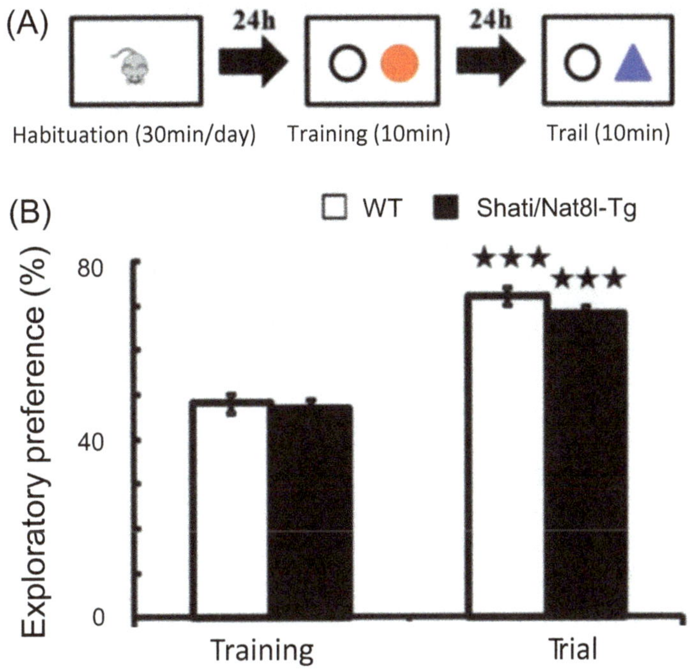

Fig. 6.12 Novel object recognition in *Shati/Nat8l*-Tg mice. (**a**) Experimental schedule of the novel object recognition test. (**b**) No difference in exploratory preference in the novel object recognition test was observed between *Shati/Nat8l*-Tg mice and wild type mice. Values are mean ± SEM (n = 10 or 14 mice/group, **P < 0.001 vs. training phase for each group, Student's t-test)

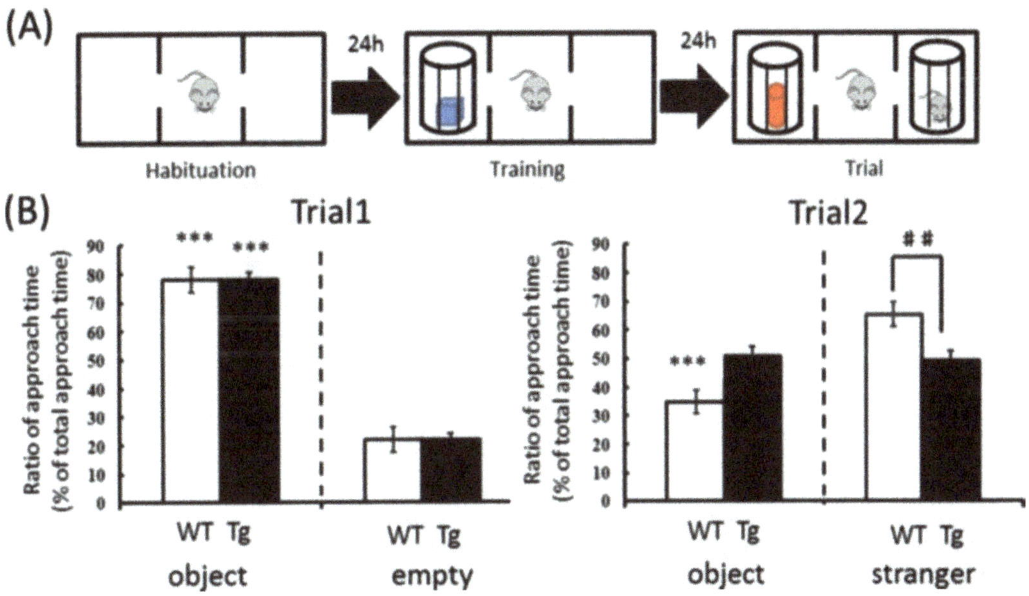

Fig. 6.13 Social interaction in *Shati/Nat8l*-Tg mice. (**a**) Experimental schedule of three chamber social interaction test. (**b**), left A novel object was placed in a wire cage on one side of the chamber, and no wire cage was placed on the other side of the chamber. Both *Shati/Nat8l*-Tg mice and wild type mice were more interested in the novel object. Values are mean ± SEM (n = 10 or 14 mice/group, ***P < 0.001 vs. empty side for each group, Student's t-test). WT: wild type, Tg: transgenic. (**b**), right Another novel object was placed in a wire cage on one side of the chamber, and an unfamiliar mouse (C57BL/6 J) was placed in a wire cage on the other side of the chamber. *Shati/Nat8l*-Tg mice were not more interested in the unfamiliar mouse than the wild type group. Values are mean ± SEM (n = 10 or 14 mice/group, ***P < 0.001 vs. unfamiliar mouse, ##P < 0.01 vs. wild type group, Student's t-test)

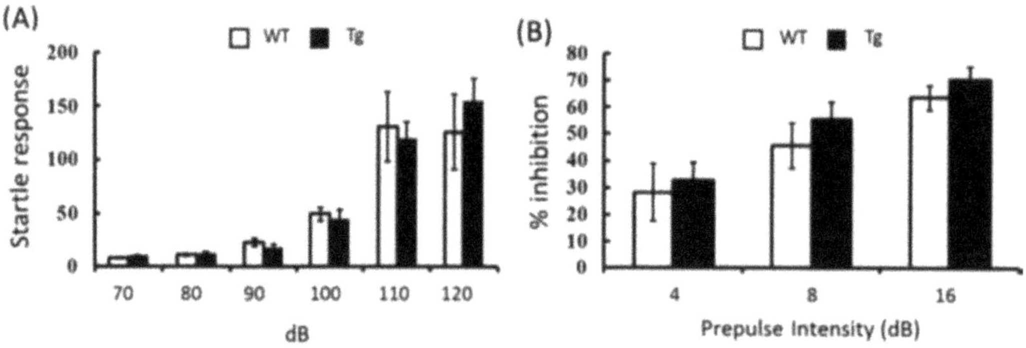

Fig. 6.14 Startle response and PPI in *Shati/Nat8l*-Tg mice. **a** Startle response was measured for 70, 80, 90, 100, 110 and 120 dB (background noise: 70 dB). Values are mean ± SEM. **b** PPI was measured with 4, 8 and 16 dB of prepulse intensity (background noise: 70 dB). Values are mean ± SEM (n = 8 or 13 mice/group)

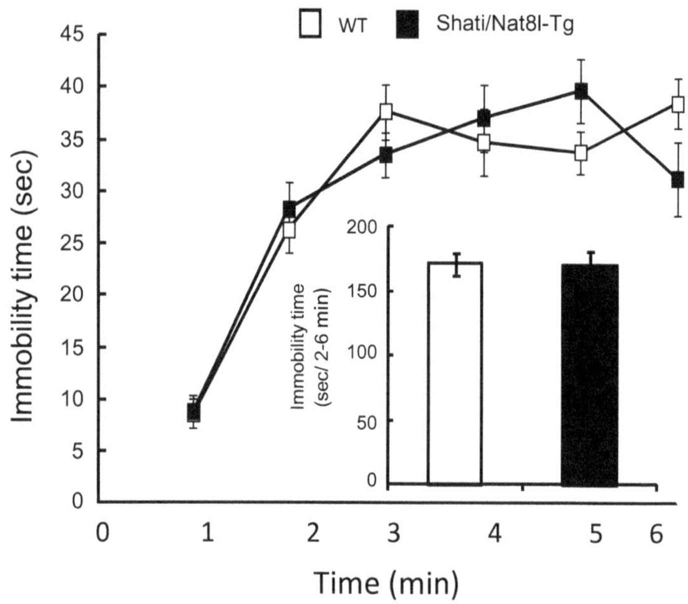

Fig. 6.15 Depressive behavior in *Shati/Nat8l*-Tg mice in the tail suspension test. No difference in immobility time was observed during the tail suspension test between *Shati/Nat8l*-Tg mice and wild type mice. Values are mean ± SEM (n = 10 or 14 mice/group)

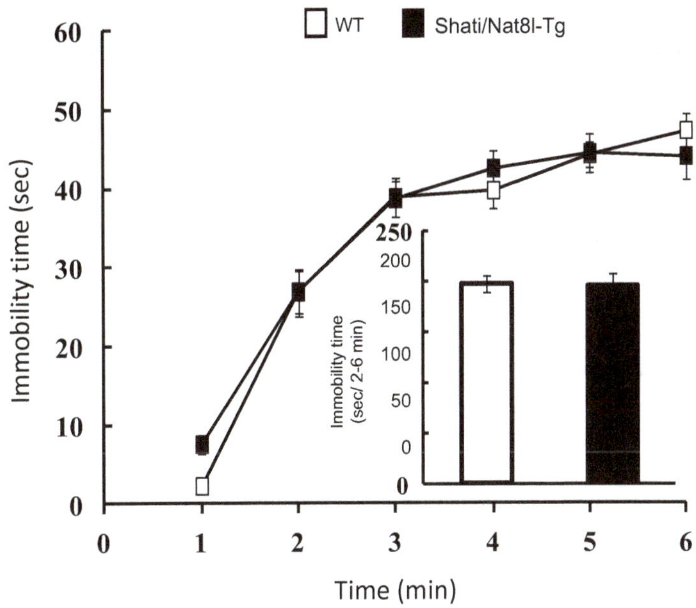

Fig. 6.16 Depressive behavior in *Shati/Nat8l*-Tg mice in the forced swimming test. No difference in immobility time was observed in the forced swimming test between *Shati/Nat8l*-Tg mice and wild type mice. Values are mean ± SEM (n = 10 or 14 mice/group)

area. Str-Shati/Nat8l mice showed no difference in methamphetamine-induced hyperactivity compared to mock-injected mice (Fig. 6.17a). Methamphetamine-induced conditioned place preference was also not changed in Str-Shati/Nat8l mice (Fig. 6.17b). Therefore, we conclude that Shati/Nat8l in the striatum does not contribute to reward effects in mice.

6.3 Shati/Nat8l in Learning and Memory

6.3.1 Hippocampal Shati/Nat8l in Learning and Memory

Shati/Nat8l produces NAA from acetyl-coA and aspartic acid, and represents one of the amino acids with the highest-concentration amino acids in the brain. Recently, a change in NAA concentration measured by MRS was proposed as a biomarker for early-stage Alzheimer's (Murray et al. 2014). This suggests that Shati/Nat8l and/or NAA are related in some way to the onset of Alzheimer's disease. However, learning ability was not changed in Y maze and novel object tests conducted in Shati/Nat8l KO mice (Furukawa-Hibi et al. 2012). We overexpressed Shati/Nat8l in the hippocampus *via* AAV injection (Hip-Shati/Nat8l), and conducted learning and memory tests. In the novel object trial session, Hip-Shati/Nat8l mice preferred to explore the novel object for a significantly prolonged time compared to mock injection mice (Fig. 6.18). This result suggests that cognitive ability might be potentiated by the overexpression of Shati/Nat8l. Murray et al. (2014) and Guo et al. (2017)

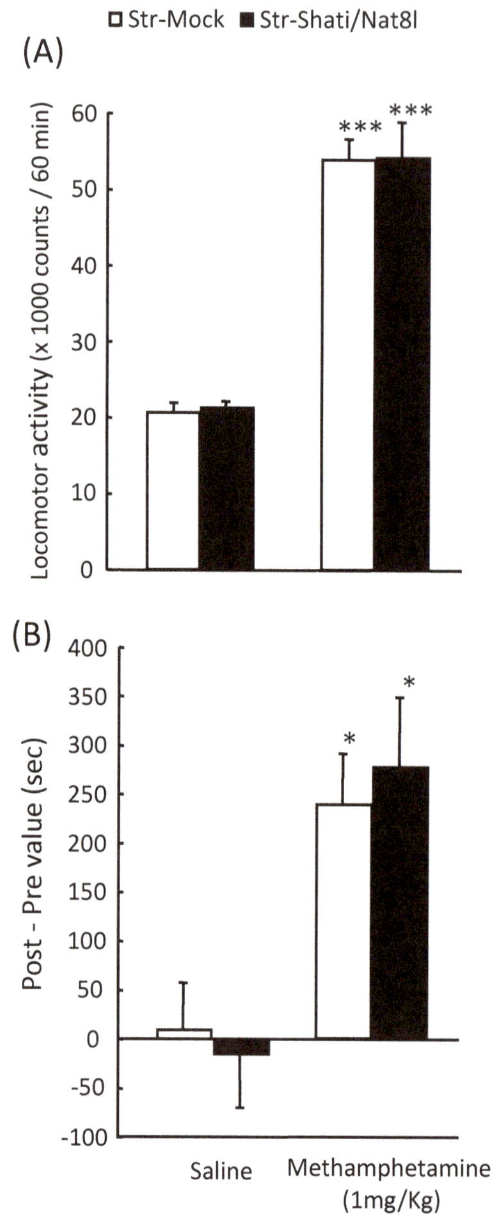

Fig. 6.17 Pharmacological changes to locomotor activity and place conditioned preference induced by methamphetamine. No difference was seen in (**a**) the locomotor activity after treatment with methamphetamine (1 mg/kg) or (**b**) conditioned place preference with methamphetamine (1 mg/kg) between Str-Mock and Str-Shati/Nat8l

demonstrated that a change in NAA level is a clinical marker for Alzheimer's disease, although these authors looked at only the posterior cingulate gyri, the inferior precunei and the posterior cingulate cortex. Proton magnetic resonance spectroscopy (^{1}H-MRS) showed low NAA/creatine ratios in the posterior cingulate cortices of patients with Alzheimer's disease, which is a typical region for the accumulation of amyloid beta. Vulnerability to shifts in NAA is not the same in all brain regions in patients with Alzheimer's disease. Our results using Hip-Shati/Nat8l mice are partly in agreement with these clinical observations. There are also other clinical studies that measure NAA levels in relation to Alzheimer's disease using the MRS technique (Zhong et al. 2014; Zhang et al. 2015). Further studies are required to

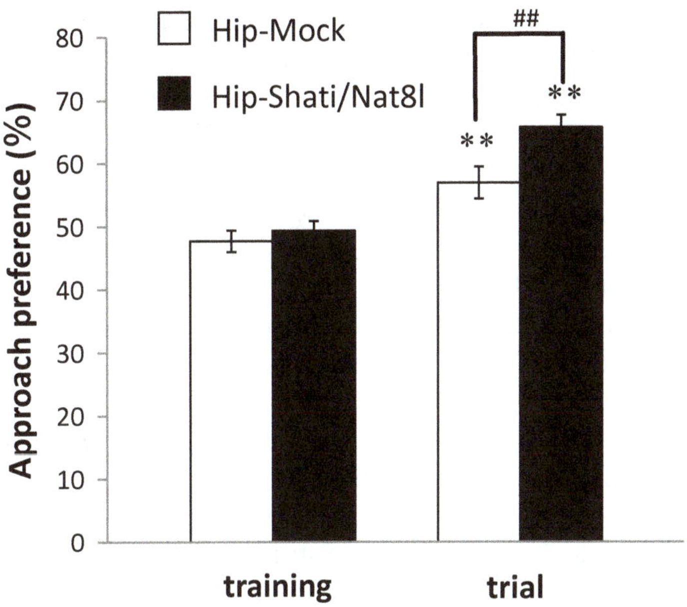

Fig. 6.18 Enhanced approach preference to novel object in Hip-Shati/Nat8l mice in the novel object recognition test. Hip-Shati/Nat8l mice significantly preferred to approach the novel object compared to Hip-mock mice. (**$P < 0.01$ vs. trial for each group, ##$P < 0.01$ vs Hip-Mock group, Student's t-test)

investigate changes in Shati/Nat8l itself in the brain of patients with Alzheimer's disease, since Shati/Nat8l has also functions, apart from being synthetase for NAA.

6.3.2 *Function of Accumbal Shati/Nat8l on Learning Memory and Emotional Behaviors*

We have shown that nicotine reversed scopolamine-induced impairment in the passive avoidance task in rats through its action on the dopaminergic neuronal system (Nitta et al. 1994). The study did not mention which brain areas are important for the nicotine-potentiated learning ability. If altered DA levels triggered by Shati/Nat8l overexpression had any effect on cognitive function, *Shati/Nat8l*-Tg mice would show potentiated cognitive function over normal mice. However, their cognitive functions were not changed in Y maze or novel object tests (Figs. 6.8 and 6.9).

6.3.3 *Function of Shati/Nat8l in Axon Outgrowth*

In vitro studies were performed to evaluate the function of Shati/Nat8l in neuronal cells, since *Shati/Nat8l* mRNA signals were observed in all brain regions of mice (Sumi et al. 2015). Especially strong signals were found in cortical pyramidal cells, dentate granule cells, hippocampal pyramidal cells, and cerebellar granule cells. Neuronal cells of all brain regions showed positive *Shati/Nat8l* mRNA signals. Hippocampal neurons were selected for their easy evaluation and high cell density. *Shati/Nat8l* mRNA positive cells colocalized with NeuN (a marker for neurons)-positive cells but not with GFAP (a marker for astrocytes)- or Iba1 (a marker for microglia)-positive cells. These results show that *Shati/Nat8l* mRNA is only expressed in neuronal cells of the mouse hippocampus. An AAV vector containing *Shati/Nat8l* was transfected into primary cultured mouse neurons. Overexpression of Shati/Nat8l in primary cultured neurons induced axonal growth but not dendrite elongation. Treatment with a selective group II mGluR antagonist did not eliminate Shati/Nat8l-induced axon outgrowth, and NAAG itself did not induce axon outgrowth. Overexpression of Shati/Nat8l also increased the ATP content in the cultured hippocampal neurons. These results suggest that neuronal Shati/Nat8l induces axon outgrowth via ATP synthesis independently of the mGluR3 signaling pathway. Shati/Nat8l is associated with microtubule structure when overexpressed in COS7 cells and primary mouse cultured neurons (Toriumi et al. 2013). On the other hand, it was also reported that Shati/Nat8l co-localizes with a mitochondrial marker in SH-SH5Y cells (Ariyannur et al. 2010), and that Shati/Nat8l is localized in the endoplasmic reticulum (Wiame et al. 2009). Shati/Nat8l may have novel functions in neuronal cells. NAA is produced in the mitochondria because it is associated with the tricarboxylic acid cycle (TCA) related to cell metabolism (Madhavarao et al. 2003). The levels of NAA and ATP were increased in primary cultured neurons overexpressed with Shati/Nat8l. The TCA cycle produces ATP molecules at the highest rate in terms of cell metabolism, and ATP in the growth cone is known to promote neurite elongation in cultured neurons (Höpker et al. 1996). Neuronal dendrite length in Shati/Nat8l KO mice was significantly shorter than in wildtype mice (Berent-Spillson et al. 2004). Shati/Nat8l appears to play a major role in ATP-induced neurite elongation. Shati/Nat8l is an indicator of the stimulation of mGluR3. However, neither NAAG nor LY341495, the endogenous agonist of mGluR3 and an antagonist of mGluR3, respectively, affected axon outgrowth. Shati/Nat8l is thus associated with neurite elongation and the ATP synthesis pathway during NAA synthesis.

6.4 Shati/Nat8l and Psychiatric Disease

6.4.1 Patients with Depression and NAA

NAA is used as a biomarker of depression in specific regions of the human brain as it is an indicator of neuronal activity in ^{1}H–MRS. NAA is significantly decreased in the anterior cingulate gyrus of patients with depression. Brain-derived neurotrophic factor (BDNF) has been reported to be one of the biomarkers for patients with depressive (Rogóż et al. 2017; Zhao et al. 2016). Anti-depressant drugs rescue the reduction in NAA, in addition to BDNF. Interestingly, *BDNF* mRNA is increased in the prefrontal cortex, the NAc and the hippocampus in the brains of Shati/Nat8l KO mice (Furukawa-Hibi et al. 2012). Therefore, the changes in Shati/Nat8l and BDNF are not parallel, but independent. Although detailed mechanisms for the roles of Shati/Nat8l and/or BDNF in depression have not been clarified, they may nevertheless serve as reliable clinical markers.

6.4.2 Shati/Nat8l and Depressive Behaviors in Mice

Miyamoto et al. (2017) also demonstrated that striatal Shati/Nat8l induces depressive behaviors. We produced mice overexpressing Shati/Nat8l in the striatum (Str-Shati/Nat8l mice) using an AAV vector, as described earlier. The Str-Shati/Nat8l mice showed depression-like behaviors in forced swimming and tail suspension tests (Miyamoto et al. 2017) as measured by prolonged immobility, indicating that Shati/Nat8l is an inducer of depression. These dysfunctions are cancelled by the anti-depressant drug, fluvoxamine, and the mGluR3 antagonist, LY341495. Shati/Nat8l levels may be a factor in the vulnerability to stress. In the psychiatric field, mental diseases are often caused by two factors, genetic background and circumstance, and striatal Shati/Nat8l might thus represent one of the genetic factors.

6.4.3 Shati/Nat8l and Postpartum Depression

Postpartum depression is observed in about 13% of postpartum women, and is defined as a depressive disorder leading to a substantial impairment of daily life. It also has large impacts on the patients' families, including the promotion of depressive tendencies in the husband, the abuse or neglect of the child and/or delayed cognitive development or increased psychopathological issues in the child (Stumbo et al. 2015).

The occurrence of postpartum depression has been related to fluctuations in the levels of steroid hormones and glucocorticoids (cortisol in humans, corticosterone in animals) occurring during pregnancy and after delivery. Mice that received chronic ultra-mild stress (CUMS, procedure described in Fig. 6.19) demonstrated similar symptoms to the depression symptoms related to pregnancy in humans. Pregnant female mice subjected to CUMS could be a model for human postpartum depression, since the mice show prolonged immobility in forced swimming and tail suspension tests and anhedonia against sucrose (Shang et al. 2016). The dams exposed to CUMS during gestation showed depression-like behavior during their postpartum period. *Shati/Nat8l* mRNA expression was increased in the striatum of the dams, but not in the NAc or the frontal cortex (Fig. 6.20). The relationship between *Shati/Nat8l* in the striatum and postpartum depression-like behavior induced by CUMS was investigated. The dams that overexpressed *Shati/Nat8l* spe-

	Morning (11:30 to 12:30)	Afternoon (14:30 to 16:30)	Night (18:30 to 8:30)
Monday	Confinement	Cage tilt (30°)	Soiled cage
Tuesday	Cage tilt	Paired housing	Overnight illumination
Wednesday	Cage tilt	Confinement	Soiled cage
Thursday	Confinement	Paired housing	Cage tilt
Friday	Confinement	Cage tilt	Reversed light/dark cycle
Weekend	Reversed light / dark cycle	Reversed light/dark cycle	Reversed light/dark cycle

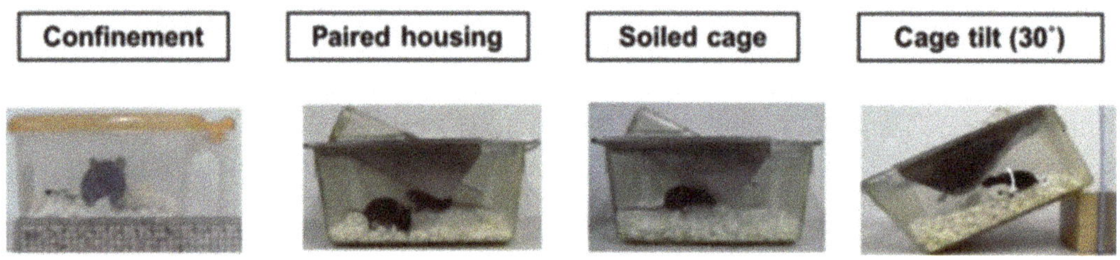

Fig. 6.19 Chronic ultramild stress protocol. The chronic ultramild stress (CUMS) regimen consisted of five ultramild stressors: period of cage tilt (30°), confinement in a small box (11 × 8 × 8 cm), paired housing, one overnight period with soiled cage (50 ml water on 1 L paper pellet) and permanent light. The animals were also placed on a reversed light/dark cycle from Friday evening through the next Monday. This procedure was scheduled over a 1-week period and repeated throughout the period from the time of separation from the male until parturition

cifically in the bilateral striatum showed increased sensitivity to stress, and exacerbated depression-like symptoms such as despair behaviors.

We also carried out a clinical study among pregnant women. Serum concentrations of Shati/Nat8l were measured in pregnant womean during late pregnancy and at 5 days and 1 month after delivery, respectively. The women were divided into two groups, a non-depressive and a depressive group, based on their score on the Edinburgh Postnatal Depression Scale (EPDS). Serum concentrations of Shati/Nat8l were higher in the depressive group than in the non-depressive group at the time point before delivery (Nitta et al. unpublished data). Serum concentrations of Shati/Nat8l at the late pregnancy stage could be one predictive biomarker for postnatal depression, and the appropriate preventive and early interventions might thus be undertaken for pregnant and postpartum women. We also measured serum concentrations of Shati/Nat8l in these women after delivery, but observed no significant differences.

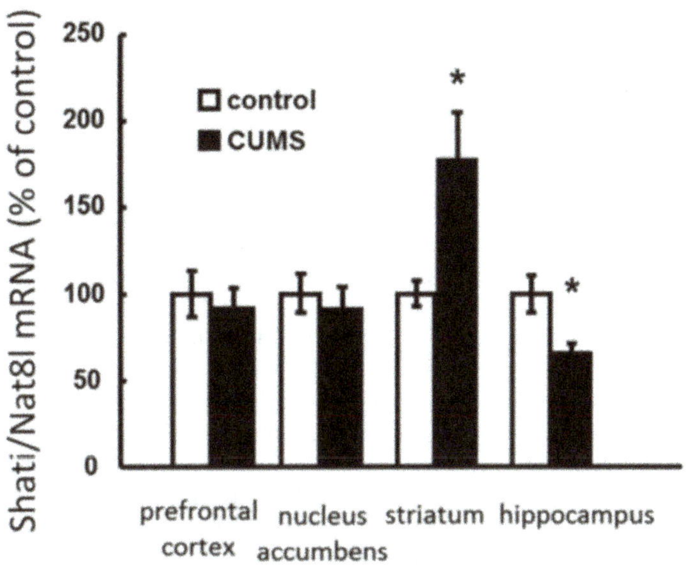

Fig. 6.20 Expression of *Shati/Nat8l* mRNA in CUMS mice. The changes in *Shati/Nat8l* mRNA expression in various brain regions of stressed postpartum mice and control mice. (*P < 0.05 vs control group in each brain region)

6.5 Conclusions

Shati/Nat8l and NAA have various functions in the central nervous system. In addition to the neuronal system, Shati/Nat8l is also highly expressed in the adipose tissue, and NAA pathway could similarly serve as an acetyl-CoA metabolizing mechanism in adipocytes (Pessentheiner et al. 2013). An increase in lipolysis followed by an activation of β-oxidation can restore acetyl-CoA back to the mitochondria. Lipid turnover can raise the oxidative potential of the brown fat cells and thereby boost the brown adipogenic phenotype. However, the physiological stimuli contributing to the regulation of the NAA pathway are unknown (Pessentheiner et al. 2013). These results suggest the possibility that Shati/Nat8l also plays a role in lifestyle diseases such as diabetes.

Because of their widespread occurrence in the human body, Shati/Nat8l and NAA have the potential to be used as treatment tools for a variety of diseases in the near future.

Conflicts of Interest The authors have declared that no competing interests exist.

Funding This study was supported by a Smoking Research Foundation Grant for Biomedical Research and Foundation, the Program for Next Generation World-Leading Researchers [NEXT Program LS047], a grant-in-aid for Scientific Research (KAKENHI) (B) [JSPS KAKENHI Grant Number, JP15H04662], a Challenging Exploratory Research grant [JSPS KAKENHI grant number, JP15K15050; 17 K19801] from the Japan Society for the Promotion of Science, a Research on Regulatory Science of Pharmaceuticals and Medical Devices grant from the Japan Agency for Medical Research and Development (AMED) [16mk0101076h0001], and the Kobayashi International Foundation.

Acknowledgments We thank Naomi Takino, Hitomi Miyauchi, and Keiko Ayabe for technical assistance in producing the AAV-Shati/Nat8l vectors.

References

Aoki Y, Abe O, Yahata N et al (2012) Absence of age-related prefrontal NAA change in adults with autism spectrum disorders. Transl Psychiatry 2:e178. https://doi.org/10.1038/tp.2012.108

Ariyannur PS, Moffett JR, Manickam P et al (2010) Methamphetamine-induced neuronal protein NAT8L is the NAA biosynthetic enzyme: implications for specialized acetyl coenzyme A metabolism in the CNS. Brain Res 1335:1–13. https://doi.org/10.1016/j.brainres.2010.04.008

Becker I, Lodder J, Gieselmann V et al (2010) Molecular characterization of N-acetylaspartylglutamate synthetase. J Biol Chem 285:29156–29164. https://doi.org/10.1074/jbc.M110.111765

Berent-Spillson A, Robinson AM, Golovoy D et al (2004) Protection against glucose-induced neuronal death by NAAG and GCP II inhibition is regulated by mGluR3. J Neurochem 89:90–99. https://doi.org/10.1111/j.1471-4159.2003.02321.x

Burri R, Steffen C, Herschkowitz N (1991) N-acetyl-L-aspartate is a major source of acetyl groups for lipid synthesis during rat brain development. Dev Neurosci 13:403–411. https://doi.org/10.1159/000112191

Bzdega T, Turi T, Wroblewska B et al (1997) Molecular cloning of a peptidase against N-acetylaspartylglutamate from a rat hippocampal cDNA library. J Neurochem 69:2270–2277. https://doi.org/10.1046/j.1471-4159.1997.69062270.x

Conn PJ, Pin JP (1997) Pharmacology and functions of metabotropic glutamate receptors. Annu Rev Pharmacol Toxicol 37:205–237. https://doi.org/10.1146/annurev.pharmtox.37.1.205

Furukawa-Hibi Y, Nitta A, Fukumitsu H et al (2012) Absence of SHATI/Nat8l reduces social interaction in mice. Neurosci Lett 526:79–84. https://doi.org/10.1016/j.neulet.2012.08.028

Guo Z, Liu X, Cao Y et al (2017) Common ^{1}H-MRS characteristics in patients with Alzheimer's disease and vascular dementia diagnosed with kidney essence deficiency syndrome: a preliminary study. Altern Ther Health Med 23:12–18. https://www.ncbi.nlm.nih.gov/pubmed/28236618

Höpker VH, Saffrey MJ, Burnstock G (1996) Neurite outgrowth of striatal neurons in vitro: involvement of purines in the growth-promoting effect of myenteric plexus explants. Int J Dev Neurosci 14:439–451. https://doi.org/10.1016/0736-5748(96)00020-2

Huang W, Wang H, Kekuda R et al (2000) Transport of N-acetylaspartate by the Na(+)-dependent high-affinity dicarboxylate transporter NaDC3 and its relevance to the expression of the transporter in the brain. J Pharmacol Exp Ther 295:392–403. http://jpet.aspetjournals.org/content/295/1/392.long

Madhavarao CN, Chinopoulos C, Chandrasekaran K et al (2003) Characterization of the N-acetylaspartate biosynthetic enzyme from rat brain. J Neurochem 86:824–835. https://doi.org/10.1046/j.1471-4159.2003.01905.x

Mazzoccoli C, Ruggieri V, Tataranni T et al (2016) N-acetylaspartate (NAA) induces neuronal differentiation of SH-SY5Y neuroblastoma cell line and sensitizes it to chemotherapeutic agents. Oncotarget 7:26235–26246. https://doi.org/10.18632/oncotarget.8454

Miyamoto Y, Ishikawa Y, Iegaki N et al (2014) Overexpression of Shati/Nat8l, an N-acetyltransferase, in the nucleus accumbens attenuates the response to methamphetamine via activation of group II mGluRs in mice. Int J Neuropsychopharmacol 17:1283–1294. https://doi.org/10.1017/S146114571400011X

Miyamoto Y, Iegaki N, Fu K et al (2017) Striatal *N*-acetylaspartate synthetase Shati/Nat8l regulates depression-like behaviors *via* mGluR3-mediated serotonergic suppression in mice. Int J Neuropsychopharmacol. https://doi.org/10.1093/ijnp/pyx078

Moffett JR, Ross C, Arun P et al (2007) N-Acetylaspartate in the CNS: from neurodiagnostics to neurobiology. Prog Neurobiol 81:89–131. https://doi.org/10.1016/j.pneurobio.2006.12.003

Murray ME, Przybelski SA, Lesnick TG et al (2014) Early Alzheimer's disease neuropathology detected by proton MR spectroscopy. J Neurosci 34:16247–16255. https://doi.org/10.1523/JNEUROSCI.2027-14.2014

Namboodiri AM, Peethambaran A, Mathew R et al (2006) Canavan disease and the role of N-acetylaspartate in myelin synthesis. Mol Cell Endocrinol 252:216–223. https://doi.org/10.1016/j.mce.2006.03.016

Neale JH, Bzdega T, Wroblewska B (2000) N-Acetylaspartylglutamate: the most abundant peptide neurotransmitter in the mammalian central nervous system. J Neurochem 75(4):43–752. https://doi.org/10.1046/j.1471-4159.2000.0750443.x

Neale JH, Olszewski RT, Zuo D et al (2011) Advances in understanding the peptide neurotransmitter NAAG and appearance of a new member of the NAAG neuropeptide family. J Neurochem 11:490–498. https://doi.org/10.1111/j.1471-4159.2011.07338.x

Nitta A, Katono Y, Itoh A et al (1994) Nicotine reverses scopolamine-induced impairment of performance in passive avoidance task in rats through its action on the dopaminergic neuronal system. Pharmacol Biochem Behav 49:807–812. https://doi.org/10.1016/0091-3057(94)90227-5

Niwa M, Nitta A, Mizoguchi H et al (2007) A novel molecule "shati" is involved in methamphetamine-induced hyperlocomotion, sensitization, and conditioned place preference. J Neurosci 27:7604–7615. https://doi.org/10.1523/JNEUROSCI.1575-07.2007

Niwa M, Nitta A, Cen X et al (2008) A novel molecule 'shati' increases dopamine uptake via the induction of tumor necrosis factor-alpha in pheochromocytoma-12 cells. J Neurochem 107:1697–1708. https://doi.org/10.1111/j.1471-4159.2008.05738.x

Pessentheiner AR, Pelzmann HJ, Walenta E et al (2013) NAT8L (N-acetyltransferase 8-like) accelerates lipid turnover and increases energy expenditure in brown adipocytes. J Biol Chem 288:36040–36051. https://doi.org/10.1074/jbc.M113.491324

Reynolds LM, Reynolds GP (2011) Differential regional N-acetylaspartate deficits in postmortem brain in schizophrenia, bipolar disorder and major depressive disorder. J Psychiatr Res 45:54–59. https://doi.org/10.1016/j.jpsychires.2010.05.001

Rogóż Z, Kamińska K, Pańczyszyn-Trzewik P et al (2017) Repeated co-treatment with antidepressants and risperidone increases BDNF mRNA and protein levels in rats. Pharmacol Rep 69:885–893. https://doi.org/10.1016/j.pharep.2017.02.022

Shang X, Shang Y, Fu J et al (2016) Nicotine significantly improves chronic stress-induced impairments of cognition and synaptic plasticity in mice. Mol Neurobiol. https://doi.org/10.1007/s12035-016-0012-2

Stumbo SP, Yarborough BJ, Paulson RI et al (2015) The impact of adverse child and adult experiences on recovery from serious mental illness. Psychiatr Rehabil J 38:320–327. https://doi.org/10.1037/prj0000141

Sumi K, Uno K, Matsumura S et al (2015) Induction of neuronal axon outgrowth by Shati/Nat8l by energy metabolism in mice cultured neurons. Neuroreport 26:74074–74076. https://doi.org/10.1097/WNR.0000000000000416

Toriumi K, Ikami M, Kondo M et al (2013) SHATI/NAT8L regulates neurite outgrowth via microtubule stabilization. J Neurosci Res 91:1525–1532. https://doi.org/10.1002/jnr.23273

Wiame E, Tyteca D, Pierrot N et al (2009) Molecular identification of aspartate N-acetyltransferase and its mutation in hypoacetylaspartia. Biochem J 425:127–136. https://doi.org/10.1042/BJ20091024

Zhang B, Ferman TJ, Boeve BF (2015) MRS in mild cognitive impairment: early differentiation of dementia with Lewy bodies and Alzheimer's disease. J Neuroimaging 25:269–274. https://doi.org/10.1111/jon.12138

Zhao G, Zhang C, Chen J et al (2016) Ratio of mBDNF to proBDNF for differential diagnosis of major depressive disorder and bipolar depression. Mol Neurobiol. https://doi.org/10.1007/s12035-016-0098-6

Zhong X, Shi H, Shen Z et al (2014) ^{1}H-proton magnetic resonance spectroscopy differentiates dementia with Lewy bodies from Alzheimer's disease. J Alzheimers Dis 40:953–966. https://doi.org/10.3233/JAD-131517

Chapter 7
Nicotinic Acetylcholine Receptors in Regulation of Pathology of Cerebrovascular Disorders

Hiroshi Katsuki and Kosei Matsumoto

Abstract Cerebrovascular disorders including ischemic stroke, intracerebral hemorrhage and subarachnoid hemorrhage are among the major clinical concerns for which effective therapies are poorly available. Accumulating lines of evidence indicate that drugs acting on nicotinic acetylcholine receptors (nAChRs) may provide therapeutic effects on these disorders, based on their neuroprotective and anti-inflammatory actions. For example, the cholinergic neurotransmission in the central nervous system via nAChRs may function as an endogenous neuroprotective system that prevents pathogenic events associated with ischemic stroke. On the other hand, exogenous administration of nicotine or nAChR agonists to experimental models of ischemic stroke has been reported to produce conflicting results (either protective or deleterious), which may be largely dependent on the different regiments of drug treatments. With regard to intracerebral hemorrhage, preclinical findings suggest that post-treatment with nAChR agonists is effective in alleviating brain tissue damage and neurological outcome. The beneficial actions of nAChR agonist have also been reported for an experimental model of subarachnoid hemorrhage, which should be confirmed by further investigations. Although smoking has been considered as an important risk factor for stroke episodes, specific targeting of the central nAChRs may prove to be an effective and novel strategy for the treatment of diverse types of cerebrovascular disorders.

Keywords Nicotine · Cerebral infarction · Hemorrhagic stroke · Neuroprotection · Neuroinflammation · Acethylcholinesterase inhibitor

---

H. Katsuki (✉) · K. Matsumoto
Department of Chemico-Pharmacological Sciences, Graduate School of Pharmaceutical Sciences, Kumamoto University, Kumamoto, Japan
e-mail: hkatsuki@gpo.kumamoto-u.ac.jp

A. Akaike et al. (eds.), *Nicotinic Acetylcholine Receptor Signaling in Neuroprotection*, https://doi.org/10.1007/978-981-10-8488-1_7

7.1 Introduction

Acetylcholine (ACh) has a long history of biomedical research as it is the first compound that has been identified as a chemical neurotransmitter. In the periphery, motor neurons release ACh from their nerve terminals that innervate skeletal muscles and transmit signals via activation of muscle type nicotinic acetylcholine receptors (nAChRs) that are heteropentamers consisting of subunits named α1, β1, δ and ε. The cell bodies of sympathetic and parasympathetic postganglionic neurons express neuronal type of nAChRs composed of subunits distinct from those contained in muscle nAChRs, such as α3α5β4 and α3α5β2β4. These nAChRs expressed in autonomic ganglia receive cholinergic inputs from preganglionic neurons. Postganglionic neurons of the parasympathetic nervous system also utilize ACh as a neurotransmitter, and various peripheral tissues receive the signals from these neurons mainly via muscarinic ACh receptors.

Cholinergic neurotransmitter system is also present in the brain, and nAChRs as well as muscarinic receptors are widely distributed throughout the central nervous system (Taly et al. 2009). A notable feature of nAChR-mediated signal transmission in the central nervous system is that it may mediate various functions in addition to the role in fast neurotransmission. That is, stimulation of nAChRs in central neurons affords cytoprotective and survival-promoting effects, as discussed in other chapters as well as in the literatures elsewhere (Akaike et al. 2010; Mudo et al. 2007). In addition, nAChR stimulation may be able to limit inflammation in the brain under pathological conditions, by directly regulating the cells involved in inflammatory reactions such as brain-resident microglia and infiltrating monocytes/macrophages (Shytle et al. 2004; Wang et al. 2003). The principal nAChR subtypes expressed in the central nervous system are homopentamers consisting of α7 subunits and heteropentamers consisting of α4 and β2 subunits, although nAChRs containing other types of subunits such as α3, α6, β3 and β4 are also expressed in a brain region-specific manner (Taly et al. 2009; Zoli et al. 2015). Differences in subunit compositions between the peripheral nAChRs (either muscle type or neuronal type) and the central nAChRs may enable drug development specifically targeted for nAChRs in the brain, thereby avoiding adverse peripheral actions.

One of the major reasons for the central nAChRs being expected to serve as drug targets is that effective pharmacotherapies are not available at present for various kinds of central nervous system disorders associated with neurodegeneration. Among these disorders are cerebrovascular diseases resulting from the disruption of circulatory system that supplies blood flow to the brain. This chapter summarizes various preclinical and clinical findings related to the functions of nAChRs in regulating pathological events associated with cerebrovascular disorders, and discusses the potentials of nAChR-related drugs as novel therapeutics combating these disorders.

7.2 Overviews on Stroke Disorders

The term “stroke” represents diverse sets of disorders associated with disrupted cerebrovascular functions, which are classified into two major categories such as ischemic stroke and hemorrhagic stroke. Ischemic stroke is featured by interception of the blood flow in the brain tissues and, depending on the causes of interception, is further categorized into several different types including atherothrombotic brain infarction, cardiogenic embolism and lacunar stroke. In either case, the consequences of hypoperfusion are shortage of supplies of oxygen and glucose to the brain parenchymal cells. Because energy demands of neurons are met almost entirely by the aerobic metabolism of glucose, even short periods of ischemic episodes may result in severe and irreversible brain tissue damage accompanied by neuron loss. Rescuing neurons from cell death is extremely difficult in the ischemic core region where oxygen/glucose supply is almost totally abolished. In contrast, in the peri-infarct or “penumbra” region where oxygen/glucose supply is decreased but not abolished, neuronal cell death displays at least in part the features of programmed cell death that occurs with a certain delay from the onset of the insults. Therefore, neuroprotection in the penumbra after ischemic insults may be possible if appropriate treatment strategies are established (Catanese et al. 2017). Practically, however, only a few drugs effective in brain tissue preservation are available at present for the treatment of ischemic stroke (Table 7.1). A powerful approach is the reestablishment of blood flow by removal of the blood clot, and for this purpose, tissue plasminogen activator that promotes fibrinolysis is administered within 4.5 h after ischemic attack. Otherwise, edaravone is the sole choice of drugs in Japan intended for neuroprotection via its free radical-scavenging action.

The major types of hemorrhagic stroke are characterized by extravasation of blood into either brain parenchyma (intracerebral hemorrhage; ICH) or subarachnoid space (subarachnoid hemorrhage; SAH), and both cases are accompanied by poor prognosis. Hemorrhagic stroke has pathological features quite distinct from those of ischemic stroke. In ICH, tissue damage is caused primarily by the blood flowing out of ruptured vessels into the brain parenchyma. Biological actions of blood constituents (particularly, proteases involved in the coagulation cascade), in addition to the physical damage of blood mass (so called the “mass effect”) are the main contributors of pathogenic events in ICH (Qureshi et al. 2009). Currently, there are no established pharmacotherapies that are applicable after the occurrence of ICH events and are effective in neuroprotection (Katsuki 2010). Drugs such as glycerol and mannitol that manipulate plasma osmotic pressure and suppress brain edema formation may be available, but they still lack solid clinical evidence that justifies their application to ICH cases (Table 7.1). Clinical practice for SAH is in a similar situation to that for ICH, in the sense that direct neuroprotective pharmacotherapies are yet unavailable. Representative drugs used for the current treatment of SAH include fasudil, a Rho kinase inhibitor that prevents post-SAH vasospasm and ozagrel, an inhibitor of thromboxane A_2 synthase that prevents platelet aggregation.

Table 7.1 Current drug therapies applicable after cerebrovascular events

Actions	Drug name	Grade	Time window
For ischemic stroke			
Thrombolytic	Tissue plasminogen activator	A	Within 4.5 h
	Urokinase	B	Within 6 h
Anticoagulant	Argatroban	B	Within 48 h
	Heparin	C1	Within 48 h
Anti-platelet	Aspirin	A	Within 48 h
	Ozagrel	B	Within 5 days
Radical scavenger	Edaravone	B	Within 24 h
Edema regulator	Glycerol or mannitol	C1	
For ICH			
Anti-hypertensive	Calcium blockers and others	B or C1	
Edema regulator	Glycerol or mannitol	C1	
Anti-fibrinolysis	Tranexamic acid	C1	
Capillary stabilizer	Carbazochrome	C1	
For SAH			
Anti-vasospasm	Fasudil	A	
Anti-platelet	Ozagrel	A	
Edema regulator	Glycerol or mannitol	C1	
Anti-hypertensive	Calcium blockers and others	C1	

According to the Japanese Guidelines for the Management of Stroke 2015 by the Japan Stroke Society. Grade A, strongly recommended; Grade B, recommended; Grade C1, may be considered for application but scientific evidence is insufficient

Overall, although cerebrovascular disorders such as ischemic stroke, ICH and SAH are among the major issues of clinical concerns in the modern world, effective drug treatment strategies are, for the most part, far from established. With these situations under consideration, the following sections summarize the findings obtained from various kinds of efforts addressing the possibility of nAChRs as drug targets for the therapies of these disorders.

7.3 Ischemic Stroke and nAChRs

7.3.1 Roles of Endogenous Cholinergic System in Regulation of Ischemic Injury

7.3.1.1 Effects of nAChR Antagonists and Allosteric Modulators

Potential involvement of endogenous ACh in regulation of the pathogenic events in ischemic brain injury has been suggested by a study addressing the effects of nAChR antagonists in neonatal rats. In 7-day-old rats that underwent permanent occlusion of left common carotid artery, subcutaneous administration of subtype non-selective nAChR antagonist mecamylamine or specific α7 nAChR antagonist methyllycaconitine just before induction of 1-h hypoxia aggravated neural damage in the hippocampus. Mecamylamine also aggravated neural damage in the cerebral cortex (Furukawa et al. 2013). On the other hand, daily treatment with mecamylamine from 24 h after induction of 45-min transient global ischemia did not clearly affect the degree of cell death-related events such as the number of dead CA1 neurons and caspase-3 activity in the hippocampus in young adult mice (Ray et al. 2014).

PNU-120596 is a positive allosteric modulator of α7 nAChRs. The drug does not activate nAChRs by itself but inhibits desensitization and enhances activation of α7 nAChRs by orthosteric agonists. In addition, the ACh degradation product choline may produce agonistic activity at nAChRs in the presence of positive allosteric modulators. Indeed, Kalappa et al. (2013) demonstrated that choline delayed oxygen/glucose deprivation-induced injury of hippocampal CA1 neurons in vitro in the presence of PNU-120596, and PNU-120596 alone was not effective in the absence of choline in these experimental settings. The combined neuroprotective effect of choline and PNU-120596 was abolished by α7 nAChR antagonist methyllycaconitine. The neuroprotective potential of PNU-120596 was also confirmed in 90-min transient focal ischemia in rats, where 3-h pretreatment or 30-min posttreatment with the drug significantly reduced the infarct volume (Kalappa et al. 2013). A companion study by the same group reported that the effective time window of PNU-120596 administered intravenously was extended to 6 h after induction of middle cerebral artery occlusion (MCAO; Sun et al. 2013). These results strongly suggest that cholinergic neurotransmission functions as an endogenous neuroprotective system against ischemic brain injury.

7.3.1.2 Effects of Acetylcholinesterase Inhibitors

The concentration of ACh in the synaptic cleft is tightly regulated by acetylcholinesterase (AChE), as ACh released from the nerve terminals is promptly degraded by this hydrolyzing enzyme. Accordingly, application of AChE inhibitors is a conventional procedure to augment cholinergic neurotransmission. Several studies have addressed the effect of AChE inhibitors in rodent models of ischemic stroke. The earliest example is a study on donepezil, a centrally acting reversible inhibitor of AChE that is prescribed for amelioration of cognitive deficits in Alzheimer disease. An oral dose of donepezil (12 mg/kg) administered 2 h before or 1 h after induction of permanent MCAO in rats significantly reduced the infarct volume. The protective effect of donepezil was abolished by mecamylamine, suggesting the involvement of nAChR activation (Fujiki et al. 2005).

Another AChE inhibitor galantamine has also been reported to exhibit neuroprotective effects where the first administration was performed 24 h before or 3 h after induction of transient global ischemia in Mongolian gerbils by occlusion of the common carotid artery. The effects included an increase in surviving neurons, a decrease in terminal deoxynucleotidyl transferase-mediated dUTP nick end labeling

(TUNEL)-positive cells/caspase-3-positive cells in hippocampal CA1 region and amelioration of spatial memory deficit, and these effects were attenuated by concurrent treatment with mecamylamine (Lorrio et al. 2007). A later examination using rat hippocampal slices subject to oxygen/glucose deprivation followed by reoxygenation revealed that a tyrosine kinase Janus kinase (Jak) 2 mediated the protective effect of galantamine by suppressing activation of nuclear factor (NF) -κB and induction of inducible nitric oxide synthase (iNOS) expression (Egea et al. 2012). Under similar experimental conditions in mouse hippocampal slices, 30-min pretreatment with nicotine (10–100 μM) reduced the extent of oxygen/glucose deprivation-induced cell injury via activation of α7 nAChRs (Egea et al. 2007).

Wang et al. (2008) reported the effect of huperzine A, yet another AChE inhibitor, in a rat model of transient focal cerebral ischemia. When administered at the onset or 6 h after transient MCAO, huperzine A restored regional cerebral blood flow, reduced infarct size and decreased neurological deficit score. Similar to the cases with galantamine, huperzine A inhibited NF-κB activation and decreased expression of proinflammatory factors such as tumor necrosis factor (TNF) -α, interleukin (IL) -1β, iNOS and cyclooxygenase (COX) -2. In addition, mecamylamine abolished the inhibitory effect of huperzine A on glial cell activation and partially reversed the reduction of infarct size by huperzine A.

Overall, these results obtained from the examinations on three different kinds of AChE inhibitors are consistent with the idea that endogenous ACh affords neuroprotective effects against ischemia and ischemia-reperfusion injury, by activating nAChRs (Fig. 7.1).

7.3.1.3 Effect of Cholinergic Neuronal Activity

Vagus nerve stimulation is known to produce several therapeutic effects, and in the case of ischemia/reperfusion injury in rats, a brief episode of vagus nerve stimulation ameliorates neurological deficits and reduces infarct volume (Sun et al. 2012). Jiang et al. (2014) addressed the mechanisms of the neuroprotective effects of vagus nerve stimulation. They confirmed that vagus nerve stimulation given at 30 min after transient focal ischemia was able to ameliorate neurological deficit and reduced the infarct volume at 24 h after reperfusion. They additionally found that the increase in the levels of several cytokines such as TNF-α, IL-1β and IL-6 in the peri-infarct region was significantly prevented by vagus nerve stimulation. Notably, vagus nerve stimulation prevented ischemia/reperfusion-induced loss of α7 nAChR expression in microglia in the penumbra region, and also reversed ischemia-induced decrease in the level of phosphorylated Akt. Although the evidence is at most indirect, these results imply the involvement of cholinergic neurotransmission pathway in the neuroprotective effect of vagus nerve stimulation.

As for microglial nAChRs, another line of findings in a positron emission tomography imaging study implicates α4β2 nAChRs in the pathology of cerebral ischemia.

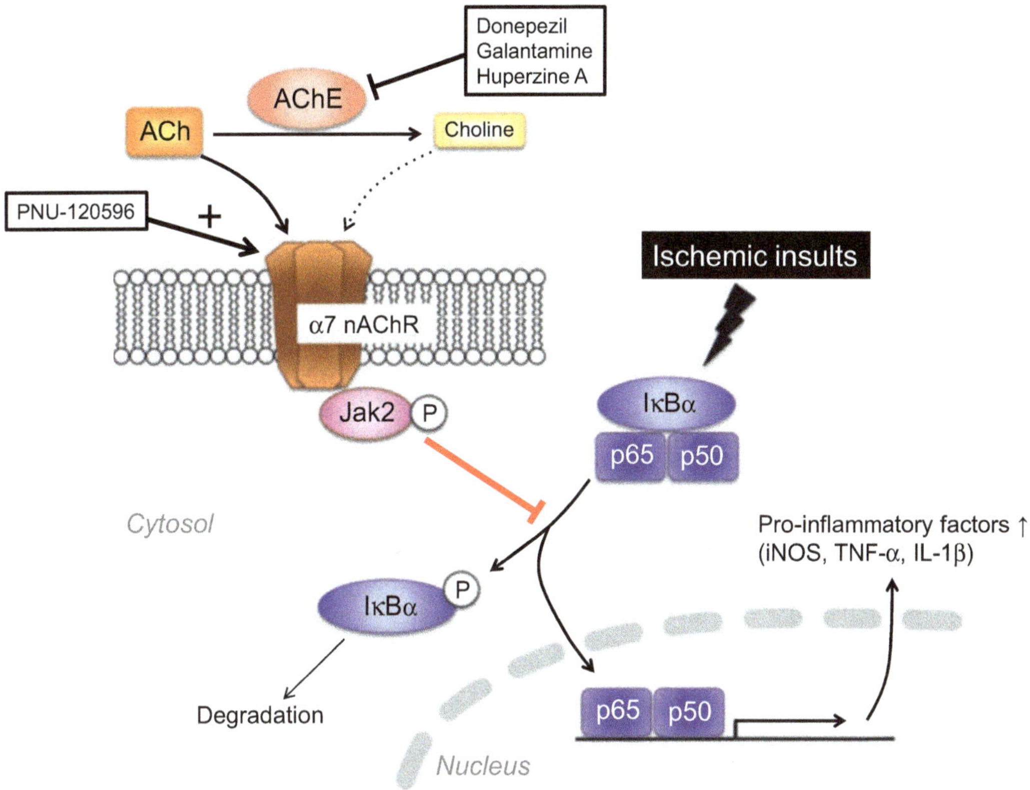

Fig. 7.1 Enhancement of endogenous cholinergic signaling suppresses ischemia-induced pathological events. Stimulation of nicotinic acetylcholine receptor (nAChR) by endogenous acetylcholine (ACh) can be enhanced either by inhibitors of acetylcholinesterase (AChE) such as donepezil that promote accumulation of extracellular ACh, or by positive allosteric modulators (PAMs) of nAChRs such as PNU-120596 that increase the affinity and/or efficacy of ACh on nAChRs. PAMs may also allow choline to exert agonistic activity on nAChRs. Stimulation of nAChRs, particularly of α7 subtype, by these drugs leads to phosphorylation/activation of a tyrosine kinase Janus kinase 2 (Jak2). Although detailed mechanisms are yet to be identified, activated Jak2 may inhibit phosphorylation of inhibitor of κB (IκB) α, prevent ischemia-induced recruitment of nuclear factor κB (NF-κB; illustrated as subunits p65 and p50), and consequently, suppress NF-κB-dependent expression of pro-inflammatory factors (See Sects. 7.3.1.1 and 7.3.1.2 for details)

That is, α4β2 nAChR binding probed by 2[^{18}F]-fluoro-A85380 and [^{11}C]PK11195 in rat brains showed a transient increase that peaked at 7 days after MCAO (Martin et al. 2015). Increased expression of α4β2 nAChRs in microglia/macrophages and astrocytes was confirmed by immunohistochemical examinations. Although the functional significance of these changes in the expression of α4β2 nAChRs is unclear, this nAChR subtype in addition to α7 nAChRs may serve as a target for regulation of pathogenic events, particularly those involving inflammatory reactions, in ischemic brain injury.

Table 7.2 Studies reporting beneficial effects of nicotine and nAChR agonists in experimental models of ischemia

Conditions of drug treatment	References
Nicotine (30–100 μg/kg, i.v.) 5 min before transient ischemia in rats	Kagitani et al. (2000)
Nicotine (0.3–1.5 mg/kg, i.p.) 30 min before transient ischemia in Monglian gerbils	Nanri et al. (1998b)
Nicotine hydrogen tartrate (1.2 mg/kg, i.p.) 2 h before transient ischemia in rats	Chen et al. (2013)
Nicotine (0.5 mg/kg, i.p.) 2, 6 or 12 h after transient ischemia followed by three times administration per day for 7 days	Guan et al. (2015)
Nicotine hydrogen tartrate (0.3 mg/kg, s.c.) twice daily for 12 days, from 2 days after focal devasularization	Gonzalez et al. (2006)
GTS-21 (1–5 mg/kg, i.p.) 30 min before, or GTS-21 (10 mg/kg, p.o.) twice daily for 2 weeks before, transient ischemia in Mongolian gerbils	Nanri et al. (1998b)
GTS-21 (1–10 mg/kg, p.o.) 24 h and 30 min before permanent ischemia in Mongolian gerbils	Nanri et al. (1998a)
PNU-282987 (10 mg/kg, i.p.) 60 min after thrombotic stroke in mice	Parada et al. (2013)
PHA-568487 (doses are not described, i.p.) immediately and 24 h after permanent ischemia in mice	Han et al. (2014b)
PHA-568487 (0.8 mg/kg, i.p.) 1 and 2 days after permanent ischemia in mice	Han et al. (2014a)

See Sect. (7.3.2.1) in the main text for details of the findings in each study
i.p. intraperitoneal, *i.v.* intravenous, *p.o.* per oral, *s.c.* subcutaneous

7.3.2 *Effects of nAChR Agonists on Ischemic Injury*

7.3.2.1 Positive Findings

As discussed in the previous section (Sect. 7.3.1), stimulation of nAChRs appears to provide neuroprotective effects against ischemia-reperfusion injury. Indeed, many lines of evidence indicate that nicotine and other compounds with direct agonistic activity on nAChRs can provide beneficial effects on experimental model of ischemic stroke (Table 7.2). Kagitani et al. (2000) reported the effect of intravenous injection of nicotine in an intermittent transient ischemia model in rats. When rats with permanent ligation of bilateral vertebral arteries received transient and intermittent occlusion (two to three times for 2 min at 2-min intervals) of bilateral carotid arteries, the blood flow in the hippocampus was substantially and reversibly decreased, and delayed death of hippocampal CA1 neurons was induced. Administration of nicotine (30–100 μg/kg) at 5 min before occlusion slightly but significantly improved hippocampal blood flow during occlusion and increased the number of surviving CA1 neurons. Kagitani et al. (2000) assume that the neuroprotecive effect of nicotine under these conditions is attributable to the vasodilative response induced by nAChR stimulation and resultant increase in regional blood flow in the hippocampus. On the other hand, the presence of nicotine during ischemic episodes may produce direct protective effects on neuronal cells. For example, in rat primary cortical cultures, 4-h hypoxia induced neuronal cell death with features of apoptosis. Application of nicotine (10–100 μM) during hypoxia prevented cell death probably via activation of both α7 nAChRs and α4β2 nAChRs, as methyllycaconitine (α7 nAChR antagonist) and dihydro-β-erythroidine (α4β2 nAChR antagonist) blocked the effect of nicotine (Hejmadi et al. 2003).

GTS-21 is a synthetic nAChR agonist with fourfold higher affinity than nicotine for α7 nAChRs. The effect of GTS-21 and nicotine was tested on an ischemia-reperfusion model of Mongolian gerbils. When the drugs were injected intraperitoneally at 30 min before 3-min forebrain ischemia, both GTS-21 (1–5 mg/kg) and nicotine (0.3–1.5 mg/kg) improved performance of animals in passive avoidance and attenuated cell death in the hippocampal CA1 region. GTS-21 (10 mg/kg) was effective also when orally administered twice daily for 2 weeks prior to ischemia (Nanri et al. 1998b). Moreover, the same group examined the effect of GTS-21 in rats with permanent occlusion of bilateral common carotid arteries (Nanri et al. 1998a). In this study, GTS-21 (1 or 10 mg/kg) was administered orally 24 h and 30 min before induction of ischemia and then once daily for 2 months. GTS-21 significantly prevented ischemia-induced histopathological changes in the cerebral cortex and in the white matter, and improved the cognitive function of rats as assessed by radial maze learning performance.

Potential involvement of endocannabinoid system in the neuroprotective effect of nicotine has been proposed by a study by Chen et al. (2013). Intraperitoneal administration of nicotine hydrogen tartrate (1.2 mg/kg) transiently increased the tissue content of endocannabinoids 2-arachidonoylglycerol and anandamide in rats, which peaked at 2 h after administration. Nicotine also increased the protein expression level of cannabinoid CB_1 receptor. Moreover, 2-h pretreatment with nicotine reduced the infarct volume and neurological deficit induced by 120-min MCAO, and these effects were significantly reversed by AM251, a CB_1 receptor antagonist.

All of these findings mentioned above were obtained by pretreatment of nicotine or nAChR agonist. However, the pretreatment regimens of drugs are not very useful for combating stroke disorders, because in almost all clinical situations the drug therapy is available only after certain delay from the onset of acute stroke episodes. With these concerns, several studies have examined the effect of therapeutic treatment with nAChR agonists on ischemic injury and indeed reported positive results. In a study by Guan et al. (2015), transient forebrain ischemia was induced in rats by four-vessel occlusion. Nicotine (0.5 mg/kg) was administered intraperitoneally at 2, 6 or 12 h after induction of 15-min ischemia, and thereafter, three times per day for 7 days. Under these conditions, nicotine significantly increased the number of surviving CA1 neurons in the hippocampus. At the same time, nicotine was found to decrease the number of microglia and to prevent ischemia-induced up-regulation of mRNAs encoding TNF-α and IL-1β in the hippocampal CA1 region. In addition, nicotine inhibited proliferation of primary cultured microglia, and this effect was blocked by α7 nAChR antagonist α-bungarotoxin. These results suggest that attenuation of proliferation and activation of microglia contribute to the neuroprotective effect of the therapeutic treatment with nicotine.

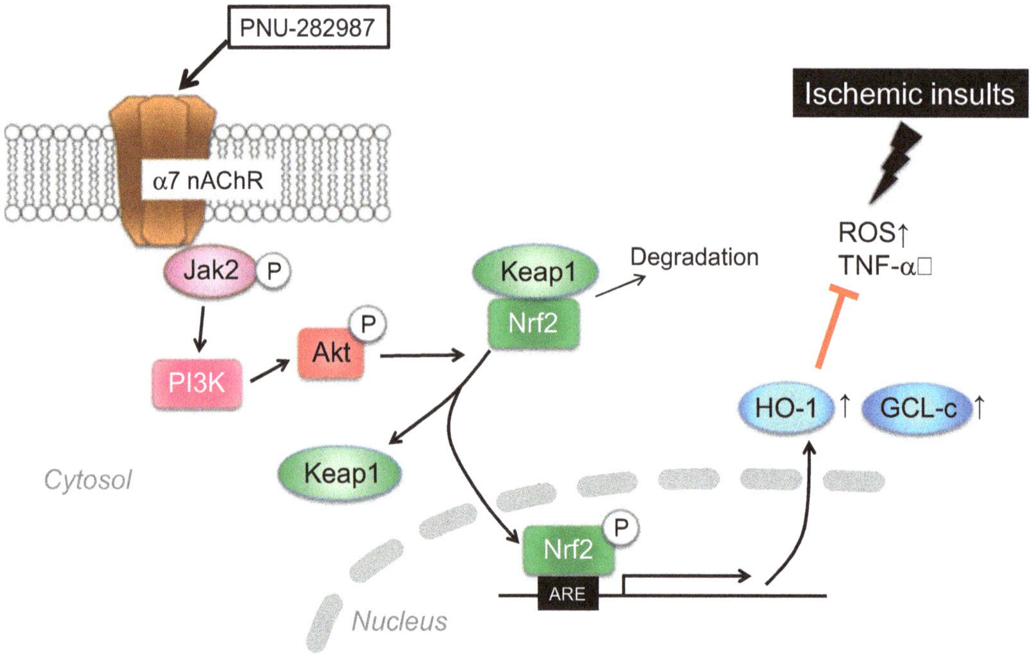

Fig. 7.2 Specific α7 nAChR agonist may afford anti-inflammatory effects via expression of heme oxygenase-1 (HO-1) in the brains after ischemic insults. According to Parada et al. (2010, 2013), application of α7 nAChR agonist such as PNU-282987 activates Jak2 in microglia/macrophages, which leads to activation of PI3-kinase (PI3K)/Akt pathway. By the action of Akt, a transcription factor Nrf2 is liberated from Keap1, escapes from degradation and binds to antioxidant response element (ARE) of the promoter regions of genes encoding phase II detoxifying enzymes such as HO-1 and the catalytic subunit of glutamate cysteine ligase (GCL-c). HO-1 induced by these signaling pathways plays a critical role in inhibiting ischemia-associated pro-inflammatory responses such as the production of reactive oxygen species (ROS) and tumor necrosis factor-α (TNF-α)

Involvement of regulation of microglia in the therapeutic effect of α7 nAChR agonist has also been demonstrated in a photothrombotic ischemia model in mice (Parada et al. 2013). That is, intraperitoneal administration of PNU-282987 (10 mg/kg) at 60 min after induction of thrombotic stroke using Rose Bengal decreased the volume of cortical infarct and diminished neurological deficits. Notably, the protective effect of PNU-282987 was abolished by concomitant treatment with heme oxygenase (HO) inhibitor or by deletion of HO-1 gene. In hippocampal slice culture preparation, PNU-282987 induced HO-1 expression, prevented cell death and attenuated production of reactive oxygen species and TNF-α resulting from oxygen/glucose deprivation and reoxygenation. The protective effect of PNU-282987 in slice cultures was abolished by application of HO inhibitor or by depletion of microglia from the slices. These results propose HO-1 as a key mediator of the neuroprotective and anti-inflammatory effect of microglial α7 nAChR stimulation (Fig. 7.2).

Using another α7 nAChR agonist PHA-568487, Han et al. (2014b) examined the role of microglia/macrophage phenotypes. Mice were treated with PHA-568487 immediately and 24 h after permanent MCAO. The treatment significantly reduced the infarct volume and partially ameliorated behavioral performance. The peri-infarct region of PHA-568487-treated mice contained a smaller number of pro-inflammatory microglia/macrophages (so called "M1" phenotype identified as $CD11b^{+}Iba\text{-}1^{+}$) and a larger number of anti-inflammatory microglia/macrophages (so called "M2" phenotype identified as $CD206^{+}Iba\text{-}1^{+}$), than that of saline-treated mice (Han et al. 2014b). Similar protective effect on neuron survival and regulatory effect on microglia/macrophage phenotypes were obtained when administration of PHA-568487 (0.8 mg/kg) was initiated at 1 day after permanent MCAO (Han et al. 2014a). These results suggest that the regulation of microglia/macrophage phenotypes underlies the neuroprotective effect of α7 nAChR agonist against ischemic injury.

The effect of repeated administration (twice daily for 12 days) of low dose nicotine (0.3 mg/kg as nicotine hydrogen tartrate) has been reported in a rat focal ischemia model prepared by unilateral devascularization in the motor cortex. The findings are notable in the sense that post-treatment started as late as 48 h after ischemic surgery was proven to be effective in promoting the recovery of motor performance. Interestingly, nicotine treatment increased the morphological complexity of dendritic processes of layer V pyramidal neurons of the cingulate cortex, both in control rats and ischemia-induced rats (Gonzalez et al. 2006). Therefore, nicotine-induced enhancement of dendritic growth of cortical neurons might facilitate the recovery of motor functions.

7.3.2.2 Negative Findings

Under several experimental conditions, nicotine has been reported to produce no effect or even worsen the outcome of ischemic events. For example, Lim et al. (2009) examined the effect of nicotine on rehabilitation following devascularization in the forelimb area of the motor cortex in rats. Oral administration of nicotine (0.3 mg/kg, twice daily for 3 weeks starting from 1 week before stroke induction) did not improve motor function recovery.

It should be noted that virtually all studies reporting the deleterious effect of nicotine on ischemic brain injury were aimed to reveal potential adverse effects of smoking on cerebrovascular disorders, and therefore that these studies generally employ long-term and/or continuous pretreatment regimen for nicotine administration (Table 7.3). An early study by Wang et al. (1997) examined the effect of nicotine (4.5 mg/kg/day) administered subcutaneously for 14 days by osmotic minipumps, prior to induction of ischemic insults in rats. Nicotine decreased the blood flow in the penumbra region during reperfusion after transient MCAO, worsened neurological deficit, and increased the injury and edema volume. Interestingly, nicotine-treated rats exhibited depletion of tissue plasminogen activator in cerebral capillaries, which might be causally relevant to the poor recovery of the blood flow after reperfusion and to the resultant exacerbation of brain tissue injury. In a more recent study, the effect of 4-week continuous treatment with nicotine (2 or 4 mg/kg/day, subcutaneously by osmotic pumps) prior to 2-h transient MCAO was examined (Li et al. 2016). Nicotine at both doses significantly increased the infarct size,

Table 7.3 Studies reporting deleterious effects of nicotine in experimental models of ischemia

Conditions of drug treatment	References
Nicotine (4.5 mg/kg/day, s.c.) continuous infusion for 14 days prior to transient ischemia in rats	Wang et al. (1997)
Nicotine (2 and 4 mg/kg/day, s.c.) continuous infusion for 4 weeks prior to transient ischemia in rats	Li et al. (2016)
Nicotine (2 mg/kg/day, s.c.) continuous infusion for 14 days prior to transient ischemia in mice	Bradford et al. (2011)
Nicotine (187.5, 562.5 or 1125 μg/kg, i.p.) 1, 3 or 6 h, respectively, before permanent ischemia in mice	Paulson et al. (2010)
Nicotine (4.5 mg/kg/day, s.c.) continuous infusion for 1 or 3 weeks prior to permanent ischemia in mice	Paulson et al. (2010)
Nicotine (1 mg/kg, i.p.) daily injection for 15 days prior to transient ischemia in female rats	Raval et al. (2009)
Nicotine (4.5 mg/kg/day, s.c.) continuous infusion for 16 days prior to transient ischemia in female rats	Raval et al. (2011)
Nicotine (4 μg/kg/min, s.c. To dams) continuous infusion from day 4 of gestation to day 10 after birth in rats	Li et al. (2012)

See Sect. 7.3.2.2 in the main text for details of the findings in each study
i.p. intraperitoneal, *s.c.* subcutaneous

although the neurological deficit seems to be ameliorated by the treatments. Authors attributed the exacerbation of pathological changes by nicotine to enhanced oxidative stress, as the cerebral cortex and the cerebral arteries in nicotine-treated rats exhibited decreased expression levels of Mn superoxide dismutase and mitochondrial uncoupling protein-2, as compared to those in control rats.

Bradford et al. (2011) examined the effect of chronic nicotine treatment with special reference to inflammatory responses. In their study, 14-day pretreatment with nicotine (0.5–2 mg/kg/day, subcutaneously by osmotic pumps) dose-dependently increased the infarct volume and brain water content at 3 days after 30-min MCAO. In addition, nicotine given at 2 mg/kg/day worsened neurological outcome and decreased the survival rate of mice. They also demonstrated that 14-day treatment with nicotine (2 mg/kg/day), either alone or in combination with ischemia/reperfusion insults, markedly increased the expression of various cytokines (including TNF-α and IL-1β) and chemokines (including CCL2 and CXCL5) in brain tissue and isolated brain microvessels. Consistent with these observations, ischemia/reperfusion-induced infiltration of neutrophils and monocytes was augmented by 14-day pretreatment with nicotine.

In a study on permanent MCAO in mice, subcutaneous delivery of 4.5 mg/kg/day for 3 weeks has been shown to exacerbate brain edema (Paulson et al. 2010). Exacerbation of brain edema was also observed when nicotine was intraperitoneally administered 1 h before MCAO. Although the precise mechanisms of action of nicotine in these experimental settings have not been addressed, the effect might be relevant to nicotine-induced altered functions of Na^+, K^+, $2Cl^-$ cotransporters in the blood-brain barrier (Paulson et al. 2006).

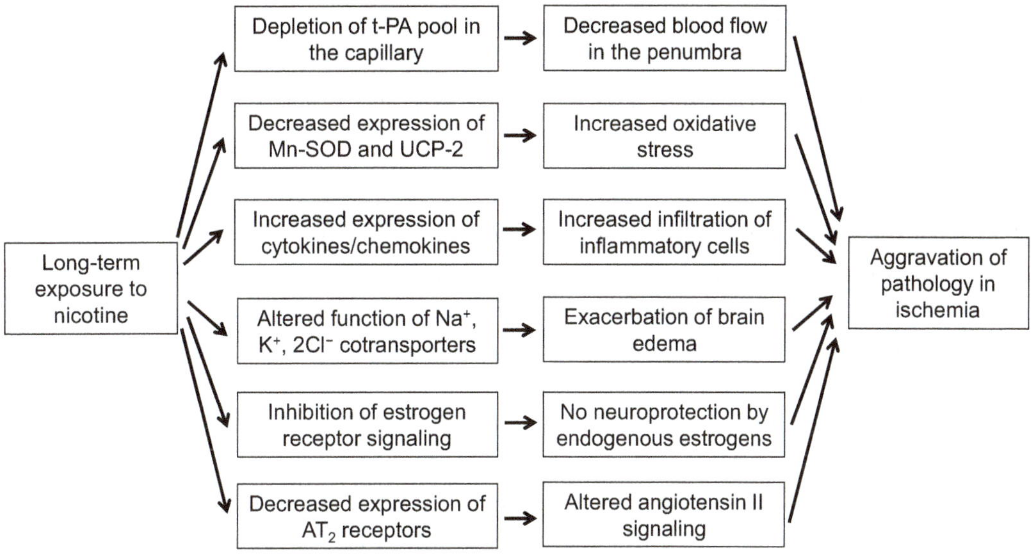

Fig. 7.3 Nicotine may produce harmful influences on ischemia-related pathological events. Long-term pretreatment with nicotine by continuous infusion is generally shown to aggravate the pathology of ischemic stroke in experimental animals. Multiple mechanisms are postulated to play important roles in these harmful consequences as summarized here (See Sect. 7.3.2.2 for details. *SOD* superoxide dismutase, *t-PA* tissue plasminogen activator, *UCP-2* uncoupling protein-2)

Potential interaction of the effect of nicotine with that of estrogen has been proposed by studies using ovariectomized rats. Daily intraperitoneal injection of 1 mg/kg nicotine for 15 days to female rats with normal menstrual cycle accelerated neuron loss in the hippocampal CA1 region at 7 days after 10-min ligation of carotid artery. In addition, ovariectomy *per se* exacerbated ischemia-induced loss of CA1 neurons and occluded the effect of repeated nicotine treatment (Ravel et al. 2009). These results suggest that the neuroprotective effect of endogenous estrogen is cancelled by nicotine. Indeed, oral contraceptives that lowered the plasma level of 17β-estradiol exacerbated ischemia-induced loss of hippocampal CA1 neurons, synergistically with 16-day treatment of nicotine. Abolishment by nicotine of the neuroprotective effect of 17β-estradiol on oxygen/glucose deprivation-induced injury, as well as attenuation by nicotine of estrogen receptor-mediated recruitment of cyclic AMP response element binding protein, was also demonstrated in rat hippocampal slice cultures (Ravel et al. 2011).

Finally, neonatal male rats continuously exposed to nicotine during the perinatal period (from day 4 of gestation to day 10 after birth) exhibited larger infarct size after hypoxic-ischemic injury than control rats. The augmented pathology may be attributable to altered angiotensin II signaling resulting from decreased expression of angiotensin II AT_2 receptors (Li et al. 2012).

Taken together, long-term continuous exposure to nicotine may aggravate the consequences of ischemic stroke, by altering expression and function of various cytoprotective proteins, pro-inflammatory factors, transporters and receptors in the brain (Fig. 7.3).

7.4 Hemorrhagic Stroke and nAChRs

7.4.1 *Effects of nAChR Agonists on Intracerebral Hemorrhage (ICH)*

ICH is initiated by the rupture of blood vessels within the brain parenchyma and bleeding from ruptured vessels. The mechanisms involved in brain tissue injury after ICH include several distinct features from those involved in ischemic brain injury. A notable feature of ICH is that blood constituents may exert specific biological actions on neurons and glial cells in the brain and make substantial contribution to the complicated pathogenic events. Thrombin, a serine protease that normally functions in the coagulation cascade, is a remarkable example because it can stimulate several members of protease-activated receptors (PARs) that are expressed in various cell types including neurons, astrocytes and microglia. Indeed, several lines of evidence indicate that thrombin may contribute to the pathogenesis of experimental ICH models. For example, a thrombin inhibitor argatroban reduces edema and inflammation associated with ICH in rats (Kitaoka et al. 2002; Nagatsuna et al. 2005).

To facilitate investigations on the pathogenic mechanisms of ICH and exploration of therapeutic drug candidates, we developed an in vitro neurodegeneration model of ICH, using organotypic brain slice cultures (Fujimoto et al. 2006). Coronal slices containing the cerebral cortex and the striatum were prepared from neonatal rats, and after cultivation for 9–11 days, they were treated with thrombin. Thrombin induced delayed neuronal cell death in the cerebral cortex and tissue shrinkage accompanied by cell death in the striatum. Results of various pharmacological interventions revealed the mechanisms involved in cell and tissue injuries in the cerebral cortex and the striatum. With regard to the tissue injury in the striatum, stimulation of PAR-1 and recruitment of mitogen-activated kinase (MAPK) families plays a critical role. In addition, thrombin-induced striatal tissue injury was abrogated by deletion of tissue microglia prior to thrombin treatment. Importantly, potential involvement of microglial MAPK activation in tissue injury was confirmed in a rat model of ICH induced in the striatum by collagenase injection (Ohnishi et al. 2007), which substantiates the validity of slice culture experiments as a model of ICH pathogenesis.

Then we examined the effect of nicotine on thrombin neurotoxicity in cortico-striatal slice cultures (Ohnishi et al. 2009). In this set of experiments, cortico-striatal slices were prepared and cultured for 11 days in serum-containing medium, maintained for 1 day in serum-free medium, and then treated with 100 U/ml thrombin in serum-free medium for 3 days. When applied to slice cultures for the entire culture period of 15 days, nicotine (3–30 μM) attenuated thrombin-induced shrinkage of striatal tissue and prevented thrombin-induced neuron loss in the cerebral cortex. Thrombin-induced increase in the number of microglia in the cortex was also attenuated by nicotine in a concentration-dependent manner. The cytoprotective effect and anti-inflammatory effect of nicotine were largely abrogated by mecamylamine (non-selective nAChR antagonist), methyllycaconitine (α7 nAChR antagonist) and dihydro-β-erythroidine (α4β2 nAChR antagonist), suggesting the involvement of both of the major central nAChR subtypes.

With these lines of evidence in vitro, we moved onto investigations in vivo to address the effect of nicotine in a mouse model of ICH prepared by injection of collagenase (that disrupts vascular basement membrane) into the striatum. Based on the findings in slice culture preparations, we initially examined the effect of long-term pretreatment of nicotine (1 mg/kg, intraperitoneally once per day for 1 week) and obtained cytoprotective effect of nicotine on striatal neurons within the hematoma assessed at 3 days after induction of ICH (our unpublished observations). However, the long-term pretreatment regimen is unrealistic for ICH pharmacotherapy in clinical practice, so we next examined the effect of nicotine in a post-treatment regimen. ICH was induced by collagenase injection into the striatum, and nicotine tartrate dehydrate (1 and 2 mg/kg as nicotine free base) was first administered intraperitoneally 3 h after ICH induction. Nicotine treatment was repeated three times in total, at 24 h intervals. Under these conditions, nicotine (2 mg/kg) partially but significantly attenuated the decrease in the number of striatal neurons in the central region of hematoma at 3 days after ICH. ICH-induced increase in TUNEL-positive cells that may represent apoptotic cell death was also inhibited by nicotine treatment. Interestingly, nicotine decreased expression of a pro-apoptotic protein Bax in the striatum and consequently increased the relative expression level of Bcl-2, an anti-apoptotic protein. Therefore, counteraction of the apoptotic cell death events may underlie the neuroprotective effect of nicotine in ICH (Fig. 7.4). In the peri-hematoma region, the pathological features were accumulation of activated microglia/macrophages and increase in oxidative stress (as revealed by nitrotyrosine immunoreactivity), both of which were significantly attenuated by nicotine treatment. Moreover, nicotine at 2 mg/kg alleviated neurological deficits observed after ICH (Hijioka et al. 2011). When the effect of α7 nAChR agonist PNU-282987 (3 and 10 mg/kg) was tested in the same treatment regimen as nicotine, the drug showed neuroprotective and anti-inflammatory effects, whereas α4β2 nAChR agonist RJR-2403 showed no significant therapeutic effect (Hijioka et al. 2012). These results suggest that α7 nAChR is the major nAChR subtype responsible for the therapeutic effect of nicotine in ICH.

Consistent with our findings, Krafft et al. (2012) reported the therapeutic effect of PNU-282987 (12 mg/kg) and another α7 nAChR agonist PHA-543613 (4 or 12 mg/kg) in a mouse model of ICH based on autologous blood infusion into the striatum. In their study, agonists were administered intraperitoneally at 1 h after ICH surgery. These drug treatments improved behavioral outcome and prevented brain edema formation at 24 h after surgery. The effect of PHA-543613 was counteracted by a phosphoinositide 3-kinase (PI3K) inhibitor wortmannin. In addition, PHA-543613 increased the level of phosphorylated Akt and prevented ICH-induced activation of glycogen synthase kinase (GSK) -3β and caspase-3, which was also cancelled by wortmannin. These results indicate that the therapeutic effect of α7 nAChR stimulation is mediated by PI3K/Akt pathway leading to inactivation of

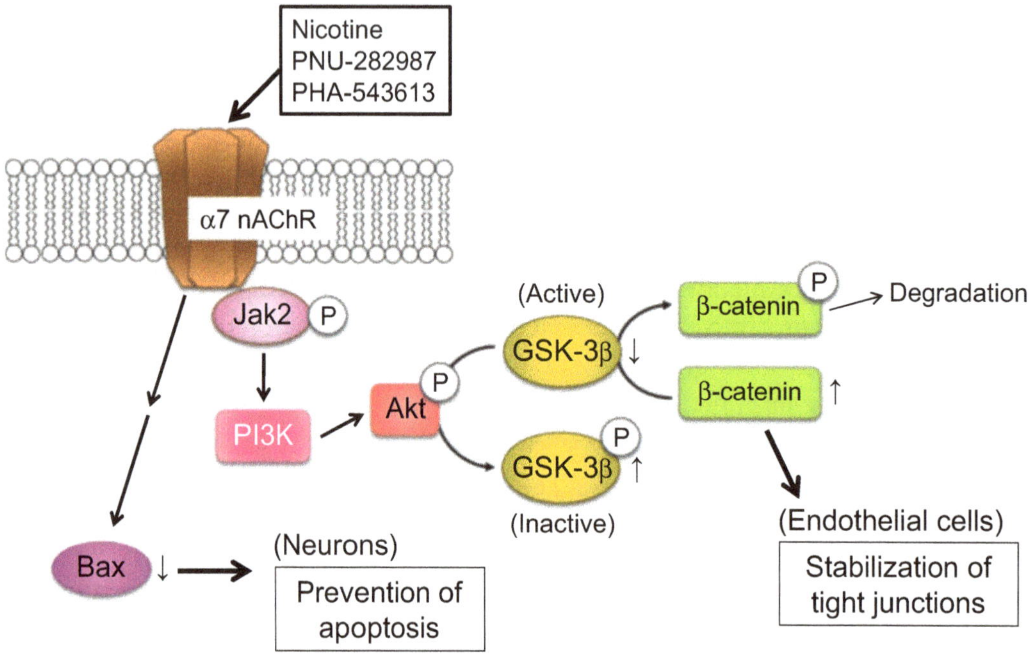

Fig. 7.4 nAChRs expressed in distinct types of cells may contribute to the therapeutic effects of nAChR agonists against brain tissue damage associated with intracerebral hemorrhage (ICH). Stimulation of nAChRs (probably α7 nAChRs) by nicotine in neurons results in decreased expression of a pro-apoptotic protein Bax, thereby inhibits ICH-induced apoptotic neuronal cell death (Hijioka et al. 2011, 2012). On the other hand, specific α7 nAChR agonists such as PNU-282987 and PHA-543613 may stimulate α7 nAChRs in endothelial cells, and recruit Jak2/PI3K/Akt pathway as in the case with Fig. 7.2. Activated Akt phosphorylates and inactivates glycogen synthase kinase-β (GSK-3β) and thereby prevents phosphorylation and degradation of β-catenin, a component of tight junctions. Stabilization of tight junctions may be relevant to the maintenance of integrity of the blood-brain barrier after hemorrhagic insults (Krafft et al. 2013)

GSK-3β and prevention of apoptotic cell death events. A follow-up study by the same group (Krafft et al. 2013) showed that PHA-543613-induced inactivation of GSK-3β led to stabilization of β-catenin and tight junction proteins such as claudin-3 and claudin-5, which may be relevant to the preservation of blood-brain barrier integrity and to the inhibition of edema formation by the drug (Fig. 7.4). A more recent study addressed the role of Jak – signal transducer and activator of transcription (STAT) signaling pathway in the effect of α7 nAChR stimulation (Krafft et al. 2017). That is, α7 nAChR agonist PHA-543613 augmented phosphorylation/activation of Jak2 and STAT3 in a mouse model of ICH by autologous blood infusion, and Jak2 inhibitor AG490 reversed the brain tissue-preserving effect of PHA-543613 in a rat model of ICH based on collagenase injection.

The main focus of the brain region in preclinical ICH studies has been the striatum (the caudate putamen), because the putamen is one of the most susceptible brain regions with regard to hypertension-associated ICH in humans, and also because this region is relatively easy of access by surgical operations in experimental animals. On the other hand, the relative incidence of non-hypertension-associated ICH that occurs in the cerebral cortex (cortical or lobar hemorrhage) has been increasing in recent years, but therapeutic approaches for cortical hemorrhage have been poorly explored. We addressed whether nicotine can provide therapeutic effect in cortical hemorrhage in mice (Anan et al. 2017). Collagenase injection into the parietal cortex induced hemorrhage, which resulted in motor deficits in mice. Daily intraperitoneal administration of nicotine (1 and 2 mg/kg), with the first injection given at 3 h after ICH induction, significantly improved motor performance. Histochemical examinations on brain sections obtained 3 days after ICH demonstrated that nicotine (2 mg/kg) significantly increased the number of surviving neurons in the hematoma and decreased the number of activated microglia/macrophages in the peri-hematoma region. Notably, the neuroprotective effect of nicotine on cortical hemorrhage was blocked by antagonists at α7 nAChRs (methyllycaconitine) and α4β2 nAChRs (dihydro-β-erythroidine). Therefore, the neuroprotective effect of nicotine in cortical hemorrhage may be mediated by both of these two receptor subtypes, unlike in the case with putaminal hemorrhage where α7 nAChR plays a dominant role.

7.4.2 *Effects of nAChR Agonists on Subarachnoid Hemorrhage (SAH)*

SAH is one of the major kinds of hemorrhagic stroke distinct from ICH. SAH is characterized by extravasation into the subarachnoid space, which mainly results from the rupture of intracranial aneurysm. At present, there is only one experimental study addressing the effect of nAChR agonist on the outcome of SAH. Duris et al. (2011) examined the effect of α7 nAChR agonist PNU-282987 on an endovascular perforation model of SAH in rats, by administering the drug intraperitoneally at 1 h after perforation surgery. They showed that PNU-282987 at 12 mg/kg ameliorated neurological function at 24 and 72 h after SAH induction, and prevented the increase in brain water content at 24 h. As in the case with ICH (Krafft et al. 2012), α7 nAChR stimulation enhanced phosphorylation/activation of Akt and prevented SAH-induced activation of caspase-3, which was abrogated by PI3K inhibitor wortmannin. Therefore, α7 nAChRs may serve as a promising drug target also for SAH therapy, although detailed pharmacological profiles of neuroprotection should be revealed by further investigations.

7.5 Nicotine, Smoking and Stroke: Potential Associations

As nicotine is the major pharmacoactive compound contained in tobacco that can directly modify the functions of the nervous system and the cardiovascular system, potential relationship between smoking and cerebrovascular disorders suggested by various epidemiological investigations may deserve considerations. It should be noted, however, that tobacco smoke contains many (over 4000) kinds of chemicals and the adverse consequences of smoking are not necessarily and solely attributable to the biological actions of nicotine.

With regard to ICH, current smoking is among the modifiable risk factors (An et al. 2017; Ariesen et al. 2003), although smoking (both current use and history of use) may be more strongly associated with ischemic lacunar stroke than with ICH (Kaplan et al. 2014). Race/population-specific influences of smoking on ICH incidence have also been reported. A study by Faigle et al. (2016) showed that smoking was one of the predictors of mortality in white populations, but not black populations, of ICH patients. In addition, meta-analyses of the risk factors for ICH and ischemic stroke suggest that smoking is a risk factor more frequent in ischemic stroke in white population but not in Chinese population (Tsai et al. 2016). In any cases, whether or not nicotine is responsible for the increased risk of ICH associated with smoking is unknown.

Several reports addressed the association of smoking and nicotine exposure with the risk and the outcome of SAH. In a case-control study on population of 18–49 years of age, exposure to nicotine in pharmaceuticals as well as current smoking has been identified as a risk factor of SAH (Broderick et al. 2003). In addition, a retrospective analysis of the size of ruptured intracranial aneurysm of SAH patients demonstrated that the average maximal aneurysm diameter in patients with combined history of hypertension and smoking was significantly smaller than in patients with hypertension only. The latter results suggest that smoking lowers the threshold of aneurysm rupture in combination with hypertension. On the other hand, a systematic review on four independent studies concerning nicotine replacement therapy for tobacco smoking in SAH patients has concluded that the therapy in the first 21 days does not appear to be associated with increased risk of poor functional outcome, death and vasospasm (Turgeon et al. 2017). Actually, there are reports showing better functional outcome (Carandang et al. 2011) and lower risk of death (Seder et al. 2011) in patients with nicotine replacement therapy than those without the therapy. These results imply the beneficial effects of nicotine against SAH pathology in humans, although more detailed and well-designed studies with larger sample size are clearly required for drawing definitive conclusion.

Current smoking has long been known as a strong risk factor for the incidence of ischemic stroke (Hawkins et al. 2002). Increased number of cigarettes smoked per day has been associated with increased risk of ischemic stroke in a study on 15–49 year-old women (Bhat et al. 2008). With regard to the disease outcome, however, "smoker's paradox" has been reported in ischemic stroke as in the case with myocardial infarction (Ovbiagele and Saver, 2005). For example, a study on 4305 cases of ischemic stroke patients, smoking was associated with lower all-cause in-hospital mortality (Ali et al. 2013). In another study on ischemic stroke patients that received thrombolytic therapy by intravenous tissue plasminogen activator, smokers had better functional outcome in addition to better recanalization and reperfusion, as compared to non-smokers (Kufner et al. 2013). A recent investigation on the potential causes of smoker's paradox showed that smokers experienced their first ever stroke 11 years younger than non-smokers, which might explain in part the association between smoking and better functional outcome (Hussein et al. 2017). Notably, subgroup analysis in the same study detected favorable outcome of current smokers in women at or older than 65 years (Hussein et al. 2017).

Overall, although smoking may be considered as an important risk factor for the occurrence of stroke episodes, contribution of nicotine to the increased risk is unclear. On the other hand, several lines of evidence indicate that smoking or nicotine treatment (as the replacement therapy) might result in favorable outcome in several particular cases of stroke.

7.6 Conclusion and Future Perspectives

The functional roles of nAChRs in the central nervous system beyond neurotransmission have been increasingly recognized. Neuroprotective and anti-inflammatory effects of nicotine and other nAChR agonists are of particular interest for the development of novel pharmacotherapies against various kinds of disorders associated with neurodegeneration. This chapter summarized preclinical and clinical findings suggesting the relationship between nicotine/nAChRs and principal types of cerebrovascular disorders such as ischemic stroke, ICH and SAH.

Several lines of experimental approaches using in vitro culture system and in vivo disease models indicated the neuroprotective and ant-inflammatory roles of endogenous cholinergic system against pathogenic events in ischemic stroke. These include exacerbation of pathology by nAChR antagonists, as well as amelioration of pathology by AChE inhibitors and positive allosteric modulators of nAChRs. In contrast, studies addressing the effects of nAChR agonists on experimental ischemic injury models gave conflicting results, where some studies reported beneficial effects but others demonstrated deleterious effects. A possible cause of these discrepancies is the different procedures employed for drug administration. Namely, virtually all studies reporting the deleterious effects of nicotine performed continuous delivery by osmotic pumps or repeated daily administration of nicotine at relatively high doses. On the other hand, studies reporting beneficial effects of nicotine and nAChR agonists generally performed daily administration of the drugs for a few times or low-dose administration in the case of long-term treatment. The complex influences of nicotine and nAChR agonists on disease consequences of experimental ischemia models might be relevant to the complicated influences of smoking on the risk and the outcome of ischemic stroke patients that include "smoker's paradox".

The number of investigations on hemorrhagic stroke is much smaller than that on ischemic stroke, but distinct lines of experimental evidence are consistent with the idea that nAChRs may serve as a target for ICH therapy. Post-treatment of animal models of striatal (putaminal) hemorrhage with nicotine or α7 nAChR agonists ameliorates neurological outcome and alleviates various neuropathological changes. Involvement of α4β2 nAChRs in addition to α7 nAChRs in neuroprotection is suggested in the case of cortical (lobar) hemorrhage model. Although smoking has been reported as a risk factor for mortality in particular populations of ICH patients, its relationship with nicotine is not evident. Accordingly, nicotine and subtype-specific nAChR agonists may be considered as novel therapeutic drugs for ICH. This proposal is particularly important because no effective pharmacotherapies for ICH directly aiming at brain tissue preservation have been established to date.

There is only one experimental study addressing the effect of nAChR agonist in SAH model, but according to the results, α7 nAChRs may serve as a promising target for therapy also for SAH. Interestingly, nicotine replacement therapy may be safely applicable to, and might produce beneficial outcome in, smokers after SAH.

An important concern at present is the shortage of information regarding the cellular and molecular mechanisms of actions of nicotine and nAChR agonists under stroke conditions, although a few studies have proposed potential involvement of several signaling pathways such as PI3K/Akt and Jak/STAT. Elucidation of the detailed mechanisms of neuroprotective and anti-inflammatory actions, in conjunction with determination of the ideal drug treatment regimens, may pave the way for developing novel strategies for treatment of distinct types of cerebrovascular disorders, by targeting nAChRs and nAChR-mediated neurotransmission.

Acknowledgments This work was supported by the Smoking Researh Foundation and JSPS KAKENHI, MEXT, Japan (Grants 16H04673 and 16 K15204).

References

Akaike A, Takada-Takatori Y, Kume T, Izumi Y (2010) Mechanisms of neuroprotective effects of nicotine and acetylcholinesterase inhibitors: role of α4 and α7 receptors in neuroprotection. J Mol Neurosci 40:211–216. https://doi.org/10.1007/s12031-009-9236-1

Ali SF, Smith EE, Bhatt DL, Fonarow GC, Schwamm LH (2013) Paradoxical association of smoking with in-hospital mortality among patients admitted with acute ischemic stroke. J Am Heart Assoc 2:e000171. https://doi.org/10.1161/JAHA.113.000171

An SJ, Kim TJ, Yoon BW (2017) Epidemiology, risk factors, and clinical features of intracerebral hemorrhage: an update. Stroke 19:3–10. https://doi.org/10.5853/jos.2016.00864

Anan J, Hijioka M, Kurauchi Y, Hisatsune A, Seki T, Katsuki H (2017) Cortical hemorrhage-associated neurological deficits and tissue damage in mice are ameliorated by therapeutic treatment with nicotine. J Neurosci Res 95:1838–1849. https://doi.org/10.1002/jnr.24016

Ariesen MJ1, Claus SP, Rinkel GJ, Algra A (2003) Risk factors for intracerebral hemorrhage in the general population: a systematic review. Stroke 34:2060–2065

Bhat VM, Cole JW, Sorkin JD, Wozniak MA, Malarcher AM, Giles WH, Stern BJ, Kittner SJ (2008) Dose-response relationship between cigarette smoking and risk of ischemic stroke in young women. Stroke 39:2439–2443. https://doi.org/10.1161/STROKEAHA.107.510073

Bradford ST, Stamatovic SM, Dondeti RS, Keep RF, Andjelkovic AV (2011) Nicotine aggravates the brain postischemic inflammatory response. Am J Physiol Heart Circ Physiol 300:H1518–H1529. https://doi.org/10.1152/ajpheart.00928.2010

Broderick JP, Viscoli CM, Brott T, Kernan WN, Brass LM, Feldmann E, Morgenstern LB, Wilterdink JL, Horwitz RI, Hemorrhagic Stroke Project Investigators (2003) Major risk factors for aneurysmal subarachnoid hemorrhage in the young are modifiable. Stroke 34:1375–1381

Carandang RA, Barton B, Rordorf GA, Ogilvy CS, Sims JR (2011) Nicotine replacement therapy after subarachnoid hemorrhage is not associated with increased vasospasm. Stroke 42:3080–3086. https://doi.org/10.1161/STROKEAHA.111.620955

Catanese L, Tarsia J, Fisher M (2017) Acute ischemic stroke therapy overview. Circ Res 120:541–558. https://doi.org/10.1161/CIRCRESAHA.116.309278

Chen Y, Nie H, Tian L, Tong L, Yang L, Lao N, Dong H, Sang H, Xiong L (2013) Nicotine-induced neuroprotection against ischemic injury involves activation of endocannabinoid system in rats. Neurochem Res 38:364–370. https://doi.org/10.1007/s11064-012-0927-6

Duris K, Manaenko A, Suzuki H, Rolland WB, Krafft PR, Zhang JH (2011) α7 nicotinic acetylcholine receptor agonist PNU-282987 attenuates early brain injury in a perforation model of subarachnoid hemorrhage in rats. Stroke 42:3530–3536. https://doi.org/10.1161/STROKEAHA.111.619965

Egea J, Rosa AO, Sobrado M, Gandía L, López MG, García AG (2007) Neuroprotection afforded by nicotine against oxygen and glucose deprivation in hippocampal slices is lost in α7 nicotinic receptor knockout mice. Neuroscience 145:866–872

Egea J, Martín-de-Saavedra MD, Parada E, Romero A, Del Barrio L, Rosa AO, García AG, López MG (2012) Galantamine elicits neuroprotection by inhibiting iNOS, NADPH oxidase and ROS in hippocampal slices stressed with anoxia/reoxygenation. Neuropharmacology 62:1082–1090. https://doi.org/10.1016/j.neuropharm.2011.10.022

Faigle R, Marsh EB, Llinas RH, Urrutia VC, Gottesman RF (2016) Race-specific predictors of mortality in intracerebral hemorrhage: differential impacts of intraventricular hemorrhage and age among blacks and whites. J Am Heart Assoc. https://doi.org/10.1161/JAHA.116.003540

Fujiki M, Kobayashi H, Uchida S, Inoue R, Ishii K (2005) Neuroprotective effect of donepezil, a nicotinic acetylcholine-receptor activator, on cerebral infarction in rats. Brain Res 1043:236–241

Fujimoto S, Katsuki H, Kume T, Akaike A (2006) Thrombin-induced delayed injury involves multiple and distinct signaling pathways in the cerebral cortex and the striatum in organotypic slice cultures. Neurobiol Dis 22:130–142

Furukawa S, Sameshima H, Yang L, Ikenoue T (2013) Activation of acetylcholine receptors and microglia in hypoxic-ischemic brain damage in newborn rats. Brain Dev 35:607–613. https://doi.org/10.1016/j.braindev.2012.10.006

Gonzalez CL, Gharbawie OA, Kolb B (2006) Chronic low-dose administration of nicotine facilitates recovery and synaptic change after focal ischemia in rats. Neuropharmacology 50:777–787

Guan YZ, Jin XD, Guan LX, Yan HC, Wang P, Gong Z, Li SJ, Cao X, Xing YL, Gao TM (2015) Nicotine inhibits microglial proliferation and is neuroprotective in global ischemia rats. Mol Neurobiol 51:1480–1488. https://doi.org/10.1007/s12035-014-8825-3

Han Z, Li L, Wang L, Degos V, Maze M, Su H (2014a) Alpha-7 nicotinic acetylcholine receptor agonist treatment reduces neuroinflammation, oxidative stress, and brain injury in mice with ischemic stroke and bone fracture. J Neurochem 131:498–508. https://doi.org/10.1111/jnc.12817

Han Z, Shen F, He Y, Degos V, Camus M, Maze M, Young WL, Su H (2014b) Activation of α-7 nicotinic acetylcholine receptor reduces ischemic stroke injury through reduction of pro-inflammatory macrophages and oxidative stress. PLoS One 9:e105711. https://doi.org/10.1371/journal.pone.0105711

Hawkins BT, Brown RC, Davis TP (2002) Smoking and ischemic stroke: a role for nicotine? Trends Pharmacol Sci 23:78–82

Hejmadi MV, Dajas-Bailador F, Barns SM, Jones B, Wonnacott S (2003) Neuroprotection by nicotine against hypoxia-induced apoptosis in cortical cultures involves activation of multiple nicotinic acetylcholine receptor subtypes. Mol Cell Neurosci 24:779–786

Hijioka M, Matsushita H, Hisatsune A, Isohama Y, Katsuki H (2011) Therapeutic effect of nicotine in a mouse model of intracerebral hemorrhage. J Pharmacol Exp Ther 338:741–749. https://doi.org/10.1124/jpet.111.182519

Hijioka M, Matsushita H, Ishibashi H, Hisatsune A, Isohama Y, Katsuki H (2012) α7 nicotinic acetylcholine receptor agonist attenuates neuropathological changes associated with intracerebral hemorrhage in mice. Neuroscience 222:10–19. https://doi.org/10.1016/j.neuroscience.2012.07.024

Hussein HM, Niemann N, Parker ED, Qureshi AI, Collaborators VISTA (2017) Searching for the smoker's paradox in acute stroke patients treated with intravenous thrombolysis. Nicotine Tob Res 19:871–876. https://doi.org/10.1093/ntr/ntx020

Jiang Y, Li L, Liu B, Zhang Y, Chen Q, Li C (2014) Vagus nerve stimulation attenuates cerebral ischemia and reperfusion injury via endogenous cholinergic pathway in rat. PLoS One 9:e102342. https://doi.org/10.1371/journal.pone.0102342

Kagitani F, Uchida S, Hotta H, Sato A (2000) Effects of nicotine on blood flow and delayed neuronal death following intermittent transient ischemia in rat hippocampus. Jpn J Physiol 50:585–595

Kalappa BI, Sun F, Johnson SR, Jin K, Uteshev VV (2013) A positive allosteric modulator of α7 nAChRs augments neuroprotective effects of endogenous nicotinic agonists in cerebral ischaemia. Br J Pharmacol 169:1862–1878. https://doi.org/10.1111/bph.12247

Kaplan EH, Gottesman RF, Llinas RH, Marsh EB (2014) The association between specific substances of abuse and subcortical intracerebral hemorrhage versus ischemic lacunar infarction. Front Neurol 5:174

Katsuki H (2010) Exploring neuroprotective drug therapies for intracerebral hemorrhage. J Pharmacol Sci 114(4):366–378

Kitaoka T, Hua Y, Xi G, Hoff JT, Keep RF (2002) Delayed argatroban treatment reduces edema in a rat model of intracerebral hemorrhage. Stroke 33:3012–3018

Krafft PR, Altay O, Rolland WB, Duris K, Lekic T, Tang J, Zhang JH (2012) α7 nicotinic acetylcholine receptor agonism confers neuroprotection through GSK-3β inhibition in a mouse model of intracerebral hemorrhage. Stroke 43:844–850. https://doi.org/10.1161/STROKEAHA.111.639989

Krafft PR, Caner B, Klebe D, Rolland WB, Tang J, Zhang JH (2013) PHA-543613 preserves blood-brain barrier integrity after intracerebral hemorrhage in mice. Stroke 44:1743–1747. https://doi.org/10.1161/STROKEAHA.111.000427

Krafft PR, McBride D, Rolland WB, Lekic T, Flores JJ, Zhang JH (2017) α7 nicotinic acetylcholine receptor stimulation attenuates neuroinflammation through JAK2-STAT3 activation in murine models of intracerebral hemorrhage. Biomed Res Int 2017:8134653. https://doi.org/10.1155/2017/8134653

Kufner A, Nolte CH, Galinovic I, Brunecker P, Kufner GM, Endres M, Fiebach JB, Ebinger M (2013) Smoking-thrombolysis paradox: recanalization and reperfusion rates after intravenous tissue plasminogen activator in smokers with ischemic stroke. Stroke 44:407–413. https://doi.org/10.1161/STROKEAHA.112.662148

Li Y, Xiao D, Dasgupta C, Xiong F, Tong W, Yang S, Zhang L (2012) Perinatal nicotine exposure increases vulnerability of hypoxic-ischemic brain injury in neonatal rats: role of angiotensin II receptors. Stroke 43:2483–2490. https://doi.org/10.1161/STROKEAHA.112.664698

Li C, Sun H, Arrick DM, Mayhan WG (2016) Chronic nicotine exposure exacerbates transient focal cerebral ischemia-induced brain injury. J Appl Physiol 120:328–333. https://doi.org/10.1152/japplphysiol.00663.2015

Lim DH, Alaverdashvili M, Whishaw IQ (2009) Nicotine does not improve recovery from learned nonuse nor enhance constraint-induced therapy after motor cortex stroke in the rat. Behav Brain Res 198:411–419. https://doi.org/10.1016/j.bbr.2008.11.038

Lorrio S, Sobrado M, Arias E, Roda JM, García AG, López MG (2007) Galantamine postischemia provides neuroprotection and memory recovery against transient global cerebral ischemia in gerbils. J Pharmacol Exp Ther 322:591–599

Martín A, Szczupak B, Gómez-Vallejo V, Domercq M, Cano A, Padro D, Muñoz C, Higuchi M, Matute C, Llop J (2015) In vivo PET imaging of the α4β2 nicotinic acetylcholine receptor as a marker for brain inflammation after cerebral ischemia. J Neurosci 35:5998–6009. https://doi.org/10.1523/JNEUROSCI.3670-14.2015

Mudo G, Belluardo N, Fuxe K (2007) Nicotinic receptor agonists as neuroprotective/neurotrophic drugs. Progress in molecular mechanisms. J Neural Transm (Vienna) 114:135–147

Nagatsuna T, Nomura S, Suehiro E, Fujisawa H, Koizumi H, Suzuki M (2005) Systemic administration of argatroban reduces secondary brain damage in a rat model of intracerebral hemorrhage: histopathological assessment. Cerebrovasc Dis 19:192–200

Nanri M, Miyake H, Murakami Y, Matsumoto K, Watanabe H (1998a) GTS-21, a nicotinic agonist, attenuates multiple infarctions and cognitive deficit caused by permanent occlusion of bilateral common carotid arteries in rats. Jpn J Pharmacol 78:463–469

Nanri M, Yamamoto J, Miyake H, Watanabe H (1998b) Protective effect of GTS-21, a novel nicotinic receptor agonist, on delayed neuronal death induced by ischemia in gerbils. Jpn J Pharmacol 76:23–29

Ohnishi M, Katsuki H, Fujimoto S, Takagi M, Kume T, Akaike A (2007) Involvement of thrombin and mitogen-activated protein kinase pathways in hemorrhagic brain injury. Exp Neurol 206:43–52

Ohnishi M, Katsuki H, Takagi M, Kume T, Akaike A (2009) Long-term treatment with nicotine suppresses neurotoxicity of, and microglial activation by, thrombin in cortico-striatal slice cultures. Eur J Pharmacol 602:288–293. https://doi.org/10.1016/j.ejphar.2008.11.041

Ovbiagele B, Saver JL (2005) The smoking-thrombolysis paradox and acute ischemic stroke. Neurology 65:293–295

Parada E, Egea J, Romero A, del Barrio L, García AG, López MG (2010) Poststress treatment with PNU282987 can rescue SH-SY5Y cells undergoing apoptosis via α7 nicotinic receptors linked to a Jak2/Akt/HO-1 signaling pathway. Free Radic Biol Med 49:1815–1821. https://doi.org/10.1016/j.freeradbiomed.2010.09.017

Parada E, Egea J, Buendia I, Negredo P, Cunha AC, Cardoso S, Soares MP, López MG (2013) The microglial α7-acetylcholine nicotinic receptor is a key element in promoting neuroprotection by inducing heme oxygenase-1 via nuclear factor erythroid-2-related factor 2. Antioxid Redox Signal 19:1135–1148. https://doi.org/10.1089/ars.2012.4671

Paulson JR, Roder KE, McAfee G, Allen DD, Van der Schyf CJ, Abbruscato TJ (2006) Tobacco smoke chemicals attenuate brain-to-blood potassium transport mediated by the Na, K, 2Cl-cotransporter during hypoxia-reoxygenation. J Pharmacol Exp Ther 316:248–254

Paulson JR, Yang T, Selvaraj PK, Mdzinarishvili A, Van der Schyf CJ, Klein J, Bickel U, Abbruscato TJ (2010) Nicotine exacerbates brain edema during in vitro and in vivo focal ischemic conditions. J Pharmacol Exp Ther 332:371–379. https://doi.org/10.1124/jpet.109.157776

Qureshi AI, Mendelow AD, Hanley DF (2009) Intracerebral hemorrhage. Lancet 373:1632–1644. https://doi.org/10.1016/S0140-6736(09)60371-8

Raval AP, Bhatt A, Saul I (2009) Chronic nicotine exposure inhibits 17β-estradiol-mediated protection of the hippocampal CA1 region against cerebral ischemia in female rats. Neurosci Lett 458:65–69. https://doi.org/10.1016/j.neulet.2009.04.021

Raval AP, Hirsch N, Dave KR, Yavagal DR, Bramlett H, Saul I (2011) Nicotine and estrogen synergistically exacerbate cerebral ischemic injury. Neuroscience 181:216–225. https://doi.org/10.1016/j.neuroscience.2011.02.036

Ray RS, Rai S, Katyal A (2014) Cholinergic receptor blockade by scopolamine and mecamylamine exacerbates global cerebral ischemia induced memory dysfunction in C57BL/6J mice. Nitric Oxide 43:62–73. https://doi.org/10.1016/j.niox.2014.08.009

Seder DB, Schmidt JM, Badjatia N, Fernandez L, Rincon F, Claassen J, Gordon E, Carrera E, Kurtz P, Lee K, Connolly ES, Mayer SA (2011) Transdermal nicotine replacement therapy in cigarette smokers with acute subarachnoid hemorrhage. Neurocrit Care 14:77–83

Shytle RD, Mori T, Townsend K, Vendrame M, Sun N, Zeng J, Ehrhart J, Silver AA, Sanberg PR, Tan J (2004) Cholinergic modulation of microglial activation by α7 nicotinic receptors. J Neurochem 89:337–343

Sun Z, Baker W, Hiraki T, Greenberg JH (2012) The effect of right vagus nerve stimulation on focal cerebral ischemia: an experimental study in the rat. Brain Stimul 5(1):1–10

Sun F, Jin K, Uteshev VV (2013) A type-II positive allosteric modulator of α7 nAChRs reduces brain injury and improves neurological function after focal cerebral ischemia in rats. PLoS One 8:e73581. https://doi.org/10.1371/journal.pone.0073581

Taly A, Corringer PJ, Guedin D, Lestage P, Changeux JP (2009) Nicotinic receptors: allosteric transitions and therapeutic targets in the nervous system. Nat Rev Drug Discov 8:733–750. https://doi.org/10.1038/nrd2927

Tsai CF, Anderson N, Thomas B, Sudlow CL (2016) Comparing risk factor profiles between intracerebral hemorrhage and ischemic stroke in Chinese and white populations: systematic review and meta-analysis. PLoS One 11:e0151743. https://doi.org/10.1371/journal.pone.0151743

Turgeon RD, Chang SJ, Dandurand C, Gooderham PA, Hunt C (2017) Nicotine replacement therapy in patients with aneurysmal subarachnoid hemorrhage: systematic review of the literature, and survey of Canadian practice. J Clin Neurosci 42:48–53. https://doi.org/10.1016/j.jocn.2017.03.014

Wang L, Kittaka M, Sun N, Schreiber SS, Zlokovic BV (1997) Chronic nicotine treatment enhances focal ischemic brain injury and depletes free pool of brain microvascular tissue plasminogen activator in rats. J Cereb Blood Flow Metab 17:136–146

Wang H, Yu M, Ochani M, Amella CA, Tanovic M, Susarla S, Li JH, Wang H, Yang H, Ulloa L, Al-Abed Y, Czura CJ, Tracey KJ (2003) Nicotinic acetylcholine receptor α7 subunit is an essential regulator of inflammation. Nature 421:384–388

Wang ZF, Wang J, Zhang HY, Tang XC (2008) Huperzine A exhibits anti-inflammatory and neuroprotective effects in a rat model of transient focal cerebral ischemia. J Neurochem 106:1594–1603. https://doi.org/10.1111/j.1471-4159.2008.05504.x

Zoli M, Pistillo F, Gotti C (2015) Diversity of native nicotinic receptor subtypes in mammalian brain. Neuropharmacology 96:302–311. https://doi.org/10.1016/j.neuropharm.2014.11.003

Chapter 8
Roles of Nicotinic Acetylcholine Receptors in the Pathology and Treatment of Alzheimer's and Parkinson's Diseases

Shun Shimohama and Jun Kawamata

Abstract Both of the two most common neurodegenerative disorders, namely Alzheimer's disease (AD) and Parkinson's disease (PD), have multiple lines of evidence, from molecular and cellular to epidemiological, that nicotinic transmission is implicated in those pathogenesis. This review presents evidences of nicotinic acetylcholine receptor (nAChR)-mediated protection against neurotoxicity induced by β amyloid (Aβ), glutamate, rotenone, and 6-hydroxydopamine (6-OHDA) and the signal transduction involved in this mechanism. Our studies clarified that survival signal transduction, α7 nAChR-Src family-PI3K-AKT pathway and subsequent upregulation of Bcl-2 and Bcl-x, would lead to neuroprotection. Recently analyzing the properties of galantamine, we clarified the neuroprotective pathway, which is mediated by enhancement of microglial α7 nAChR resulting in upregulation of Aβ phagocytosis. Galantamine sensitizes microglial α7 nAChRs to choline and induce Ca^{2+} influx into microglia. The Ca^{2+}-induced intracellular signaling cascades may then stimulate Aβ phagocytosis through the actin reorganization. This discovery would facilitate further investigation of possible nAChRs enhancing drugs targeting not only neuronal but also microglial nAChRs.

Keywords Alzheimer's disease · Parkinson's disease · Nicotine · nAChR · β amyloid · Glutamate · Microglia · Phagocytosis

8.1 Introduction

Alzheimer's disease (AD) pathology is characterized by the presence of two hallmarks, senile plaques (SP) and neurofibrillary tangles (NFT), and by extensive neuronal loss (Giannakopoulos et al. 1996). β amyloid (Aβ) is a major element of SP and one of the candidates for the cause of the neurodegeneration found in AD. It has

S. Shimohama (✉) · J. Kawamata
Department of Neurology, School of Medicine, Sapporo Medical University, Sapporo, Hokkaido, Japan
e-mail: shimoha@sapmed.ac.jp

A. Akaike et al. (eds.), *Nicotinic Acetylcholine Receptor Signaling in Neuroprotection*, https://doi.org/10.1007/978-981-10-8488-1_8

been shown that the accumulation of Aβ precedes other pathological changes and causes neurodegeneration and neuronal death in vivo (Yankner et al. 1990). Several mutations of the Aβ precursor protein (APP) are found in familial AD, and these mutations are involved in amyloidogenesis (Citron et al. 1992). Also, familial AD mutations of presenilin 1 (PS-1) enhance the generation of Aβ 1-42 (Tomita et al. 1997). The cerebral cortex contains a dense plexus of cholinergic axon terminals that arise from the cells of the basal forebrain including the nucleus basalis of Meynert (Bigl et al. 1982; Mesulam et al. 1983). Degeneration of this cholinergic projection is recognized as one of the most prominent pathological changes in AD brain (Whitehouse et al. 1981; Rosser et al. 1982). In AD, the cholinergic system is affected, and a reduction in the number of nicotinic acetylcholine receptor (nAChR) has been reported (Shimohama et al. 1986; Whitehouse and Kalaria 1995). ACh receptors are classified into two groups; nAChRs and muscarinic ACh receptors (mAChRs). In the brain, nAChRs show additional complexity, as there are multiple receptor subtypes with differing properties and functions (Clarke et al. 1985; Lindstrom et al. 1995). At least nine α subunits (α2–α7, α9, and α10 in mammals; α8 in chicks) and three β subunits (β2–β4) have been identified in the brain. Both α and β subunits are required to form functional heteropentametric receptors, with the exception of α7–10 subunits, which apparently form functional homopentameric receptors. In the brain, α7 homometric and α4β2 heterometric nAChRs are the two major subtypes. Both α4β2 and α7 subtypes have been implicated in the mechanism of neuroprotection provided by nicotine (Kihara et al. 1998, 2001). It is also known that Aβ binds very strongly to α7 nicotinic acetylcholine receptor (nAChR) (Wang et al. 2000) and up-regulation of α7 nAChR is observed in transgenic mice co-expressing mutant (A246E) human presenilin 1 and (K670N/M671L) APP (Dineley et al. 2002). Multiple lines of evidence show that neuronal nAChRs are involved in synaptic plasticity as well as in neuronal survival and neuroprotection. Moreover, presynaptic nAChRs can modulate the release of many neurotransmitters, including dopamine (DA), noradrenaline, serotonin, ACh, γ-aminobutyric acid (GABA), and glutamate. These neurotransmitter systems play an important role in cognitive and non-cognitive functions such as learning, memory, attention, locomotion, motivation, reward, reinforcement, and anxiety. Thus, nAChRs are considered promising therapeutic targets for new treatments of neurodegenerative disorders. It is also known that α4 and β2 nAChR genes, *CHRNA4* and *CHRNB2*, are causative genes of autosomal dominant nocturnal frontal lobe epilepsy (ADNFLE) (Steinlein et al. 1995; De Fusco et al. 2000). Analyzing the polymorphism of the nAChRs genes in AD patients and controls, we showed that genetic polymorphisms of the neuronal nAChR genes might be related to the pathogenesis of sporadic AD (Kawamata and Shimohama 2002). This, in conjunction with the memory-enhancing activity of nicotine and selective nAChR agonists such as the α7 nAChR agonist, 3-(2,4)-dimethoxybenzylidene anabaseine (DMXBA) (Meyer et al. 1997), suggests a significant role of nAChRs in learning and memory. Therefore, it is generally recognized that the down-regulation of nAChRs is involved in the intellectual dysfunction in AD. Our studies showed that nAChR stimulation protected neurons from Aβ- and glutamate-induced neurotoxicity. This allowed us to hypothesize that nAChRs are involved in a neuroprotective cascade (Kihara et al. 1997, 1998, 2001; Akaike et al. 1994) as described in the following sections.

Parkinson's disease (PD) is the second most common progressive neurodegenerative disorder next to AD. It is characterized by relatively selective degeneration of dopaminergic neurons in the substantia nigra and loss of dopamine in the striatum resulting in resting tremor, rigidity, bradykinesia and postural instability (Shimohama et al. 2003; Obeso et al. 2010). Although the pathogenesis of PD is still unclear, it is thought that the interaction of gene and the environment plays roles in causing the multi-factorial disease. Rural residency, pesticides and intrinsic toxic agents were reported as environmental risk factors for sporadic PD. Recent studies revealed several mutations in familial PD genes such as *α-synuclein, parkin, PINK1, LRRK2, DJ-1, UCHL1, ATP13A2 and GBA* (glucocerebrocidase) (Hardy 2010; Sidransky et al. 2009). The most reproducible epidemiological relevant factor against Parkinson's disease (PD) is cigarette smoking habits (Dorn 1959; Quik 2004). Epidemiological studies suggest that the use of pesticides increases the risk of PD, possibly via reduced activity of complex I in the mitochondrial respiratory chain in the substantia nigra (Parker et al. 1989; Mann et al. 1992; Mizuno et al. 1998). Grady et al. examined mouse brain using in situ hybridization to characterize the mRNA expression pattern of nAChRs. The ventral tegmental area (VTA) and substantia nigra expressed high concentrations of α4 and α6 and β2, and β3 mRNAs, intermediate levels of α5 mRNA, and low levels of the α3 and α7 mRNAs. No signal for α2 and β4 mRNA was detected (Le Novère et al. 1996; Grady et al. 2007). They reviewed the subtypes of nAChRs on dopaminergic terminals of mouse striatum reporting five nAChR subtypes that expressed on dopaminergic nerve terminals, three of which are α6 containing subunits, namely α4α6β2β3, α6β2β3, and α6β2. The remaining two subtypes, α4β2, α4α5β2, are more numerous than the α6-containg subtypes. The α6 containing nAChRs, which do not contribute to dopamine release induced by nicotine, are mainly located on dopaminergic neuronal terminals and probably mediating the endogenous cholinergic modulation of dopamine release at the terminal level. In contrast, α4β2 nAChR represent the majority of functional heteromeric nAChRs on dopaminergic neuronal soma. α7 nAChRs are present on dopaminergic neuronal soma, contributing to nicotine reinforcement (Champtiaux et al. 2003). There are several studies analyzing the decline of specific nAChRs in PD patients. Court et al. reported the decline of α3 subunits and no change of α7 subunits. Gotti et al. and Court et al. reported decreased level of α4 subunits but Guan et al. reported not (Court et al. 2000; Gotti et al. 1997; Guan et al. 2002). Bordia et al. reported the decline of α6 subunits in caudate and putamen. They further specified that the most vulnerable subtype in striatum of MPTP-treated mice and monkeys is α6α4β2β3 rather than α6β2β3 and further identified the specific loss of α6α4β2β3 subtype in PD brains (Bordia et al. 2007). These results seem to indicate that the decline of nigrostriatal specific α6 subtypes is highly specific and relevant to the PD pathogenesis but not is α7 subtype. Functional studies on α6 nAChRs should be undertaken to confirm its pathological importance in PD. For this purpose, Drenan et al. (2008) generated the gain-of-function α6 nAChR transgenic mouse, which turned to present locomotive hyperactivity. With low dose of nicotine by the way of stimulating dopamine but not GABA, its phenotype was exaggerated and hyperdopaminergic state in vivo was observed. Current drug therapy against PD is limited to supplementing DA or enhancing dopaminergic effect. Some may have neuroprotective effects, but their effects remain controversial (Quik 2004; Du et al. 2005; Iravani et al. 2006). It has also been reported that smokers have a lower risk for PD (De Reuck et al. 2005; Wirdefeldt et al. 2005), and nAChRs were decreased in the brains of PD patients (Fujita et al. 2006) and model animals (Quik et al. 2006a). Nicotine may upregulate DA release at striatum from nigral dopaminergic neurons (Morens et al. 1995), followed by stimulation of $\alpha 4\beta 2$ nAChRs (Champtiaux et al. 2003). Furthermore, nicotine could protect mitochondria and had protective effect from oxidative stress (Cormier et al. 2003; Xie et al. 2005). In studies made in vivo, stimulation of nAChRs resulted in neuroprotection in PD model animals (Parain et al. 2003). Although several clinical trials to evaluate possible therapeutic effect of nicotine to PD patients have been conducted, whether nicotine has therapeutic effects on PD is still controversial. The relatively high dose transdermal nicotine administration might have therapeutic effect on PD patients (Villafane et al. 2007). In the following we present evidence for nAChR-mediated neuroproptection in PD models based mainly on our studies.

8.2 Alzheimer's Disease and nAChRs

8.2.1 nAChR Enhancement Shows Neuroprotection Against Glutamate Toxicity

Glutamate cytotoxicity is one of the most suspected causative pathways in neurodegenerative process, namely in AD and PD. To give examples, it is also assumed that glutamate plays an important role in the neurodegeneration observed in hypoxic-ischemic brain injury (Choi 1988; Meldrum and Garthwaite 1990). Several investigators have also suggested that cortical neurodegeneration in AD is attributable to glutamate (Maragos et al. 1986; Mattson 1988). Moreover, brief glutamate exposure induces delayed cell death in cultured neurons from certain brain regions, such as the cerebral cortex and hippocampus. In these brain regions, the N-methyl-D-aspartate (NMDA) glutamate receptor subtype plays a crucial role in glutamate neurotoxicity. Several studies have indicated the existence of nitric oxide (NO) synthase in the CNS, including the cerebral cortex. NMDA receptor stimulation induces Ca^{2+} influx into cells through ligand-gated ion channels, thereby triggering NO formation. NO is also thought to diffuse to the adjacent cells, resulting in the appropriate physiological response and/or glutamate-related cell death (Choi 1988; Hartley and Choi 1989; Dawson et al. 1991).

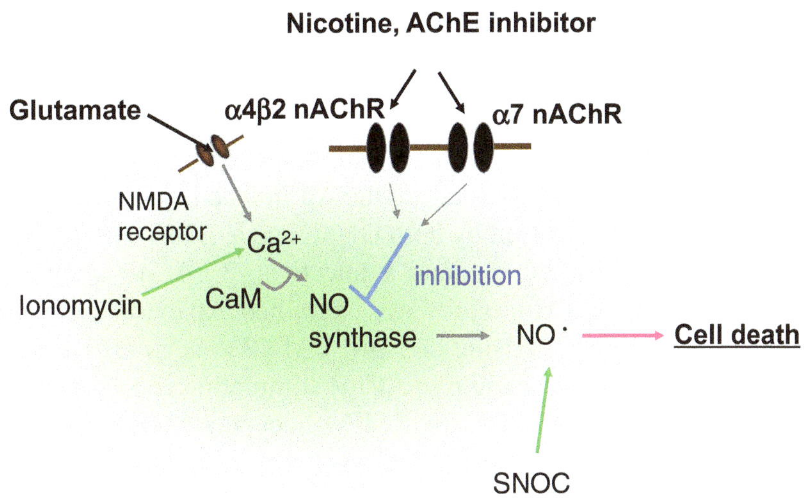

Fig. 8.1 Proposed hypothesis for the mechanism of nAChR-mediated survival signal transduction against glutamate-Iinduced necrosis. The NMDA glutamate receptor subtype plays a crucial role in glutamate neurotoxicity. NMDA receptor stimulation induces Ca^{2+} influx into cells through ligand-gated ion channels, thereby triggering NO formation. NO would diffuse to the adjacent cells, resulting in the appropriate physiological response and/or glutamate-related cell death

We examined the effects of nicotine on glutamate-induced neurotoxicity using primary cultures of rat cortical neurons. Cell viability was decreased by treatment with 1 mM glutamate for 10 min followed by incubation in glutamate-free medium for 1 h. Incubating the cultures with 10 μM nicotine for 24 h prior to glutamate exposure significantly reduced glutamate cytotoxicity. To investigate whether nicotine-induced neuroprotection is due to a specific effect mediated by nAChRs, the effects of cholinergic antagonists were examined. An addition of dihydro-β-erythroidine (DHβE), an α4β2 nAChR antagonist, or α-BTX, an α7 nAChR antagonist, to the medium containing nicotine reduced the protective effect of nicotine. We also examined the protection of nicotine against the effects of ionomycin, a calcium ionophore, and SNOC, an NO-generating agent. Incubating the cultures for 10 min in either 3 μM ionomycin- or 300 μM SNOC-containing medium markedly reduced cell viability. A 24-h pretreatment with nicotine significantly attenuated the ionomycin cytotoxicity, but did not affect the SNOC cytotoxicity (Akaike et al. 1994; Shimohama et al. 1996; Kaneko et al. 1997) (Fig. 8.1).

We have also shown that nicotinic α7 nAChRs protect against glutamate neurotoxicity and neuronal ischemic damage in vivo. The α7 nAChR agonist, dimethoxybenzylidene anabaseine (DMXBA), protected rat neocortical neurons against excitotoxicity administered 24 h before, but not concomitantly with, NMDA. This action was blocked by nicotinic but not muscarinic antagonists. DMXBA (1 mg/kg i.p.) also reduced infarct size in rats when injected 24 h before, but not during, focal ischemic insults. In a mecamylamine-sensitive manner, α7 nAChRs appear neuroprotective in non-apoptotic model (Shimohama et al. 1998).

8.2.2 *Nicotine Protects Neurons Against Aβ Toxicity In Vitro*

A 48-h exposure to 20 μM neurotoxic Aβ25–35 caused a significant reduction in the neuronal cells of rat fetal primary culture. Simultaneous incubation of the cultures with nicotine and Aβ significantly reduced the Aβ-induced cytotoxicity. The protective effect of nicotine was reduced by both DHβE and α-BTX. The effect of a selective α4β2 nAChR agonist, cytisine, and a selective α7 nAChR agonist, DMXBA (Hunter et al. 1994), on Aβ cytotoxicity was examined. Aβ cytotoxicity was significantly reduced when 10 μM cytisine or 1 μM DMXB was co-administered. These findings suggest that both α4β2 and α7 nAChR stimulation is protective against Aβ cytotoxicity. In addition, MK-801, an NMDA receptor antagonist, inhibited Aβ cytotoxicity when administrated simultaneously with Aβ, suggesting that Aβ cytotoxicity is mediated via the NMDA receptor, or via glutamate in cultured cortical neurons (Kihara et al. 1997, 1998, 2001).

Although it is regarded that PS-1 mutations enhance the generation of Aβ1–42, it is controversial whether Aβ is directly toxic to neurons. We found that Aβ25–35-induced neurotoxicity was inhibited by MK801. It can therefore be hypothesized that Aβ might modulate or enhance glutamate-induced cytotoxicity. Indeed, Aβ causes a reduction in glutamate uptake in cultured astrocytes (Harris et al. 1996), indicating that, to some extent, Aβ-induced cytotoxicity might be mediated via glutamate cytotoxicity.

In our study (Kihara et al. 2000), incubation of the cortical neurons with both Aβ1–40 (1 nM) and Aβ1–42 (100 pM) for 7 days did not induce cell death. These are the concentrations of Aβ in the cerebrospinal fluid (CSF) of AD patients (Jensen et al. 1999). Although 20 μM glutamate alone did not significantly induce cell death, exposure to 20 μM glutamate for 24 h caused a significant reduction in the neuronal cells in the Aβ-treated group, showing that Aβ itself is not toxic at low concentrations, but makes neurons vulnerable to glutamate. Conversely, co-incubation of the cultures with nicotine (50 μM for 7 days) and Aβ significantly reduced Aβ-enhanced glutamate cytotoxicity (Akaike et al. 1994; Shimohama et al. 1996; Kaneko et al. 1997).

To investigate the mechanism of the protective effect of nicotine, we focused on the phosphatidylinositol 3-kinase (PI3K) pathway because PI3K had been shown to protect cells from apoptosis (del Peso et al. 1997). Long exposure to low concentrations of glutamate (50 μM for 24 h) induced cytotoxicity. Incubating the cultures with nicotine (10 μM for 24 h) prior to glutamate exposure significantly suppressed glutamate cytotoxicity. Simultaneous application of LY294002, a PI3K inhibitor, with nicotine cancelled the protective effect of nicotine. α-BTX blocked the protection provided by nicotine and DMXB. Furthermore, this DMXBA-induced protection was also reduced by LY294002. Although α4β2 nAChR stimulation also had a protective effect on Aβ- and glutamate-induced cytotoxicity, this effect was not inhibited by LY294002, suggesting PI3K system is not directly involved in α4β2 nAChR-mediated neuroprotection. PD98059, a mitogen-activated protein (MAP) kinase kinase (MEK) inhibitor, did not reduce the protective effect of nicotine, also suggesting that the MEK/ERK pathway is not directly involved in the protective

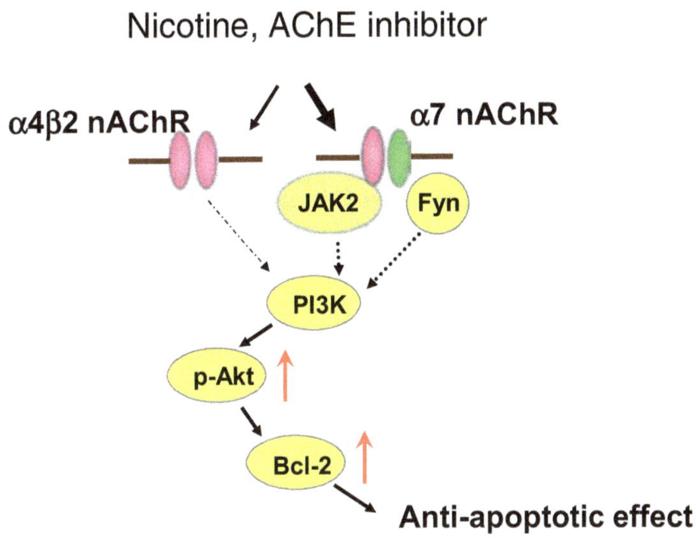

Fig. 8.2 Proposed hyposis for the mechanism of nAChR-mediated survival signal transduction against Aβ-induced apoptosis. Nicotine-induced neuroprotection is mediated via nAChRs, especially through α7 and α4β2 receptors, and inhibited by a PI3K inhibitor and an Akt/PKB inhibitor. This means that nicotine activates the PI3K-Akt/PKB pathways and increase survival of neurons. JAK2 and Fyn are key molecules trigger activation of the PI3K-Akt/PKB pathways which lead to subsequent upregulation of Bcl-2 and neuroprotection

effect of nicotine. A non-receptor tyrosine kinase inhibitor, PP2, did reduce the protective effect of nicotine, suggesting that Src is involved in the mechanism of the protective effect. Cycloheximide also inhibited the protection, implying that some protein synthesis is necessary for this effect.

AKT is a serine/threonine protein kinase and a putative effector of PI3K. To investigate the activation of AKT by nicotine through PI3K, we examined the level of phosphorylated AKT using an anti-phospho-specific AKT antibody. The phosphorylated form of AKT appeared immediately after the application of nicotine. Nicotine-induced AKT phosphorylation was blocked by simultaneous application of LY294002, but not of PD98059, indicating that PI3K, but not MAPK is involved. The AKT phosphorylation is blocked by α-BTX, but not by DHβE, implying that nicotine-induced AKT phosphorylation is mediated by α7 but not by α4β2 nAChRs. PP2 also blocked AKT phosphorylation, which suggests the involvement of tyrosine kinase. The level of total AKT protein which was detected with anti-AKT antibody remained unchanged.

Bcl-2 and Bcl-x proteins are anti-apoptotic proteins that can prevent cell death induced by a variety of toxic attacks (Zhong et al. 1993). It has been reported that AKT activation leads to the overexpression of Bcl-2 (Matsuzaki et al. 1999). Because nicotine can activate AKT via PI3K, we examined the protein levels of Bcl-2 and Bcl-x. We found that treatment with nicotine for 24 h increased the levels of Bcl-2 and Bcl-x, and this was inhibited by LY294002, which indicates the involvement of the PI3K pathway in nicotine-induced Bcl-2 and Bcl-x upregulation. These results suggest that nAChR stimulation protects neurons from glutamate-induced cytotoxicity by activating PI3K, which in turn activates AKT and upregulates Bcl-2 and Bcl-x (Kihara et al. 2001) (Fig. 8.2).

8.2.3 Galantamine Acts As an Allosteric Potentiating Ligand (APL) of nAChRs and Blocks Aβ-Enhanced Glutamate Toxicity In Vitro

Galantamine is an acetylcholinesterase inhibitor (AChEI) that is currently used for the treatment of AD. Although its AChEI activity appears to be much weaker than other clinically available AChEIs, its therapeutic effects on cognitive function in AD are comparable with the other agents. Furthermore, the long term extension clinical trial of galantamine suggested that the cognitive benefits of galantamine are sustained for at least 36 months (Raskind et al. 2004). In addition to the inhibition of AChE, galantamine binds to nAChRs and allosterically potentiates their synaptic transmission. Consequently, galantamine is called an allosteric potentiating ligand (APL) of nAChRs. This APL effect is present on both α7 and α4β2 nAChRs (Maelicke et al. 2001). Thus, galantamine could stimulate cholinergic transmission in two ways: (1) by inhibiting AChE and increasing AChs, and (2) by potentiating cholinergic transmission through the APL effect. We demonstrated that galantamine protected cortical neurons against Aβ-enhanced glutamate toxicity by, at least partially, the α7 nAChR-PI3K-AKT pathway (Kihara et al. 2004).

8.2.4 Galantamine-Induced Aβ Clearance Mediated via Stimulation of Microglial nAChRs

We found that in human AD brain, microglia accumulates on Aβ deposits and expresses α7 nAChRs including the APL-binding site, which is recognized specifically with FK1 antibody. Treatment of rat microglia with galantamine significantly enhanced microglial Aβ phagocytosis, and acetylcholine competitive angatonists as well as FK1 antibody inhibited the enhancement.

We further demonstrated that galantamine treatment facilitated Aβ clearance in brains of rodent AD models. We investigate effect of daily intraperitoneal galantamine (1 or 5 mg/kg) administration on Aβ clearance in rat that had received intrahippocampal Aβ42 (1 μg) injection. The amount of Aβ was significantly reduced by galantamine in a dose-dependent manner, compared with the vehicle-treated rats. This result suggests that galantamine may enhance microglial Aβ phagocytosis and promote the Aβ clearance from the Aβ-injected rat brain.

Hemizygous APdE9 mice is expressing chimeric mouse/human amyloid precursor protein APPswe (mouse APP695 harboring a human Aβ domain and mutations K594N and M595L linked to Swedish familial AD pedigrees) and human mutated presenilin 1-dE9 (deletion of exon 9), and present a weak decline in spatial learning and memory at 9 months of age. We had administrated the mice galantamine (1 or 5 mg/kg) from 9 months of age for 7 weeks and evaluated spatial learning and memory using water maze testing at 11 months of age. Both low and high dose galantamine significantly improved the performance in the 11 months old APdE9 mice.

Pathological evaluation also revealed that the Aβ burden in the brains of APdE9 mice treated with galantamine show less Aβ plaque. The measurement of amount of insoluble Aβ40 and Aβ42 in formic acid-extracted fraction of the brain revealed a significant decrease in galantamine-treated mice compared to sham treated mice.

Using primary-cultured rat microglia, we evaluated the microglial Aβ phagocytosis. We treated rat microglia with 1 μM Aβ42 in the presence or absence of galantamine or nicotine. Galantamine enhanced microglial Aβ phagocytosis in a concentration-dependent manner and phagocytosis reached the peak at 1 μM galantamine. Nicotine also increased Aβ phagocytosis at the concentration of 1000 μM. These effects were inhibited by pretreatment with the blockage of APL-binding site by FK1 antibody as well as with nAChR antagonists. Although galantamine-enhanced microglial Aβ phagocytosis was significantly inhibited by FK1 antibody, Fk1 antibody alone did not influence the magnitude of Aβ phagocytosis in the absence of galantamine. From these findings, we can assume that the galantamine-enhanced microglial Aβ phagocytosis requires the combined actions of an acetylcholine competitive agonist and the APL for nAChRs. In fact, depletion of choline, an acetylcholine-competitive α7 nAChR agonist, from the culture medium impedes the enhancement.

We investigated whether the Ca^{2+} influx correlates with enhanced microglial Aβ phagocytosis. In the absence of galantamine or nicotine, the levels of microglial Aβ phagocytosis were almost the same in Ca^{2+} (−) or Ca^{2+} (+) DMEM. Galantamine and nicotine significantly enhanced microglial Aβ phagocytosis in Ca^{2+} (+) DMEM, but not in Ca^{2+} (−) condition. Similarly, inhibition of the calmodulin-dependent pathways for the actin reorganization by 20 μM W-7, an inhibitor of calmodulin, or 10 μM KN93, an inhibitor of Ca^{2+}/CaM-dependent protein kinase II (CaMKII), abolished the enhancement. We evaluated other signaling cascades including JAK2-PI3K-AKT cascade, Fyn-PI3K-AKT cascade, MAPKK (MEK) cascade, using each inhibitor and concluded that they are not involved in galantamine enhanced microglial Aβ phagocytosis. These results suggest that Ca^{2+} influx through nAChRs and subsequent activation of CaM-CaMKII signaling cascade were involved in enhanced microglial Aβ phagocytosis through the actin reorganization (Takata et al. 2010) (Fig. 8.3).

8.2.5 Donepezil Promotes Internalization of NMDA Receptors by Stimulating α7 nAChRs and Attenuates Glutamate Cytotoxicity

Donepezil is one of the most widely prescribed AChEI for the treatment of AD and related dementias. Our group reported that in addition to up-regulating the PI3K-AKT pathway, there is another mechanism underlying neuroprotection by donepezil, showing decreases glutamate toxicity through down-regulation of NMDA receptors, following stimulation of α7 nAChRs in primary rat neuron cultures (Shen et al. 2010).

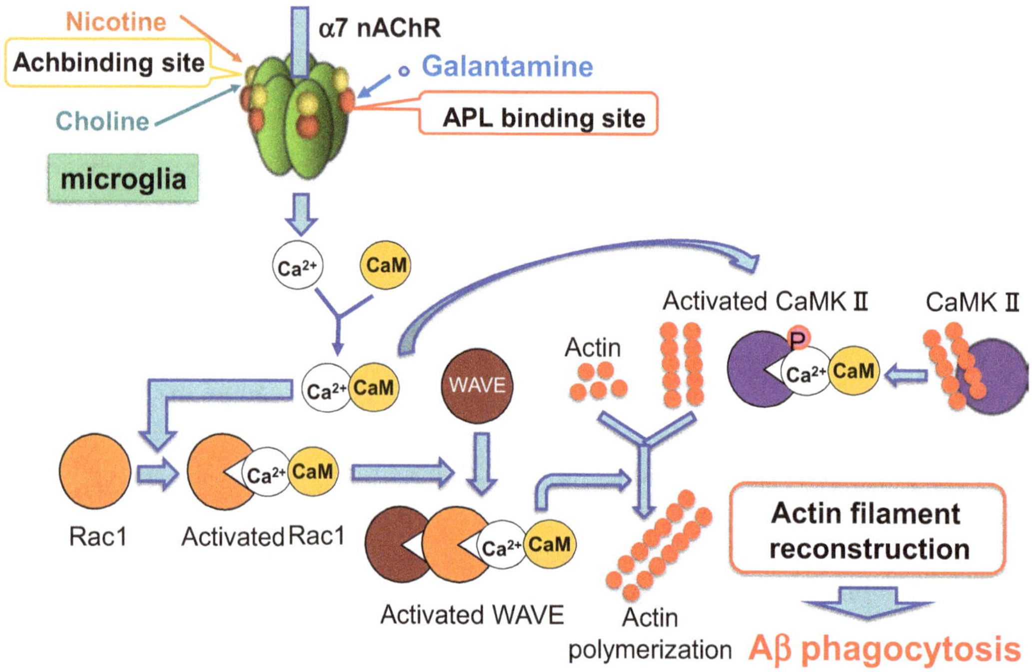

Fig. 8.3 Proposed pathway for microglial CaM/CaMKII/Aβ phagocytosis. Ca^{2+} influx through nAChRs and subsequent activation of CaM-CaMKII signaling cascade are involved in enhanced microglial Aβ phagocytosis through the actin reorganization

8.2.6 Donepezil Directly Acts on Microglia to Inhibit Its Inflammatory Activation

Hwang et al. reported that 5–20 μM donepezil attenuates microglial production of nitric oxide and tumor necrosis factor (TNF)-α, and suppressed the gene expression of inducible nitric oxide synthase, inteleukin-1β, and TNF-α in the microglia cultures. They also confirmed donepezil inhibit inflammatory NF-kB signaling in microglial cell line (Hwang et al. 2010).

8.2.7 Temporal Changes of CD68 and α7nAChR Expression in Microglia in AD-Like Mouse Models

As shown above, activated microglia are involved in Aβ clearance and that stimulation of α7nAChR in microglia enhances Aβ clearance. Nevertheless, how microglia and α7 nAChR in microglia are affected in AD remains unknown. The study aimed to collect fundamental data for considering whether microglia are potential targets for AD treatment and the appropriate timing of therapeutic intervention, by evaluating the temporal changes of Aβ, microglia, neurons, presynapses, and α7 nAChR by immunohistochemical studies in mouse models of AD. In an Aβ-injected AD mouse model, we observed early accumulation of CD68-positive microglia at Aβ deposition sites and gradual reduction of Aβ. Microglia were closely associated with Aβ deposits, and were confirmed to participate in clearing Aβ. In a transgenic mouse model of AD, we observed an increase in Aβ deposition from 6 months of age, followed by a gradual increase in microglial accumulation at Aβ deposit sites. Activated microglia in APdE9 mice showed two-step transition: a CD68-negative activated form at 6–9 months and a CD68-positive form from 12 months of age. In addition, α7 nAChR in microglia increased markedly at 6 months of age when activated microglia appeared for the first time, and decreased gradually coinciding with the increase of Aβ deposition. These findings suggest that early microglial activation is associated with α7 nAChR upregulation in microglia in APdE9 mice. These novel findings are important for the development of new therapeutic strategy for AD (Matsumura et al. 2015).

8.3 Parkinson's Disease and nAChRs

8.3.1 nAChR Enhancement Shows Dopaminergic Neuronal Protection Against Rotenone Cytotoxicity

Rotenone is a naturally occurring complex ketone pesticide derived from the roots of *Lonchocarpus* species. It can rapidly cross over cellular membranes without the aid of transporters, including the blood brain barrier (BBB). Rotenone is a strong inhibitor of complex I, which is located at the inner mitochondrial membrane and protrudes into the matrix. In 2000, Betarbet et al. (2000) demonstrated with rat model that chronic systemic exposure to rotenone causes many features of PD, including slow-progressive dopamine neuronal loss in nigrostriatal dopaminergic system, and Lewy body-like particles, which are primarily aggregations of α-synuclein (Mizuno et al. 1998; Inden et al. 2007). Rotenone works as a mitochondrial complex I inhibitor. Acute lethal doses of rotenone eliminate the mitochondrial respiratory system of the cell, resulting in an anoxic status that immediately causes cell death. At sub-lethal doses it causes partial inhibition of mitochondrial complex I, and in this situation mitochondrial dysfunction leads to increased oxidative stress, decreased ATP production, increased aggregation of unfolded proteins, and then activated apoptotic pathway(s) that result in neuronal cell death (Betarbet et al. 2000), resembling dopaminergic neurodegeneration in PD.

In cultures of rat fetus mesencephalic neurons, 48 h exposure to rotenone caused dose-dependent neurotoxicity, more evident in dopaminergic neurons than in other neuronal cells. This result showed that dopaminergic neurons were more vulnerable to rotenone-induced neurotoxicity. Simultaneous administration of nicotine resulted in a dose-dependent increase of the viability of dopaminergic neurons. This neuroprotective effect was inhibited by 100 μM mecamylamine, a broad-spectrum nAChR antagonist, 100 nM αBuTx and 1 μM DHβE. Nicotine-induced neuroprotection was therefore shown to occur via nAChRs, especially through α7 and α4β2 receptors. Furthermore, nicotinic neuroprotection is inhibited by LY294002, a PI3K inhibitor, and triciribine, an AKT/PKB inhibitor. This means that nicotine could activate the PI3K-AKT/PKB pathways and increase the survival of mesencephalic dopaminergic cells against rotenone-induced cell death (Takeuchi et al. 2009). From our previous studies, it is known that the PI3K-AKT/PKB pathways would lead to subsequent upregulation of Bcl-2 and neuroprotection (Akaike et al. 2010; Shimohama 2009).

We confirmed that orally rotenone (30 mg/kg for 28 days)-treated mouse model showed motor deficits, dopaminergic cell death in the substantia nigra, and nerve terminal/axonal loss in the striatum. These findings are relevant to some previous reports on rotenone PD models (Schmidt and Alam 2006; Ravenstijn et al. 2008). Simultaneous subcutaneous administration of nicotine (0.21 mg/kg/day) prevented both motor deficits and dopaminergic neuronal cell loss in the substantia nigra of rotenone-treated mice.

8.3.2 nAChR Enhancement Show Dopaminergic Neuronal Protection Against 6-OHDA- Induced Hemiparkinsonian Rodent Model

6-hydroxydopamine (6-OHDA)'s strong neurotoxic effects were described by Ungerstedt in 1971, in a study presenting the first example of using a chemical agent to produce an animal model of PD (Ungerstedt 1971). Since 6-OHDA cannot cross over the BBB, systemic administration fails to induce parkinsonism. This induction model requires 6-OHDA to be injected into the SN, medial forebrain bundle, and striatum. The intrastriatal injection of 6-OHDA causes progressive retrograde neuronal degeneration in the VTA and substantia nigra.

Costa et al. evaluated the neuroprotection of nicotine in 6-OHDA-induced hemiparkinsonian rat model. They injected 6 μg 6-OHDA in the SN, and confirmed that the dopamine level in the corpus striatum was decreased nearly by half. Repeated subcutaneous nicotine administration at 4 h before and 20, 44 and 68 h after 6-OHDA injection significantly prevented the striatal dopamine loss and the protection reverted by nAChR antagonist. The protective effect was not achieved by one-off administration of nicotine before or after 6-OHDA injection (Costa et al. 2001).

Using rat 6-OHDA-induced hemiparkinsonian model, the neuroprotective effects of galantamine and nicotine were evaluated. 32 nmol 6-OHDA with or without 4–120 nmol galantamine and/or 120 nmol nicotine were injected into unilateral SN of rats. Although methamphetamine-stimulated rotational behavior and dopaminergic neuronal loss induced by 6-OHDA were not inhibited by galantamine alone, those were moderately inhibited by nicotine alone. In addition, 6-OHDA-induced neuronal loss and rotational behavior were synergistically inhibited by co-injection of galantamine and nicotine. These protective effects were abolished by mecamyla-

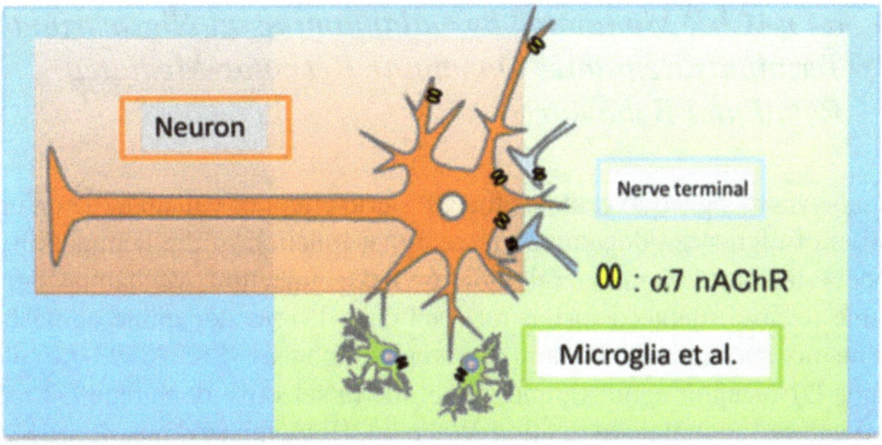

Fig. 8.4 Proposed pathway for nAChR-mediated neuronal protection: direct effect to neurons and indirect effect to microglia against 6-OHDA-induced hemiparkinsonian rodent model. We hypothesize that DMXBA simultaneously affects microglia and dopaminergic neurons and that both actions lead to dopaminergic neuroprotection

mine, a nAChR antagonist. α7nAChR was expressed on both dopaminergic and non-dopaminergic neurons in the rat substantia nigra pars compacta (SNpc). A combination of galantamine and nicotine greatly suppressed 6-OHDA-induced reduction of α7nAChR- immunopositive dopaminergic neurons. These results suggest that galantamine synergistically enhances the neuroprotective effect of nicotine against 6-OHDA-induced dopaminergic neuronal loss through an allosteric modulation of α7nAChR activation (Yanagida et al. 2008).

To explore a novel therapy against PD through enhancement of α7 nAChR, we evaluated the neuroprotective effects of DMXBA in a rat 6-OHDA-induced hemiparkinsonian model. Microinjection of 6-OHDA into the nigrostriatal pathway of rats destroys dopaminergic neurons selectively. DMXBA dose-dependently inhibited methamphetamine-stimulated rotational behavior and dopaminergic neuronal loss induced by 6-OHDA. The protective effects were abolished by methyllycaconitine citrate salt hydrate, an α7 nAChR antagonist. Immunohistochemical study confirmed abundant α7 nAChR expression in the cytoplasm of dopaminergic neurons. These results indicate that DMXBA prevented 6-OHDA-induced dopaminergic neuronal loss through stimulating α7 nAChR in dopaminergic neurons. Injection of 6-OHDA elevated immunoreactivities to glial markers such as ionized calcium binding adaptor molecule 1, CD68, and glial fibrillary acidic protein in the substantia nigra pars compacta of rats. In contrast, these immunoreactivities were markedly inhibited by comicroinjection of DMXBA. Microglia also expressed α7 nAChR in both resting and activated states. Hence, we hypothesize that DMXBA simultaneously affects microglia and dopaminergic neurons and that both actions lead to dopaminergic neuroprotection. The findings that DMXBA attenuates 6-OHDA-induced dopaminergic neurodegeneration and glial activation in a rat model of PD raise the possibility that DMXBA could be a novel therapeutic compound to prevent PD development (Suzuki et al. 2013) (Fig. 8.4).

8.3.3 α4 nAChR Modulated by Galantamine on Nigrostriatal Terminals Regulates Dopamine Receptor-Mediated Rotational Behavior

This study was designed to evaluate the allosteric effect of galantamine on nAChR regulation of nigrostrial dopaminergic neuronal function in the hemiparkinsonian rat model established by unilateral nigral 6-OHDA injection. Methamphetamine, a dopamine releaser, induced ipsilateral rotation, whereas dopamine agonists apomorphine (a non-selective dopamine receptor agonist), SKF38393 (a selective dopamine D1 receptor agonist), and quinpirole (a selective dopamine D2 receptor agonist) induced contralateral rotation. When 6-OHDA-injected rats were co-treated with nomifensine, a dopamine transporter inhibitor, a more pronounced and a remarkable effect of nicotine and galantamine was observed. Under these conditions, the combination of nomifensine with nicotine or galantamine induced the ipsilateral rotation similar to the methamphetamine-induced rotational behavior, indicating that nicotine and galantamine also induce dopamine release from striatal terminals. Both nicotine- and galantamine-induced rotations were significantly blocked by flupenthixol (an antagonist of both D1 and D2 dopamine receptors) and mecamylamine (an antagonist of nAChRs), suggesting that galantamine modulation of nAChRs on striatal dopaminergic terminals regulates dopamine receptor-mediated movement. Immunohistochemical staining showed that α4 nAChRs were highly expressed on striatal dopaminergic terminals, while no α7 nAChRs were detected. Pretreatment with DHβE significantly inhibited nicotine- and galantamine-induced rotational behaviors, whereas pretreatment with methyllycaconitine was ineffective. Moreover, the α4 nAChR agonist ABT-418 induced ipsilateral rotation, while the α7nAChR agonist PNU282987 had no significant effect on rotational behavior. These results suggest that galantamine can enhance striatal dopamine release through allosteric modulation of α4 nAChRs on nigrostriatal dopaminergic terminals (Inden et al. 2016).

8.3.4 Neuroprotective Effect of Nicotine in MPTP-Induced Parkinsonian Model

In 1979 and 1983, MPTP was initially identified as a strong neurotoxin when heroin addicts accidentally self-administered MPTP and developed an acute form of parkinsonism that was indistinguishable from idiopathic PD (Davis et al. 1979; Langston et al. 1983). The tragic results of MPTP poisoning in the heroin addicts led to the development of MPTP-induced rodent and non-human primate animal models of PD. Jeyarasasingam et al. reported exposure of rat primary mesencephalic cultures to 10^{-7} and 10^{-4} M nicotine partially protect against dopaminergic neurotoxicity induced by 1-methyl-4-phenylpyridinium (MPP^{+}). The optimal protective effect was observed when pre-exposure to nicotine for 24 h before administration of

MPP^+. They also showed the nicotine protection was mediated by non-α7 nAChR stimulation but not through α7 nAChR stimulation (Jeyarasasingam et al. 2002). Junyent et al. reported comparison of two prosurvival pathways, AKT pathway and JAK2/STAT3 pathway, in MPP^+ treated cerebellar granule cell culture. Their data indicated that the treatment of cerebellar granule cell with MPP^+ decreased both survival pathways. Loss of STAT3 could be a signal pathway involved in neuroprotection against the MPP^+, whereas AKT activation, using a PTEN inhibitor, did not play a prominent role in neuroprotection (Junyent et al. 2010).

In MPTP-induced animal model, the neuroprotective effect of nicotine is not consistent probably due to different experimental methods. Besides small number of negative reports (Behmand and Harik 1992), several independent groups confirmed the neuroprotective effects of nicotine against MPTP in rodents. The pretreatment of nicotine is essential and post treatment did not show any neuroprotective effect in MPTP-induced rat as well as in primate models. There are many reports attributing the neuroprotective effect of cigarette smoking against MPTP cytotoxicity to inhibition of monoamine oxidase B (MAO-B), which converts MPTP to active MPP^+. But because of the fact that nicotine does not inhibit brain MAO-B, the nicotinic neuroprotection against MPTP cytotoxicity is not mediated through MAO-B inhibition. A blockade of MPP^+ uptake into the dopaminergic cells via increased dopamine release may be the reason of the protective effect. Jasons et al. (1992) reported the chronic infusion of nicotine via minipumps produced a dose-related enhancement of MPTP-induced dopaminergic neurotoxicity in mouse, which might be caused by a failure of nAChRs to desensitized to the chronic nicotine exposure (Parain et al. 2001, 2003). Regarding to primate model, there have been only several papers from one group examining the nicotine-induced neuronal protection in MPTP-induced primate PD motor deficit model (Quik et al. 2006a, b; Bordia et al. 2006; Huang et al. 2009). In their reports, neuroprotection was observed only when nicotine is given orally before the MPTP exposure. Decamp and Schneider established stable cognitive deficit primate model injecting low dose of MPTP (0.025–0.10 mg/kg) over a period ranging from 98 to 158 days, without the confounding effect of significant motor impairment. They examined the effect of nicotine, l-dopa, and SIB-1553A, α4β4 nAChR agonist, on spatial delayed response task performance and reported that nicotine and SIB-1153A improved performance whereas l-dopa impaired (Decamp and Schneider 2009).

8.4 Neuroprotective Enhancement of nAChRs Through Four Pathways (Kawamata and Shimohama 2011)

1. PI3K/AKT pathway

Our studies showed that nAChR stimulation protected neurons from Aβ-, glutamate-, rotenone-, and 6-OHDA-induced neurotoxicity. From the experimental data, our hypothesis for the mechanism of nAChR-mediated survival signal transduction is as follows: activation of α7 nAChRs stimulates the Src family, which in turn activates PI3K. PI3K phosphorylates AKT, which causes upregulation of Bcl-2 and Bcl-x. α4β2 nAChR stimulation also causes neuroprotection cascade without direct involvement of PI3K system.

2. JAK2/STAT3 pathway

Other properties of nicotine proposed by other groups are anti-inflammatory potentials and modulating innate immune pathways mainly via α7 nAChR. Nicotine exerts its anti-inflammatory effect in activated immune cells, macrophages and microglia as well as neurons, by interacting α7 nAChR. Activated α7 nAChR binds directory to JAK2 and triggers the JAK2/STAT3 pathway to interfere with the activation of TLR-induced NF-κB, which is responsible for pro-inflammatory cytokine transcription (Cui and Li 2010).

3. MEK/ERK pathway

Importance of the MEK/ERK pathway in nicotinic neuroprotection has also been emphasized by several groups (Buckingham et al. 2009; Wang et al. 2003). Dajas-Bailador et al. reported nicotine stimulation leads to PKA activation through α7 nAChR and further Raf-1/MEK/ERK signaling pathway (Dajas-Bailador et al. 2002). Other group showed that stepwise activation of Ras/Raf-1/MEK/ERK cascade provides for an increased cytoplasmic concentration of STAT3 due to an up-regulated expression (Arredondo et al. 2006) activating the JAK2/STAT3 pathway in human oral keratonocytes.

4. Microglial CaM/CaMKII/Aβ phagocytosis pathway

In addition to known three neuroprotective pathways in neurons, we showed microglial Aβ clearance effect mediated through nAChRs enhancement should have special importance especially in AD therapy (Takata et al. 2010).

8.5 Conclusion

Targeting enhancement of nAChRs is one of the most practical therapeutic alternatives against AD to date. Based on epidemiological and experimental findings, clinical application of nicotinic enhancement against PD is also believed to be promising strategy different from ongoing dopamine replenish therapies. The underlying mechanisms of the neuroprotective effect induced by nicotinic stimulation were studied vigorously and three neuronal survival signal transductions have been elucidated as reviewed here. Recently microglial CaM/CaMKII/Aβ phagocytosis pathway is proved to be additional important neuroprotective pathway in AD models. Combined with other therapeutic methods under development, the enhancement of nAChRs would keep its position as safe and practical therapeutic alternatives against the progress of neurodegenerative disorders such as AD and PD.

Acknowledgements This work was supported in part by the Japan Society for the Promotion of Science (JSPS) KAKENHI Grant Number 15K09840 (J.K.) and 16H05279 (S.S.), the Orange-MCI from the Japan Agency for Medical Research and Development (AMED)(S.S.), and the Smoking Research Foundation (No. 1503837, S.S.).

References

Akaike A, Tamura Y, Yokota T, Shimohama S, Kimura J (1994) Nicotine-induced protection of cultured cortical neurons against N-methyl-D-aspartate receptor-mediated glutamate cytotoxicity. Brain Res 644:181–187

Akaike A, Takada-Takatori Y, Kume T, Izumi Y (2010) Mechanisms of neuroprotective effects of nicotine and acetylcholinesterase inhibitors: role of α4 and α7 receptors in neuroprotection. J Mol Neurosci 40:211–216

Arredondo J, Chernyavsky AI, Jolkovsky DL, Pinkerton KE, Grando SA (2006) Receptor-mediated tobacco toxicity: cooperation of the Ras/Raf-1/MEK1/ERK and JAK-2/STAT-3 pathways downstream of alpha7 nicotinic receptor in oral keratinocytes. FASEB J 20:2093–2101

Behmand RA, Harik SI (1992) Nicotine enhances 1-methyl-4-phenyl- 1,2,3,6- tetrahydropyridine neurotoxicity. J Neurochem 58:776–779

Betarbet R, Sherer TB, MacKenzie G, Garcia-Osuna M, Panov AV, Greenamyre JT (2000) Chronic systemic pesticide exposure reproduces features of Parkinson's disease. Nat Neurosci 3:1301–1306

Bigl V, Woolf NJ, Butcher LL (1982) Cholinergic projections from the basal forebrain to frontal, parietal, temporal, occipital, and cingulate cortices: a combined fluorescent tracer and acetylcholinesterase analysis. Brain Res Bull 8:205–211

Bordia T, Parameswaran N, Fan H, Langston JW, McIntosh JM, Quik M (2006) Partial recovery of striatal nicotinic receptors in 1-methyl-4-phenyl-1,2,3,6-tetrahydropyridine (MPTP)-lesioned monkeys with chronic oral nicotine. J Pharmacol Exp Ther 319:285–292

Bordia T, Grady SR, McIntosh JM, Quik M (2007) Nigrostriatal damage preferentially decreases a subpopulation of α6β2* nAChRs in mouse, monkey, and Parkinson's disease striatum. Mol Pharmacol 72:52–61

Buckingham SD, Jones AK, Brown LA, Sattelle DB (2009) Nicotinic acetylcholine receptor signalling: roles in Alzheimer's disease and amyloid neuroprotection. Pharmacol Rev 61:39–61

Champtiaux N, Gotti C, Cordero-Erausquin M, David DJ, Przybylski C, Léna C, Clementi F, Moretti M, Rossi FM, Le Novère N, McIntosh JM, Gardier AM, Changeux JP (2003) Subunit composition of functional nicotinic receptors in dopaminergic neurons investigated with knock-out mice. J Neurosci 23:7820–7829

Choi DW (1988) Calcium-mediated neurotoxicity: relationship to specific channel types and role in ischemic damage. Trends Neurosci 11:465–469

Citron M, Oltersdorf T, Haass C, McConlogue L, Hung AY, Seubert P, Vigo-Pelfrey C, Lieberburg I, Selkoe DJ (1992) Mutation of the β-amyloid precursor protein in familial Alzheimer's disease increases β-protein production. Nature 360:672–674

Clarke PB, Schwartz RD, Paul SM, Pert CB, Pert A (1985) Nicotinic binding in rat brain: autoradiographic comparison of [^{3}H]acetylcholine, [^{3}H]nicotine, and [^{125}I]-α-bungarotoxin. J Neurosci 5:1307–1315

Cormier A, Morin C, Zini R, Tillement J, Lagrue G (2003) Nicotine protects rat brain mitochondria against experimental injuries. Neuropharmacology 44:642–652

Costa G, Abin-Carriquiry JA, Dajas F (2001) Nicotine prevents striatal dopamine loss produced by 6-hydroxydopamine lesion in the substantia nigra. Brain Res 888:336–342

Court JA, Martin-Ruiz C, Graham A, Perry E (2000) Nicotinic receptors in human brain: topography and pathology. J Chem Neuroanat 20:281–298

Cui WY, Li MD (2010) Nicotinic modulation of innate immune pathways via α7 nicotinic acetylcholine receptor. J Neuroimmune Pharmacol 5:479–488

Dajas-Bailador FA, Soliakov L, Wonnacott S (2002) Nicotine activates the extracellular signal-regulated kinase 1/2 via the alpha7 nicotinic acetylcholine receptor and protein kinase A, in SH-SY5Y cells and hippocampal neurones. J Neurochem 80:520–530

Davis GC, Williams AC, Markey SP, Ebert MH, Caine ED, Reichert CM, Kopin IJ (1979) Chronic Parkinsonism secondary to intravenous injection of meperidine analogues. Psychiatry Res 1:249–254

Dawson VL, Dawson TM, London ED, Bredt DS, Snyder SH (1991) Nitric oxide mediates glutamate neurotoxicity in primary cortical cultures. Proc Natl Acad Sci U S A 88:6368–6371

De Fusco M, Becchetti A, Patrignani A, Annesi G, Gambardella A, Quattrone A, Ballabio A, Wanke E, Casari G (2000) The nicotinic receptor β2 subunit is mutant in nocturnal frontal lobe epilepsy. Nat Genet 26:275–276

De Reuck J, De Weweire M, Van Maele G, Santens P (2005) Comparison of age of onset and development of motor complications between smokers and non-smokers in Parkinson's disease. J Neurol Sci 231:35–39

Decamp E, Schneider JS (2009) Interaction between nicotinic and dopaminergic therapies on cognition in a chronic Parkinson model. Brain Res 1262:109–114

del Peso L, Gonzalez-Garcia M, Page C, Herrera R, Nunez G (1997) Interleukin-3-induced phosphorylation of BAD through the protein kinase Akt. Science 278:687–689

Dineley KT, Xia X, Bui D, Sweatt JD, Zheng H (2002) Accelerated plaque accumulation, associative learning deficits, and up-regulation of α7 nicotinic receptor protein in transgenic mice co-expressing mutant human presenilin 1 and amyloid precursor proteins. J Biol Chem 277:22768–22780

Dorn HF (1959) Tobacco consumption and mortality from cancer and other diseases. Public Health Rep 74:581–593

Drenan RM, Grady SR, Whiteaker P, McClure-Begley T, McKinney S, Miwa JM, Bupp S, Heintz N, McIntosh JM, Bencherif M, Marks MJ, Lester HA (2008) In vivo activation of midbrain dopamine neurons via sensitized, high-affinity α6 nicotinic acetylcholine receptors. Neuron 60:123–136

Du F, Li R, Huang Y, Li X, Le W (2005) Dopamine D3 receptor-preferring agonists induce neurotrophic effects on mesencephalic dopamine neurons. Eur J Neurosci 22:2422–2430

Fujita M, Ichise M, Zoghbi SS, Liow JS, Ghose S, Vines DC, Sangare J, Lu JQ, Cropley VL, Iida H, Kim KM, Cohen RM, Bara-Jimenez W, Ravina B, Innis RB (2006) Widespread decrease of nicotinic acetylcholine receptors in Parkinson's disease. Ann Neurol 59:174–177

Giannakopoulos P, Hof PR, Kövari E, Vallet PG, Herrmann FR, Bouras C (1996) Distinct patterns of neuronal loss and Alzheimer's disease lesion distribution in elderly individuals older than 90 years. J Neuropathol Exp Neurol 55:1210–1220

Gotti C, Fornasari D, Clementi F (1997) Human neuronal nicotinic receptors. Prog Neurobiol 53:199–237

Grady SR, Salminen O, Laverty DC, Whiteaker P, McIntosh JM, Collins AC, Marks MJ (2007) The subtypes of nicotinic acetylcholine receptors on dopaminergic terminals of mouse striatum. Biochem Pharmacol 74:1235–1246

Guan ZZ, Nordberg A, Mousavi M, Rinne JO, Hellström-Lindahl E (2002) Selective changes in the levels of nicotinic acetylcholine receptor protein and of corresponding mRNA species in the brains of patients with Parkinson's disease. Brain Res 956:358–366

Hardy J (2010) Genetic analysis of pathways to Parkinson disease. Neuron 68:201–206

Harris ME, Wang Y, Pedigo NWJ, Hensley K, Butterfield DA, Carney JM (1996) Amyloid β peptide (25–35) inhibits Na^+-dependent glutamate uptake in rat hippocampal astrocyte cultures. J Neurochem 67:277–286

Hartley DM, Choi DW (1989) Delayed rescue of *N*-methyl-D-aspartate receptor-mediated neuronal injury in cortical culture. J Pharmacol Exp Ther 250:752–758

Huang LZ, Parameswaran N, Bordia T, Michael McIntosh J, Quik M (2009) Nicotine is neuroprotective when administered before but not after nigrostriatal damage in rats and monkeys. J Neurochem 109:826–837

Hunter BE, de Fiebre CM, Papke RL, Kem WR, Meyer EM (1994) A novel nicotinic agonist facilitates induction of long-term potentiation in the rat hippocampus. Neurosci Lett 168:130–134

Hwang J, Hwang H, Lee HW, Suk K (2010) Microglia signaling as a target of donepezil. Neuropharmacology 58:1122–1129

Inden M, Kitamura Y, Takeuchi H, Yanagida T, Takata K, Kobayashi Y, Taniguchi T, Yoshimoto K, Kaneko M, Okuma Y, Taira T, Ariga H, Shimohama S (2007) Neurodegeneration of mouse nigrostriatal dopaminergic system induced by repeated oral administration of rotenone is prevented by 4-phenylbutyrate, a chemical chaperone. J Neurochem 101:1491–1504

Inden M, Takata K, Yanagisawa D, Ashihara E, Tooyama I, Shimohama S, Kitamura Y (2016) α4 nicotinic acetylcholine receptor modulated by galantamine on nigrostriatal terminals regulates dopamine receptor-mediated rotational behavior. Neurochem Int 94:74–81

Iravani M, Haddon C, Cooper J, Jenner P, Schapira A (2006) Pramipexole protects against MPTP toxicity in non-human primates. J Neurochem 96:1315–1321

Janson AM, Fuxe K, Goldstein M (1992) Differential effects of acute and chronic nicotine treatment on MPTP-(1-methyl-4-phenyl-1,2,3,6-tetrahydropyridine) induced degeneration of nigrostriatal dopamine neurons in the black mouse. Clin Investig 70:232–238

Jensen M, Schröder J, Blomberg M, Engvall B, Pantel J, Ida N, Basun H, Wahlund LO, Werle E, Jauss M, Beyreuther K, Lannfelt L, Hartmann T (1999) Cerebrospinal fluid Aβ42 is increased early in sporadic Alzheimer's disease and declines with disease progression. Ann Neurol 45:504–511

Jeyarasasingam G, Tompkins L, Quik M (2002) Stimulation of non-α7 nicotinic receptors partially protects dopaminergic neurons from 1-methyl-4-phenylpyridinium-induced toxicity in culture. Neuroscience 109:275–285

Junyent F, Alvira D, Yeste-Velasco M, de la Torre AV, Beas-Zarate C, Sureda FX, Folch J, Pallàs M, Camins A, Verdaguer E (2010) Prosurvival role of JAK/STAT and Akt signaling pathways in MPP^+-induced apoptosis in neurons. Neurochem Int 57:774–782

Kaneko S, Maeda T, Kume T, Kochiyama H, Akaike A, Shimohama S, Kimura J (1997) Nicotine protects cultured cortical neurons against glutamate-induced cytotoxicity via α7-neuronal receptors and neuronal CNS receptors. Brain Res 765:135–140

Kawamata J, Shimohama S (2002) Association of novel and established polymorphisms in neuronal nicotinic acetylcholine receptors with sporadic Alzheimer's disease. J Alzheimers Dis 4:71–76

Kawamata J, Shimohama S (2011) Stimulating nicotinic receptors trigger multiple pathways attenuating cytotoxicity in models of Alzheimer's and Parkinson's diseases. J Alzheimers Dis 24(Suppl 2):95–109

Kihara T, Shimohama S, Sawada H, Kimura J, Kume T, Kochiyama H, Maeda T, Akaike A (1997) Nicotinic receptor stimulation protects neurons against β-amyloid toxicity. Ann Neurol 42:159–163

Kihara T, Shimohama S, Urushitani M, Sawada H, Kimura J, Kume T, Maeda T, Akaike A (1998) Stimulation of α4β2 nicotinic acetylcholine receptors inhibits β-amyloid toxicity. Brain Res 792:331–334

Kihara T, Shimohama S, Honda K, Shibasaki H, Akaike A (2000) Neuroprotective effect of nicotinic agonists via PI3 kinase cascade against glutamate cytotoxicity enhanced by β amyloid. Neurology 54(Suppl 3):A367

Kihara T, Shimohama S, Sawada H, Honda K, Nakamizo T, Shibasaki H, Kume T, Akaike A (2001) α7 nicotinic receptor transduces signals to phosphatidylinositol 3-kinase to block A β-amyloid-induced neurotoxicity. J Biol Chem 276:13541–13546

Kihara T, Sawada H, Nakamizo T, Kanki R, Yamashita H, Maelicke A, Shimohama S (2004) Galantamine modulates nicotinic receptor and blocks Aβ-enhanced glutamate toxicity. Biochem Biophys Res Commun 325:976–982

Langston JW, Ballard P, Tetrud JW, Irwin I (1983) Chronic Parkinsonism in humans due to a product of meperidine-analog synthesis. Science 219:979–980

Le Novère N, Zoli M, Changeux JP (1996) Neuronal nicotinic receptor α 6 subunit mRNA is selectively concentrated in catecholaminergic nuclei of the rat brain. Eur J Neurosci 8:2428–2439

Lindstrom J, Anand R, Peng X, Gerzanich V, Wang F, Li Y (1995) Neuronal nicotinic receptor subtypes. Ann N Y Acad Sci 757:100–116

Maelicke A, Samochocki M, Jostock R, Fehrenbacher A, Ludwig J, Albuquerque EX, Zerlin M (2001) Allosteric sensitization of nicotinic receptors by galantamine, a new treatment strategy for Alzheimer's disease. Biol Psychiatry 49:279–288

Mann V, Cooper J, Krige D, Daniel S, Schapira A, Marsden C (1992) Brain, skeletal muscle and platelet homogenate mitochondrial function in Parkinson's disease. Brain 115(Pt. 2):333–342

Maragos WF, Greenamyre JT, Penney JB, Young AB (1986) Glutamate dysfunction in Alzheimer's disease: an hypothesis. Trends Neurosci 10:65–68

Matsumura A, Suzuki S, Iwahara N, Hisahara S, Kawamata J, Suzuki H, Yamauchi A, Takata K, Kitamura Y, Shimohama S (2015) Temporal changes of CD68 and α7 nicotinic acetylcholine receptor expression in microglia in Alzheimer's disease-like mouse models. J Alzheimers Dis 44:409–423

Matsuzaki H, Tamatani M, Mitsuda N, Namikawa K, Kiyama H, Miyake S, Tohyama M (1999) Activation of Akt kinase inhibits apoptosis and changes in Bcl-2 and Bax expression induced by nitric oxide in primary hippocampal neurons. J Neurochem 73:2037–2046

Mattson MP (1988) Neurotransmitters in the regulation of neuronal cytoarchitecture. Brain Res Rev 13:179–212

Meldrum B, Garthwaite J (1990) Excitatory amino acid neurotoxicity and neurodegenerative disease. Trends Pharmacol Sci 11:379–387

Mesulam MM, Mufson EJ, Levey AI, Wainer BH (1983) Cholinergic innervation of cortex by the basal forebrain: cytochemistry and cortical connections of the septal area, diagonal band nuclei, nucleus basalis (substantia innominata) and hypothalamus in the rhesus monkey. J Comp Neurol 214:170–197

Meyer EM, Tay ET, Papke RL, Meyers C, Huang GL, de Fiebre CM (1997) 3-[2,4-Dimethoxybenzylidene]anabaseine (DMXB) selectively activates rat α7 receptors and improves memory-related behaviors in a mecamylamine-sensitive manner. Brain Res 768:49–56

Mizuno Y, Yoshino H, Ikebe S, Hattori N, Kobayashi T, Shimoda-Matsubayashi S, Matsumine H, Kondo T (1998) Mitochondrial dysfunction in Parkinson's disease. Ann Neurol 44(3 Suppl 1):S99–S109

Morens D, Grandinetti A, Reed D, White L, Ross G (1995) Cigarette smoking and protection from Parkinson's disease: false association or etiologic clue? Neurology 45:1041–1051

Obeso JA, Rodriguez-Oroz MC, Goetz CG, Marin C, Kordower JH, Rodriguez M, Hirsch EC, Farrer M, Schapira AH, Halliday G (2010) Missing pieces in the Parkinson's disease puzzle. Nat Med 16:653–661

Parain K, Marchand V, Dumery B, Hirsch E (2001) Nicotine, but not cotinine, partially protects dopaminergic neurons against MPTP-induced degeneration in mice. Brain Res 890:347–350

Parain K, Hapdey C, Rousselet E, Marchand V, Dumery B, Hirsch EC (2003) Cigarette smoke and nicotine protect dopaminergic neurons against the 1-methyl-4-phenyl-1,2,3,6-tetrahydropyridine Parkinsonian toxin. Brain Res 984:224–232

Parker W Jr, Boyson S, Parks J (1989) Abnormalities of the electron transport chain in idiopathic Parkinson's disease. Ann Neurol 26:719–723

Quik M (2004) Smoking, nicotine and Parkinson's disease. Trends Neurosci 27:561–568

Quik M, Chen L, Parameswaran N, Xie X, Langston J, McCallum SE (2006a) Chronic oral nicotine normalizes dopaminergic function and synaptic plasticity in 1-methyl-4-phenyl-1,2,3,6-tetrahydropyridine-lesioned primates. J Neurosci 26:4681–4689

Quik M, Parameswaran N, McCallum SE, Bordia T, Bao S, McCormack A, Kim A, Tyndale RF, Langston JW, Di Monte DA (2006b) Chronic oral nicotine treatment protects against striatal degeneration in MPTP-treated primates. J Neurochem 98:1866–1875

Raskind MA, Peskind ER, Truyen L, Kershaw P, Damaraju CV (2004) The cognitive benefits of galantamine are sustained for at least 36 months: a long-term extension trial. Arch Neurol 61:252–256

Ravenstijn PG, Merlini M, Hameetman M, Murray TK, Ward MA, Lewis H, Ball G, Mottart C, de Ville de Goyet C, Lemarchand T, van Belle K, O'Neill MJ, Danhof M, de Lange EC (2008) The exploration of rotenone as a toxin for inducing Parkinson's disease in rats, for application in BBB transport and PK-PD experiments. J Pharmacol Toxicol Methods 57:114–130

Rosser MN, Svendsen C, Hunt SP, Mounjoy CQ, Roth M, Iversen LL (1982) The substantia innominata in Alzheimer's disease: a histochemical and biochemical study of cholinergic marker enzymes. Neurosci Lett 28:217–222

Schmidt WJ, Alam M (2006) Controversies on new animal models of Parkinson's disease pro and con: the rotenone model of Parkinson's disease (PD). J Neural Transm Suppl 70:273–276

Shen H, Kihara T, Hongo H, Wu X, Kem WR, Shimohama S, Akaike A, Niidome T, Sugimoto H (2010) Neuroprotection by donepezil against glutamate excitotoxicity involves stimulation of α7 nicotinic receptors and internalization of NMDA receptors. Br J Pharmacol 161:127–139

Shimohama S (2009) Nicotinic receptor-mediated neuroprotection in neurodegenerative disease models. Biol Pharm Bull 32:332–336

Shimohama S, Taniguchi T, Fujiwara M, Kameyama M (1986) Changes in nicotinic and muscarinic cholinergic receptors in Alzheimer-type dementia. J Neurochem 46:288–293

Shimohama S, Akaike A, Kimura J (1996) Nicotine-induced protection against glutamate cytotoxicity. Nicotinic cholinergic receptor-mediated inhibition of nitric oxide formation. Ann N Y Acad Sci 777:356–361

Shimohama S, Greenwald DL, Shafron DH, Akaika A, Maeda T, Kaneko S, Kimura J, Simpkins CE, Day AL, Meyer EM (1998) Nicotinic α7 receptors protect against glutamate neurotoxicity and neuronal ischemic damage. Brain Res 779:359–363

Shimohama S, Sawada H, Kitamura Y, Taniguchi T (2003) Disease model: Parkinson's disease. Trends Mol Med 9:360–365

Sidransky E, Nalls MA, Aasly JO, Aharon-Peretz J, Annesi G, Barbosa ER, Bar-Shira A, Berg D, Bras J, Brice A, Chen CM, Clark LN, Condroyer C, De Marco EV, Dürr A, Eblan MJ, Fahn S, Farrer MJ, Fung HC, Gan-Or Z, Gasser T, Gershoni-Baruch R, Giladi N, Griffith A, Gurevich T, Januario C, Kropp P, Lang AE, Lee-Chen GJ, Lesage S, Marder K, Mata IF, Mirelman A, Mitsui J, Mizuta I, Nicoletti G, Oliveira C, Ottman R, Orr-Urtreger A, Pereira LV, Quattrone A, Rogaeva E, Rolfs A, Rosenbaum H, Rozenberg R, Samii A, Samaddar T, Schulte C, Sharma M, Singleton A, Spitz M, Tan EK, Tayebi N, Toda T, Troiano AR, Tsuji S, Wittstock M, Wolfsberg TG, Wu YR, Zabetian CP, Zhao Y, Ziegler SG (2009) Multicenter analysis of glucocerebrosidase mutations in Parkinson's disease. N Engl J Med 361:1651–1661

Steinlein OK, Mulley JC, Propping P, Wallace RH, Phillips HA, Sutherland GR, Scheffer IE, Berkovic SF (1995) A missense mutation in the neuronal nicotinic acetylcholine receptor α4 subunit is associated with autosomal dominant nocturnal frontal lobe epilepsy. Nat Genet 11:201–203

Suzuki S, Kawamata J, Matsushita T, Matsumura A, Hisahara S, Takata K, Kitamura Y, Kem W, Shimohama S (2013) 3-[(2,4-Dimethoxy)benzylidene]-anabaseine dihydrochloride protects against 6-hydroxydopamine-induced parkinsonian neurodegeneration through α7 nicotinic acetylcholine receptor stimulation in rats. J Neurosci Res 91:462–471

Takata K, Kitamura Y, Saeki M, Terada M, Kagitani S, Kitamura R, Fujikawa Y, Maelicke A, Tomimoto H, Taniguchi T, Shimohama S (2010) Galantamine-induced amyloid-β clearance mediated via stimulation of microglial nicotinic acetylcholine receptors. J Biol Chem 285:40180–40191

Takeuchi H, Yanagida T, Inden M, Takata K, Kitamura Y, Yamakawa K, Sawada H, Izumi Y, Yamamoto N, Kihara T, Uemura K, Inoue H, Taniguchi T, Akaike A, Takahashi R, Shimohama

S (2009) Nicotinic receptor stimulation protects nigral dopaminergic neurons in rotenone-induced Parkinson's disease models. J Neurosci Res 87:576–585
Tomita T, Maruyama K, Saido TC, Kume H, Shinozaki K, Tokuhiro S, Capell A, Walter J, Grünberg J, Haass C, Iwatsubo T, Obata K (1997) The presenilin 2 mutation (N141I) linked to familial Alzheimer disease (Volga German families) increases the secretion of amyloid β protein ending at the 42nd (or 43rd) residue. Proc Natl Acad Sci U S A 94:2025–2030
Ungerstedt U (1971) Postsynaptic supersensitivity after 6-hydroxy-dopamine induced degeneration of the nigro-striatal dopamine system. Acta Physiol Scand 367(Suppl):69–93
Villafane G, Cesaro P, Rialland A, Baloul S, Azimi S, Bourdet C, Le Houezec J, Macquin-Mavier I, Maison P (2007) Chronic high dose transdermal nicotine in Parkinson's disease: an open trial. Eur J Neurol 12:1313–1316
Wang HY, Lee DH, D'Andrea MR, Peterson PA, Shank RP, Reitz AB (2000) β-Amyloid(1-42) binds to α7 nicotinic acetylcholine receptor with high affinity. Implications for Alzheimer's disease pathology. J Biol Chem 275:5626–5632
Wang HY, Li W, Benedetti NJ, Lee DH (2003) α7 nicotinic acetylcholine receptors mediate β-amyloid peptide-induced tau protein phosphorylation. J Biol Chem 278:31547–31553
Whitehouse PJ, Kalaria RN (1995) Nicotinic receptors and neurodegenerative dementing diseases: basic research and clinical implications. Alzheimer Dis Assoc Disord 9:3–5
Whitehouse PJ, Price DL, Clark AW, Coyle TT, Delong M (1981) Alzheimer's disease: evidence for a selective loss of cholinergic neurons in the nucleus basalis. Ann Neurol 10:122–126
Wirdefeldt K, Gatz M, Pawitan Y, Pedersen N (2005) Risk and protective factors for Parkinson's disease: a study in Swedish twins. Ann Neurol 57:27–33
Xie Y, Bezard E, Zhao B (2005) Investigating the receptor-independent neuroprotective mechanisms of nicotine in mitochondria. J Biol Chem 280:32405–32412
Yanagida T, Takeuchi H, Kitamura Y, Takata K, Minamino H, Shibaike T, Tsushima J, Kishimoto K, Yasui H, Taniguchi T, Shimohama S (2008) Synergistic effect of galantamine on nicotine-induced neuroprotection in hemiparkinsonian rat model. Neurosci Res 62:254–261
Yankner BA, Duffy LK, Kirschner DA (1990) Neurotrophic and neurotoxic effects of amyloid β protein: reversal by tachykinin neuropeptides. Science 250:279–282
Zhong LT, Kane DJ, Bredesen DE (1993) BCL-2 blocks glutamate toxicity in neural cell lines. Mol Brain Res 19:353–355

Chapter 9
SAK3-Induced Neuroprotection Is Mediated by Nicotinic Acetylcholine Receptors

Kohji Fukunaga and Yasushi Yabuki

Abstract Cholinergic neurotransmission plays a critical role in neuronal plasticity and cell survival in the central nervous system (CNS). Two types of acetylcholine receptors (AChRs), muscarinic AChRs (mAChRs) and nicotinic AChRs (nAChRs), trigger intracellular signaling through G protein activity and ion influx, respectively. To assess mechanisms underlying neuroprotection through nAChRs, we developed SAK3, a novel modulator of nAChR activity. Recently, we found that SAK3 enhances T-type calcium channel activity, promoting ACh release in the hippocampal CA1 region of olfactory-bulbectomized mice. Here, we observed potent SAK3 neuroprotective activity in mice with 20-min bilateral common carotid artery occlusion (BCCAO) or hypothyroidism. Treatment of mice with the α7 nAChR-selective inhibitor methyllycaconitine (0.5 mg/kg/day, p.o.) antagonized SAK3-mediated neuroprotection and memory improvement in BCCAO mice. Single administration of the anti-Graves' disease therapeutic methimazole (MMI) to female mice disrupted olfactory bulb (OB) glomerular structure, and cholinergic neurons largely disappeared in the medial septum followed by memory loss. Chronic SAK3 (0.5–1 mg/kg, p.o.) administration significantly rescued the number of cholinergic medial septum neurons in MMI-treated mice and improved cognitive deficits seen in those mice. Overall, our study suggests that, in mice, the novel nAChR modulator SAK3 can rescue neurons impaired by transient ischemia and hypothyroidism. We also address mechanisms common to SAK3-induced neuroprotection in both conditions.

Keywords Nicotinic acetylcholine receptor · T-type calcium channel · Neuroprotection · Ischemia · Hypothyroidism · Methimazole · Memory · Alzheimer's disease

---

K. Fukunaga (✉) · Y. Yabuki
Department of Pharmacology, Graduate School of Pharmaceutical Sciences, Tohoku University, Sendai, Japan
e-mail: kfukunaga@m.tohoku.ac.jp

A. Akaike et al. (eds.), *Nicotinic Acetylcholine Receptor Signaling in Neuroprotection*, https://doi.org/10.1007/978-981-10-8488-1_9

Abbreviations

Aβ	Amyloid-β
ACh	Acetylcholine
Akt	Protein kinase B
BCCAO	Bilateral common carotid artery occlusion
CNS	Central nervous system
DhβE	Dihydro-β-erythroidine
ERK	Extracellular signal-regulated kinase
HO-1	Heme-oxygenase 1
JAK2	Janus-activated kinase 2
MEC	Mecamylamine
MMI	Methimazole
MLA	Methyllycaconitine
mAChR	Muscarinic ACh receptor
nAChR	Nicotinic ACh receptor
OBX	Olfactory-bulbectomized
PI3K	Phosphatidylinositol 3 kinase
PKC	Protein kinase C
RGC	Retinal ganglion cell
SAK3	Ethyl 8'-methyl-2',4-dioxo-2- (piperidin-1-yl)-2'H-spiro[cyclopentane-1,3'-imidazo[1,2-a]pyridin]-2-ene-3-carboxylate
ST101	Spiro[imidazo[1,2-a] pyridine-3,2-indan]-2(3H)-one

9.1 Introduction

Acetylcholine (ACh) is a major neurotransmitter in the central nervous system (CNS) and transduces signals via two types of ACh receptors (AChRs): muscarinic (mAChRs) and nicotinic (nAChRs). While mAChRs are G-protein-coupled, nAChRs are ligand-gated cation channels consisting of five subunits (Zdanowski et al. 2015). Both AChR pathways function in learning and memory (Melancon et al. 2013; Pandya and Yakel 2013) and play a critical role in cell survival in in vitro and in vivo models (Akaike et al. 2010; Tan et al. 2014; Zdanowski et al. 2015). Drugs that enhance ACh concentration in the CNS, including the acetylcholine esterase (AChE) inhibitors donepezil, galantamine and rivastigmine, are among widely used therapeutics used to treat early stage Alzheimer's Disease (AD). However, it remains unclear whether the effects of AChE inhibitors are mediated by nAChRs or mAChRs in human brain. We recently developed the lead compound of the AD therapeutic SAK3 (ethyl 8′-methyl-2′,4-dioxo-2-(piperidin-1-yl)-2′H-spiro[cyclopentane-1,3′-imidazo[1,2 a]pyridin] -2-ene-3-carboxylate) (Yabuki et al. 2017a, b). SAK3 primarily stimulates T-type voltage gated Ca^{2+} channels in brain, and importantly it enhances ACh release in hippocampus, thereby improving memory in olfactory-bulbectomized (OBX) mice. We found that SAK3 effects on ACh release and memory improvement were antagonized by nAChR inhibitors, suggesting that SAK3 modulates nAChR. This review focuses primarily on SAK3 neuroprotective activity mediated by nicotinic cholinergic pathways.

9.2 Neuroprotection Mediated by mAChRs

Subchronic treatment with the acetylcholinesterase inhibitor galantamine (3.5 mg/kg, i.p.) prevents cell death and axonal injury after ocular hypertension surgery in rat retinal ganglion cells (RGCs), an effect blocked by the non-selective mAChR antagonist scopolamine, the M1-type mAChR antagonist pirenzepine, or the M4-type mAChR antagonist tropicamide, but not by nAChR inhibitors (Almasieh et al. 2010). In agreement with these results, the M1-type mAChR agonist pilocarpine protects RGCs from glutamate-induced neurotoxicity and ischemia/reperfusion injury in rat primary retinal cultures and in rat retina (Tan et al. 2014). M1-type mAChR activation in PC12 cells promotes protein kinase C (PKC) activity and inhibits glycogen synthase kinase-3β (GSK-3β) activity, thereby increasing levels of NF-E2-related factor-2 (Nrf2) protein, which regulates transcription of the gene encoding the anti-oxidant protein hemeoxygenase I (HO-1) (Espada et al. 2009; Ma et al. 2013). Therefore, activation of that anti-oxidant pathway through Nrf2 stimulation likely underlies mAChR-dependent neuroprotection. Likewise, the M1-type mAChR-selective agonist AF267B rescues rat primary hippocampal neurons exposed to amyloid-β (Aβ) from cell death by inhibiting increases in GSK-3β (Farías et al. 2004). On the other hand, the mAChR antagonist scopolamine does not block neuroprotection by acetylcholinesterase inhibitors on glutamate (1 mM) toxicity in primary rat cortical neurons (Takada-Takatori et al. 2009). Thus, how mAChRs promote neuroprotection is not entirely clear.

9.3 Neuroprotective Action Mediated by nAChRs

Nine different nAChR subunits (α2-7 and β2-4) are expressed in mammalian brain, and in mouse brain major nAChRs are comprised of homomeric α7 AChR and heteromeric α4β2 complexes (Dani and Bertrand 2007; Dineley et al. 2015; Yakel 2013). Many studies in cultured neurons support the idea that nAChRs have neuroprotective effects. For example, nicotine (10 μM) treatment protects cultured rat primary cortical neurons from cell death by glutamate (1 mM) exposure by activating α4β2 and α7 nAChRs (Kaneko et al. 1997). In addition, the α4β2 inhibitor dihydro-β-erythroidine (DHβE) and α7 inhibitor methyllycaconitine (MLA) both block neuroprotective effects of acetylcholinesterase inhibitors on glutamate (1 mM)-induced excitotoxicity in cultured neurons, an effect not seen following treatment of cells with the mAChR antagonist scopolamine (Takada-Takatori et al.

2009). In vivo, galantamine treatment prevents death of gerbil hippocampal CA1 pyramidal neurons following transient bilateral common carotid artery occlusion (BCCAO), an effect blocked by the non-selective nAChR inhibitor mecamylamine (MEC) (Lorrio et al. 2007). Combined neostigmine and anisodamine treatment are neuroprotective against middle cerebral artery occlusion in wild type- but not in α7 nAChR knock-out mice (Qian et al. 2015). We recently observed that the acetylcholinesterase inhibitor donepezil antagonizes loss of cholinergic neurons in the medial septum (MS) of OBX mice through nAChR stimulation (Yamamoto and Fuknaga 2013). In addition, Hijioka et al. (2012) reported that the α7-specific agonist PNU-282987 but not the α4-specific agonist RJR-2403 blocks neuronal loss following intracerebral hemorrhage in mouse striatum. Since MEC, DHβE and MLA do not block neuroprotective effects of galantamine following ocular hypertension surgery in rat RGCs, neuroprotection mediated by nAChRs may play a more predominant role in CNS than in peripheral neurons. We previously reported that galantamine stimulates glutamatergic and GABAnergic synaptic transmission via nAChR stimulation in rat cortical neurons (Moriguchi et al. 2009). Interestingly, galantamine increases hippocampal insulin-like growth factor 2 expression via the α7 nAChR in mice (Kita et al. 2013). Similarly, stimulation of α7 by the selective agonist PHA-543613 or galantamine treatment enhances α7 channel activity and improves Aβ-induced cognitive deficits in mice (Sadigh-Eteghad et al. 2015). In addition, galantamine treatment promotes survival of newborn neurons in the hippocampal dentate gyrus (DG) viaα7 nAChR but not via M1 mAChR activity (Kita et al. 2014). Taken together, the neuroprotective effect of galantamine is mediated both by mAChRs and nAChRs in the CNS.

9.4 Development of the Novel nAChR Modulator SAK3

T-type calcium channels, which are encoded by the *CACNA1G* (Cav3.1), *CACNA1H* (Cav3.2) and *CACNA1I* (Cav3.3), are voltage-gated calcium channels that give rise to low-threshold calcium spikes, which in turn trigger burst firing mediated by sodium channels in many neurons (Huguenard 1996; Perez-Reyes 2003). Recently, we found that a novel AD therapeutic candidate, ST101 (spiro[imidazo[1,2-a] pyridine-3,2-indan]-2(3H)-one), increases Cav3.1 T-type calcium channel currents (Moriguchi et al. 2012). ST101 accelerated ACh release in the hippocampus of OBX mice, an effect inhibited by the T-type calcium channel blocker mibefradil and by nAChR inhibitors (Yamamoto et al. 2013). Moreover, intraventricular injection of mecamylamine inhibited ST101-elicited neurogenesis in the hippocampal DG of OBX mice (Shioda et al. 2010), suggesting that ST101 may activate nAChR and promote ACh release. However, clinical trials showed that administration of ST101 alone was not sufficient to improve memory deficits in AD patients (Gauthier et al. 2015). Therefore, we sought a more potent Cav3.1 and Cav3.3 T-type calcium channel enhancer, resulting in development of SAK3 (Yabuki et al. 2017b). We found that SAK3 promoted more potent ACh release in mouse hippocampal CA1 than did ST101 (Yabuki et al. 2017b).

9.5 SAK3-Induced Neuroprotection in Brain Ischemia

We confirmed SAK3 neuroprotection using a 20-min BCCAO mouse model. To do so, we administered SAK3 (at 0.1, 0.5 or 1.0 mg/kg, p.o.) orally to mice 24 h after BCCAO ischemia. SAK3 administration at 0.5 or 1.0 mg/kg/day significantly blocked loss of hippocampal CA1 neurons and memory deficits seen in BCCAO mice. Treatment with the α7 nAChR-selective inhibitor methyllycaconitine (MLA: 6.0 mg/kg/day, i.p.) antagonized both neuroprotection and memory improvement seen in SAK3 (0.5 mg/kg/day, p.o.)-treated mice (Fig. 9.1). Since excess calcium influx enhances excitotoxic and proapoptotic pathways to induce ischemic neuronal death (Berliocchi et al. 2005; Bano and Nicotera 2007), the impact of T-type channel regulators on neuroprotection is unclear. For example, intraventricular injection of mibefradil and pimozide 6 h before 10-min BCCAO ischemia antagonizes hippocampal injury in rats (Bancila et al. 2011). Other T-type calcium channel blockers, such as U-92032 and flunarizine, administered 1 h prior to BCCAO inhibit delayed neuronal death in the gerbil hippocampal CA1 region (Ito et al. 1994). Such varied effects of T-type calcium channel blockers may be due to differences in timing of drug administration. We administered SAK3 to animals 24 h after BCCAO, whereas others have administered T-type calcium channel blockers before brain ischemia (Bancila et al. 2011; Ito et al. 1994). Moreover, some T-type calcium channel inhibitors, such as mibefradil and flunarizine have affinities to other channel types such as L-type calcium, sodium or potassium channels (Liu et al. 1999; Bloc et al. 2000; McNulty and Hanck 2004). Therefore, SAK3 is neuroprotective against brain ischemia by a mechanism that differs from that of other drugs.

9.6 SAK3 Ameliorates Methimazole-Induced Cholinergic Neuronal Damage

The drug methimazole (MMI) is widely used to antagonize hyperthyroidism and manage Graves' disease, an autoimmune condition promoting hyperthyroidism (Cano-Europa et al. 2011; Wu et al. 2013). Biochemically, MMI acts by preventing iodine incorporation into the thyroid hormone precursor, thyroglobulin, and thus interferes with conversion of thyroxine (T4) to triiodothyronine (T3) (Cooper 1984; Amara et al. 2012; Parisa and Fahimeh 2015). Importantly, treatment with moderate doses of MMI reportedly impairs olfactory function in rats, while high doses cause complete destruction of the olfactory epithelium (OE) (Genter et al. 1995). The OE is a critical site of regeneration of physically- or chemically-injured olfactory sensory neurons (OSNs) (Schwob et al. 1992; Suzukawa et al. 2011). Thyroid hormone deficiency also causes significantly reduced levels of choline acetyltransferase (ChAT), a marker of cholinergic neurons, in various brain regions (Kojima et al. 1981; Oh et al. 1991; Sawin et al. 1998). Since cholinergic neurons in the MS innervate the olfactory bulb and hippocampus (Mesulam et al. 1983a), olfactory

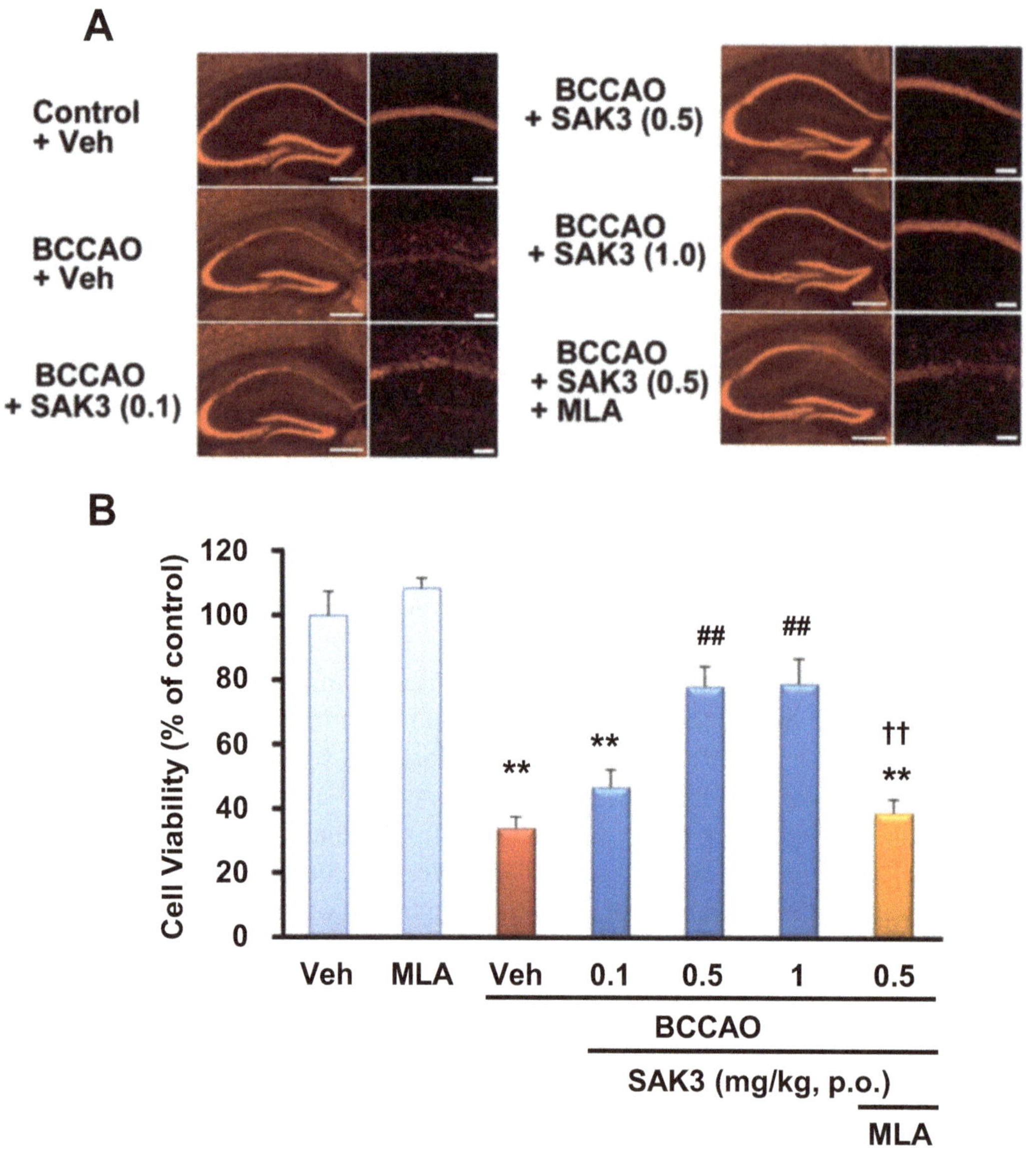

Fig. 9.1 Oral SAK3 administration antagonizes loss of CA1 neurons after BCCAO through α7 nAChR stimulation. (**a**) Representative histological sections of hippocampus in control, vehicle-administered BCCAO, SAK3 (0.1, 0.5 or 1.0 mg/kg, p.o.)-administered BCCAO mice or SAK3 (0.5 mg/kg, p.o.)-administered BCCAO mice treated with MLA. Mice were sacrificed 11 days after BCCAO for histopathological analysis. *Scale bars*: low magnification, 500 μm; high magnification, 100 μm. (**b**) Cell viability is expressed as a percent of the average number of viable hippocampal CA1 cells from control mice (n = 12–23 per group). *Error bars* represent SEM. ** $p < 0.01$ vs. control mice. ## $p < 0.01$ vs. vehicle-administered BCCAO mice. †† $p < 0.01$ vs. SAK3 (0.5 mg/kg, p.o.)-administered BCCAO mice. MLA, methllycaconitine (6.0 mg/kg, i.p.) treatment; SAK3 (0.1), SAK3 (0.1 mg/kg, p.o.) administration; SAK3 (0.5), SAK3 (0.5 mg/kg, p.o.) administration; SAK3 (1.0), SAK3 (1.0 mg/kg, p.o.) administration; and Veh, vehicle administration. (Modified from Yabuki et al. 2017a)

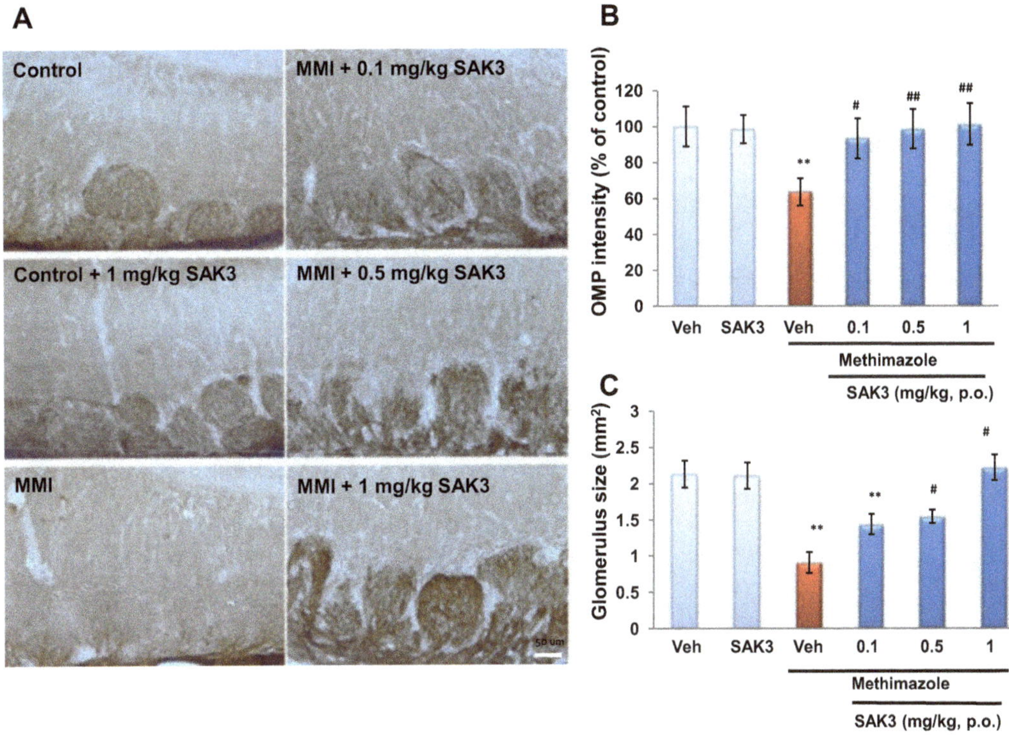

Fig. 9.2 MMI-induced decreases in OMP expression in olfactory bulb glomeruli are antagonized by SAK3 administration. (**a**) Coronal sections of olfactory bulb from indicated control (c), MMI-treated, or MMI-treated and SAK3-treated (0.1, 0.5 and 1 mg/kg) mice were incubated with OMP antibody. (**b**) SAK3 treatment significantly restored OMP staining intensity (**b**) and increased glomerulus size (**c**) in the OB glomerular layer. Scale bar, 50 μm. Error bars represent S.E.M. (**$p < 0.01$ vs control, #$p < 0.05$ and ##$p < 0.01$ vs MMI). n = 7 per group. (Modified from Noreen et al. 2017)

bulbectomy leads to anterograde degeneration of MS cholinergic neurons and concomitant loss of hippocampal cholinergic nerve terminals (Han et al. 2008). Loss of MS cholinergic neurons is also associated with cognitive deficits seen in Alzheimer's disease (Robinson et al. 2011). Indeed, single administration of MMI (75 mg/kg, i.p.) promotes hypothyroidism in mice, and SAK3 treatment prevents hypothyroidism-induced loss of MS cholinergic neurons, thereby improving memory deficits seen in MMI-treated mice (Noreen et al. 2017). In humans, adult onset hypothyroidism is associated with impaired spatial memory performance and cognitive function (Tong et al. 2007; Artis et al. 2012), although mechanisms underlying these impairments remain unclear.

Our recent analysis of MMI-treated mice showed that SAK3 may be neuroprotective and antagonize these cognitive deficits (Fig. 9.2). We found that perturbation of OSN maturation by a single dose of MMI is accompanied by a decrease in the number of MS cholinergic neurons (Fig. 9.3), a loss that likely causes memory and cognitive deficits seen in these mice. Importantly, SAK3 administration to MMI-treated mice rescued degeneration of MS cholinergic neurons and improved deficits in spatial reference memory and cognition.

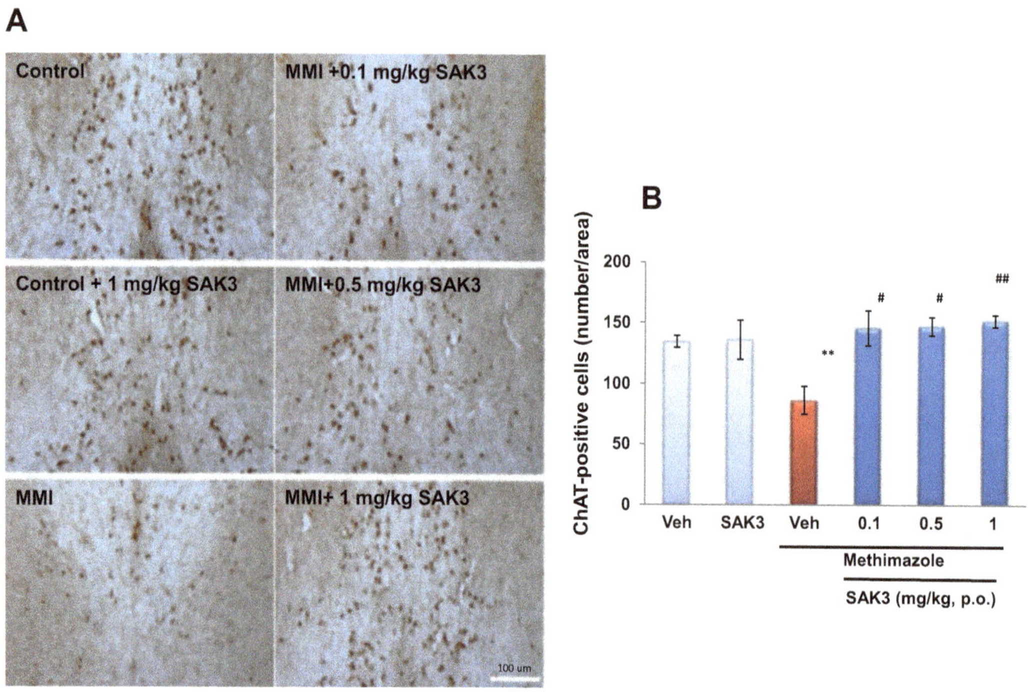

Fig. 9.3 SAK3 administration rescues MMI-induced decreases in the number of ChAT-positive cells in the medial septum. Photomicrographs showing anti-ChAT staining in the medial septum (MS) area. (**b**) ChAT-positive cells were counted in the MS of control or MMI-treated mice with or without SAK3 administration (0.1, 0.5 and 1 mg/kg). *Scale bar*, 100 μm. Error bars represent S.E.M. (**$p < 0.01$ vs control, #$p < 0.05$ and ##$p < 0.01$ vs MMI). n = 7 per group. (Modified from Noreen et al. 2017)

9.7 SAK3 Is Neuroprotective Via nAChRs

Several reports indicate that nAChR neuroprotective activity requires activation of protein kinase B (Akt) signaling, a critical cell survival pathway (Davis and Pennypacker 2016; Fan et al. 2017). The α7 but not the α4 nAChR subunit interacts with the non-receptor-type tyrosine kinase Fyn and janus-activated kinase 2 (JAK2) (Kihara et al. 2001; Shaw et al. 2002), and α7 nAChR stimulation triggers activation of both kinases and subsequently upregulates phosphatidylinositol 3 kinase (PI3K) (Kihara et al. 2001; Shaw et al. 2002). Activated PI3K in turn promotes Akt activity and downstream survival signaling, including Nrf2/HO-1 signaling in neurons (Franke et al. 1997; Kihara et al. 2001; Navarro et al. 2015; Niture and Jaiswal 2012; Shaw et al. 2002). By contrast, α7 nAChR activation in microglia and/or astrocytes is neuroprotective by promoting release of anti-inflammatory cytokines and blocking release of inflammatory cytokines (Di Cesare et al. 2015; Shin and Dixon 2015). The observation that both SAK3-induced ACh release and SAK3-induced neuroprotection are blocked by α7 nAChR inhibitors supports the idea that SAK3 effects are in large part mediated by nAChRs. SAK3-induced neuroprotection is closely associated with enhanced Akt rather than ERK activities (Yabuki et al. 2017a, b) (Fig. 9.4). In this context, α7 nAChR activation by SAK3 administration is critical for neuroprotection.

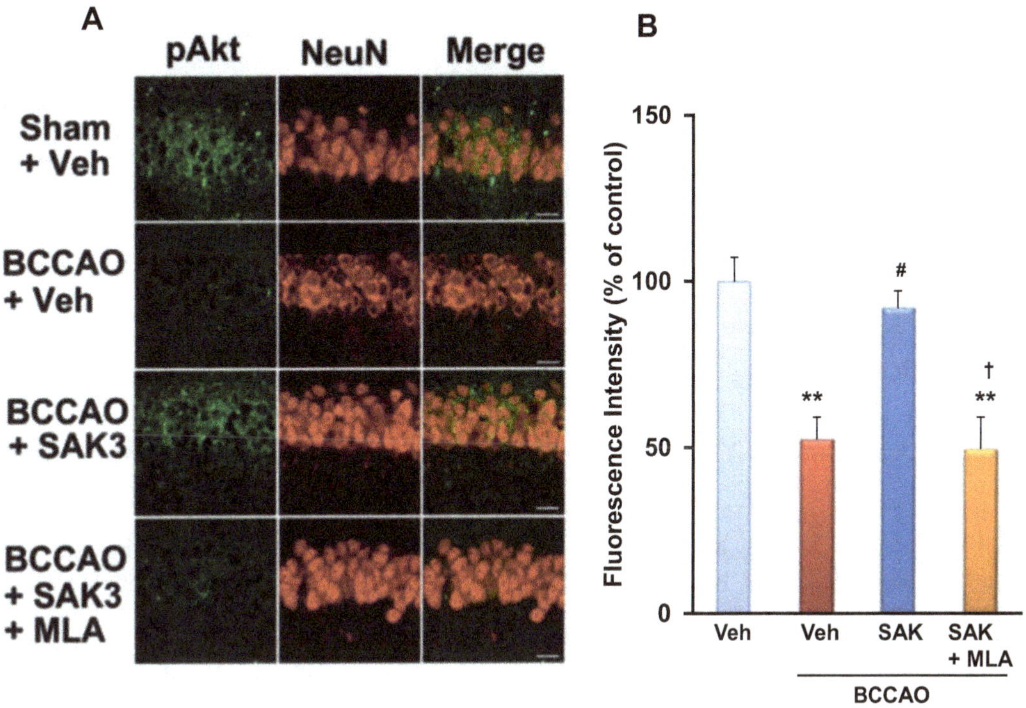

Fig. 9.4 Acute SAK3 administration rescues Akt phosphorylation in CA1 pyramidal neurons of BCCAO mice through α7 nAChR stimulation. (**a**) Representative images showing fluorescent immunostaining with phospho-Akt (Ser-473: green) and NeuN (red) antibodies. Phosphorylated Akt immunoreactivity decreased in CA1 NeuN-positive neurons 24 h after BCCAO. Treatment with MLA (6.0 mg/kg, i.p.) blocked SAK3-dependent increases in Akt phosphorylation in NeuN-positive neurons. Scale bars: 20 μm. (**b**) Fluorescence intensity of Akt phosphorylation was measured in the hippocampal CA1 region. Immunofluorescence intensity of phosphorylated Akt significantly decreased in CA1 pyramidal cells (n = 4–5 per group). Error bars represent SEM. ** $p < 0.01$ vs. control mice. # $P < 0.05$ vs. vehicle-administered BCCAO mice. † $p < 0.05$ vs. SAK3 (0.5 mg/kg, p.o.)-administered BCCAO mice. MLA, methllycaconitine (6.0 mg/kg, i.p.) treatment; SAK3 (0.5), SAK3 (0.5 mg/kg, p.o.) administration; and Veh, vehicle administration. (Modified from Yabuki et al. 2017a)

9.8 Conclusion

Here, we have discussed neuroprotective activity of AChR signaling based on analysis of the novel modulator SAK3. SAK3 enhances activity of T-type calcium channels, promoting ACh release and activating hippocampal nAChRs, which are critical for memory formation. However, off-target analysis is required to determine whether SAK3 modulates nAChRs directly or indirectly. Since SAK3 activity in the CNS differs from that of cholinesterase inhibitors and from the nAChR modulator memantine, SAK3 is an attractive candidate to antagonize CNS neurodegenerative disorders such as Alzheimer's or Lewy body Diseases.

Disclosure/Conflict of Interest The authors have no conflict of interest.

Acknowledgments This work was supported in part by grants-in-aid for Scientific Research from the Ministry of Education, Science, Sports and Culture of Japan (Kakenhi 25293124 and 26102704 to K.F., and 15H06036 to Y.Y.), a Project of Translational and Clinical Research Core Centers from the Japan Agency for Medical Research and Development (AMED) (to K.F.), and the Smoking Research Foundation (to K.F.).

References

Akaike A, Takada-Takatori Y, Kume T, Izumi Y (2010) Mechanisms of neuroprotective effects of nicotine and acetylcholinesterase inhibitors: role of alpha4 and alpha7 receptors in neuroprotection. J Mol Neurosci 40(1–2):211–216

Almasieh M, Zhou Y, Kelly ME, Casanova C, Di Polo A (2010) Structural and functional neuroprotection in glaucoma: role of galantamine-mediated activation of muscarinic acetylcholine receptors. Cell Death Dis 1:e27

Amara IB, Troudi A, Soudani N, Guermazi F, Zeghal N (2012) Toxicity of methimazole on femoral bone in suckling rats: alleviation by selenium. Exp Toxicol Pathol 64:187–195

Artis AS, Bitiktas S, Taşkın E, Dolu N, Liman N, Suer C (2012) Experimental hypothyroidism delays field excitatory post-synaptic potentials and disrupts hippocampal long-term potentiation in the dentate gyrus of hippocampal formation and Y-maze performance in adult rats. J Neuroendocrinol 24:422–433

Bancila M, Copin JC, Daali Y, Schatlo B, Gasche Y, Bijlenga P (2011) Two structurally different T-type Ca^{2+} channel inhibitors, mibefradil and pimozide, protect CA1 neurons from delayed death after global ischemia in rats. Fundam Clin Pharmacol 25(4):469–478

Bano D, Nicotera P (2007) Ca^{2+} signals and neuronal death in brain ischemia. Stroke 38(2 Suppl):674–676

Berliocchi L, Bano D, Nicotera P (2005) Ca^{2+} signals and death programmes in neurons. Philos Trans R Soc Lond B Biol Sci 360(1464):2255–2258

Bloc A, Cens T, Cruz H, Dunant Y (2000) Zinc-induced changes in ionic currents of clonal rat pancreatic -cells: activation of ATP-sensitive K+ channels. J Physiol 529(Pt 3):723–734

Cano-Europa E, Blas-Valdivia V, Franco-Colin M, Gallardo-Casa CA, Ortiz-Butron R (2011) Methimazole-induced hypothyroidism causes cellular damage in the spleen, heart, liver, lung and kidney. Acta Histochem 113:1–5

Cooper DS (1984) Antithyroid drugs. N Engl J Med 311:1353–1362

Dani JA, Bertrand D (2007) Nicotinic acetylcholine receptors and nicotinic cholinergic mechanisms of the central nervous system. Annu Rev Pharmacol Toxicol 47:699–729

Davis SM, Pennypacker KR (2016) Targeting antioxidant enzyme expression as a therapeutic strategy for ischemic stroke. Neurochem Int 107:3–32. In press

Di Cesare Mannelli L, Tenci B, Zanardelli M, Failli P, Ghelardini C (2015) α7 nicotinic receptor promotes the neuroprotective functions of astrocytes against oxaliplatin neurotoxicity. Neural Plast 2015:396908

Dineley KT, Pandya AA, Yakel JL (2015) Nicotinic ACh receptors as therapeutic targets in CNS disorders. Trends Pharmacol Sci 36(2):96–108

Espada S, Rojo AI, Salinas M, Cuadrado A (2009) The muscarinic M1 receptor activates Nrf2 through a signaling cascade that involves protein kinase C and inhibition of GSK-3beta: connecting neurotransmission with neuroprotection. J Neurochem 110(3):1107–1119

Fan YY, Hu WW, Nan F, Chen Z (2017) Postconditioning-induced neuroprotection, mechanisms and applications in cerebral ischemia. Neurochem Int 107:43–56. In press

Farías GG, Godoy JA, Hernández F, Avila J, Fisher A, Inestrosa NC (2004) M1 muscarinic receptor activation protects neurons from beta-amyloid toxicity. A role for Wnt signaling pathway. Neurobiol Dis 17(2):337–348

Franke TF, Kaplan DR, Cantley LC (1997) PI3K: downstream AKTion blocks apoptosis. Cell 88:435–437

Gauthier S, Rountree S, Finn B, LaPlante B, Weber E, Oltersdorf T (2015) Effects of the acetylcholine release agents ST101 with donepezil in Alzheimer's disease: a randomized phase 2 study. J Alzhemiers Dis 48(2):473–481

Genter MB, Deamer NJ, Blake BL, Wesley DS, Levi PE (1995) Olfactory toxicity of methimazole: dose–response and structure–activity studies and characterization of flavincontaining monooxygenase activity in the Long-Evans rat olfactory mucosa. Toxicol Pathol 23:477–486

Han F, Shioda N, Moriguchi S, Qin ZH, Fukunaga K (2008) The vanadium (IV) compound rescues septohippocampal cholinergic neurons from neurodegeneration in olfactory bulbectomized mice. Neuroscience 151:671–679

Hijioka M, Matsushita H, Ishibashi H, Hisatsune A, Isohama Y, Katsuki H (2012) α7 Nicotinic acetylcholine receptor agonist attenuates neuropathological changes associated with intracerebral hemorrhage in mice. Neuroscience 222:10–19

Huguenard JR (1996) Low-threshold calcium currents in central nervous system neurons. Annu Rev Physiol 58:329–348

Ito C, Im WB, Takagi H, Takahashi M, Tsuzuki K, Liou SY, Kunihara M (1994) U-92032, a T-type Ca^{2+} channel blocker and antioxidant, reduces neuronal ischemic injuries. Eur J Pharmacol 257(3):203–210

Kaneko S, Maeda T, Kume T, Kochiyama H, Akaike A, Shimohama S, Kimura J (1997) Nicotine protects cultured cortical neurons against glutamate-induced cytotoxicity via alpha7-neuronal receptors and neuronal CNS receptors. Brain Res 765(1):135–140

Kihara T, Shimohama S, Sawada H, Honda K, Nakamizo T, Shibasaki H, Kume T, Akaike A (2001) Alpha 7 nicotinic receptor transduces signals to phosphatidylinositol 3-kinase to block A beta-amyloid-induced neurotoxicity. J Biol Chem 276(17):13541–13546

Kita Y, Ago Y, Takano E, Fukuda A, Takuma K, Narsuda T (2013) Galantamine increases hippocampal insulin-like growth factor 2 expression via a7 nicotinic acetylcholine receptors in mice. Psychopharmacologia 225(3):543–551

Kita Y, Ago Y, Higashino K, Asada K, Takano E, Takuma K, Matsuda T (2014) Galantamine promotes adult hippocampal neurogenesis via M1 muscarinic and α7 nicotinic receptors in mice. Int J Neuropsychopharmacol 17(12):1957–1968

Kojima M, Kim JS, Uchimurea H, Hirano M, Nakahara T, Matsumoto T (1981) Effect of thyroidectomy on choline acetyltransferase in rat hypothalamic nuclei. Brain Res 209:227–230

Liu JH, Bijlenga P, Occhiodoro T, Fischer-Lougheed J, Bader CR, Bernheim L (1999) Mibefradil (Ro 40-5967) inhibits several Ca^{2+} and K^{+} currents in human fusion-competent myoblasts. Br J Pharmacol 126(1):245–250

Lorrio S, Sobrado M, Arias E, Roda JM, García AG, López MG (2007) Galantamine postischemia provides neuroprotection and memory recovery against transient global cerebral ischemia in gerbils. J Pharmacol Exp Ther 322(2):591–599

Ma K, Yang LM, Chen HZ, Lu Y (2013) Activation of muscarinic receptors inhibits glutamate-induced GSK-3β overactivation in PC12 cells. Acta Pharmacol Sin 34(7):886–892

McNulty MM, Hanck DA (2004) State-dependent mibefradil block of Na+ channels. Mol Pharmacol 66(6):1652–1661

Melancon BJ, Tarr JC, Panarese JD, Wood MR, Lindsley CW (2013) Allosteric modulation of the M1 muscarinic acetylcholine receptor: improving cognition and a potential treatment for schizophrenia and Alzheimer's disease. Drug Discov Today 18(23–24):1185–1199

Mesulam MM, Mufson EJ, Wainer BH, Levey AI (1983) Central cholinergic pathway in the rat: an overview based on an alternative nomenclature (Ch1-Ch6). Neuroscience 10:1185–1201

Moriguchi S, Zhao X, Marszalec W, Yeh JZ, Fukunaga K, Narahashi T (2009) Nefiracetam and galantamine modulation of excitatory and inhibitory synaptic transmission via stimulation of neuronal nicotinic acetylcholine receptors in rat cortical neurons. Neuroscience 160(2):484–491

Moriguchi S, Shioda N, Yamamoto Y, Tagashira H, Fukunaga K (2012) The T-type voltage-gated calcium channel as a molecular target of the novel cognitive enhancer ST101: enhancement of long-term potentiation and CaMKII autophosphorylation in rat cortical slices. J Neurochem 121:44–53

Navarro E, Buendia I, Parada E, León R, Jansen-Duerr P, Pircher H, Egea J, Lopez MG (2015) Alpha7 nicotinic receptor activation protects against oxidative stress via heme-oxygenase I induction. Biochem Pharmacol 97(4):473–481

Niture SK, Jaiswal AK (2012) Nrf2 protein up-regulates antiapoptotic protein Bcl-2 and prevents cellular apoptosis. J Biol Chem 287(13):9873–9886

Noreen H, Yabuki Y, Fukunaga K (2017) Novel spiroimidazopyridine derivative SAK3 improves methimazole-induced cognitive deficits in mice. Neurochem Int 108:91–99. In press

Oh JD, Butcher LL, Woolf NJ (1991) Thyroid hormone modulates the development of cholinergic terminal fields in the rat forebrain relation to nerve growth factor receptor. Brain Res Dev Brain Res 59:133–142

Pandya AA, Yakel JL (2013) Effects of neuronal nicotinic acetylcholine receptor allosteric modulators in animal behavior studies. Biochem Pharmacol 86(8):1054–1062

Parisa SD, Fahimeh J (2015) Sensitive amperometric determination of methimazole based on the electrocatalytic effect of rutin/multi-walled carbon nanotube film. Bioelectrochemistry 101:66–74

Perez-Reyes E (2003) Molecular physiology of low-voltage-activated t-type calcium channels. Physiol Rev 83(1):117–161

Qian J, Zhang JM, Lin LL, Dong WZ, Cheng YQ, Su DF, Liu AJ (2015) A combination of neostigmine and anisodamine protects against ischemic stroke by activating α7nAChR. Int J Stroke 10(5):737–744

Robinson L, Platt B, Riedel G (2011) Involvement of the cholinergic system in conditioning and perceptual memory. Behav Brain Res 221:443–465

Sadigh-Eteghad S, Talebi M, Mahnoudi J, Babri S, Shanehbandi D (2015) Selective activation of a7 nicotinic acetylcholine receptor by PHA-543613 improves Aβ25-35-mediated cognitive deficits in mice. Neuroscience 298:81–93

Sawin S, Brodish P, Carter CS, Stanton ME, Lau C (1998) Development of cholinergic neurons in rat brain regions: dose-dependent effects of propylthiouracil-induced hypothyroidism. Neurotoxicol Teratol 20:627–635

Schwob JE, Szumowski KEM, Stasky AA (1992) Olfactory sensory neurons are trophically dependent on the olfactory bulb for their prolonged survival. J Neurosci 12:3896–3919

Shaw S, Bencherif M, Marrero MB (2002) Janus kinase 2, an early target of alpha 7 nicotinic acetylcholine receptor-mediated neuroprotection against Abeta-(1-42) amyloid. J Biol Chem 277(47):44920–44924

Shin SS, Dixon CE (2015) Targeting α7 nicotinic acetylcholine receptors: a future potential for neuroprotection from traumatic brain injury. Neural Regen Res 10(10):1552–1554

Shioda N, Yamamoto Y, Han F, Moriguchi S, Yamaguchi Y, Hino M, Fukunaga K (2010) A novel cognitive enhancer, ZSET1446/ST101, promotes hippocampal neurogenesis and ameliorates depressive behavior in olfactory bulbectomized mice. J Pharmacol Exp Ther 333(1):43–50

Suzukawa K, Kondo K, Kanaya K, Sakamoto T, Watanabe K, Ushio M, Kaga K, Yamasoba T (2011) Age-related changes of the regeneration mode in the mouse peripheral olfactory system following olfactotoxic drug methimazole-induced damage. J Comp Neurol 519:2154–2174

Takada-Takatori Y, Kume T, Izumi Y, Ohgi Y, Niidome T, Fujii T, Sugimoto H, Akaike A (2009) Roles of nicotinic receptors in acetylcholinesterase inhibitor-induced neuroprotection and nicotinic receptor up-regulation. Biol Pharm Bull 32(3):318–324

Tan PP, Yuan HH, Zhu X, Cui YY, Li H, Feng XM, Qiu Y, Chen HZ, Zhou W (2014) Activation of muscarinic receptors protects against retinal neurons damage and optic nerve degeneration in vitro and in vivo models. CNS Neurosci Ther 20(3):227–236

Tong H, Chen GH, Liu RY, Zhou JN (2007) Age-related learning and memory impairments in adult-onset hypothyroidism in Kunming mice. Physiol Behav 91:290–298

Wu X, Liu H, Zhu X, Shen J, Shi Y, Liu Z, Gu M, Song Z (2013) Efficacy and safety of methimazole ointment for patients with hyperthyroidism. Environ Toxicol Pharmacol 36:1109–1112

Yabuki Y, Jing X, Fukunaga K (2017a) The T-type calcium channel enhancer SAK3 inhibits neuronal death following transient brain ischemia via nicotinic acetylcholine receptor stimulation. Neurochem Int 108:272–281. https://doi.org/10.1016/j.neuint.2017.04.015

Yabuki Y, Matsuo K, Izumi H, Haga H, Yoshida T, Wakamori M, Kakehi A, Sakimura K, Fukuda T, Fukunaga K (2017b) Pharmacological properties of SAK3, a novel T-type voltage-gated Ca^{2+} channel enhancer. Neuropharmacology 117:1–13

Yakel JL (2013) Cholinergic receptors: functional role of nicotinic ACh receptors in brain circuits and disease. Pflugers Arch 465(4):441–450

Yamamoto Y, Fuknaga K (2013) Donepezil rescues the medial septum cholinergic neurons via nicotinic ACh receptor stimulation in olfactory bulbectomized mice. Adv Alzheimer's Dis 2(4):161–170

Yamamoto Y, Shioda N, Han F, Moriguchi S, Fukunaga K (2013) Novel cognitive enhancer ST101 enhances acetylcholine release in mouse dorsal hippocampus through T-type voltage-gated calcium channel stimulation. J Pharmacol Sci 121:212–226

Zdanowski R, Krzyżowska M, Ujazdowska D, Lewicka A, Lewicki S (2015) Role of α7 nicotinic receptor in the immune system and intracellular signaling pathways. Cent Eur J Immunol 40(3):373–379

Chapter 10
Removal of Blood Amyloid As a Therapeutic Strategy for Alzheimer's Disease: The Influence of Smoking and Nicotine

Nobuya Kitaguchi, Kazunori Kawaguchi, and Kazuyoshi Sakai

Abstract Accumulation of amyloid β protein (Aβ) in the brain causes cognitive impairment in Alzheimer's disease (AD). The nature of the relationship between smoking and AD or dementia has been controversial. However, a recent meta-analysis revealed that smoking is a risk factor for AD. With regard to nicotinic acetylcholinergic receptors (nAChRs), both AD and control patients that smoke have been reported to show an increase in ^{3}H-cytisine (an α4β4 nAChR agonist) binding in the temporal cortex. The α7 nAChR is also a key factor in AD pathology, particularly in relation to internalization of Aβs. Furthermore, there are many reports showing the neuroprotective effects of nicotine. The internalization of Aβ may lead to Aβ clearance in the brain.

We hypothesized that an extracorporeal system that rapidly removes Aβ from the blood may accelerate Aβ clearance from the brain. We have reported that (1) several medical materials including hemodialyzers can effectively remove blood Aβ, (2) the concentrations of blood Aβs decreased during hemodialysis, (3) removal of blood Aβ enhanced Aβ influx into the blood (ideally from the brain), resulting in maintenance or improvement of cognitive function, and (4) Aβ deposition in the brain of hemodialysis patients was significantly lower than in controls. Smoking affected blood Aβ removal efficiencies and brain atrophy. We believe this Extracorporeal Blood Aβ Removal Systems (E-BARS) may contribute as a therapy for AD.

Keywords Alzheimer's disease · Amyloid β · Aβ · Blood purification · Hemodialysis · Dialyzer · HDC · E-BARS

N. Kitaguchi (✉) · K. Kawaguchi · K. Sakai
Faculty of Clinical Engineering, School of Health Science, Fujita Health University, Toyoake, Japan
e-mail: nkitaguc@fujita-hu.ac.jp

A. Akaike et al. (eds.), *Nicotinic Acetylcholine Receptor Signaling in Neuroprotection*, https://doi.org/10.1007/978-981-10-8488-1_10

10.1 Introduction: Amyloid β Protein in Alzheimer's Disease

One of the major pathological changes associated with Alzheimer's disease (AD) is the deposition of amyloid β protein (Aβ) as senile plaques and an increase in Aβ peptides in the brain (Kuo et al. 1996; Selkoe 2001). There are several Aβ species in the brain and plasma that are approximately 4 kDa in weight such as the 40-amino acid $A\beta_{1-40}$ and the 42-amino acid $A\beta_{1-42}$. $A\beta_{1-42}$ aggregates more easily and is more toxic (Hung et al. 2008), forming soluble Aβ oligomers that can cause synapse loss and affect long-term potentiation in hippocampal neurons (Walsh et al. 2002). One mechanism proposed to underlie the increase in brain Aβ is reduced Aβ clearance rather than enhanced Aβ production, particularly in sporadic AD cases. Aβ production in the brains of AD patients was reported to be similar to that of normal subjects, yet Aβ clearance from AD brains was approximately 30% lower than in controls (Mawuenyega et al. 2010). In other words, it may be possible to treat AD by increasing Aβ clearance from the brain.

Recently, an anti-Ab monoclonal antibody that selectively targets aggregated forms of Aβ, aducanumab, was reported to be effective in improving cognitive function and reducing the brain Aβ burden, as measured by brain Aβ imaging (Sevigny et al. 2016). Similarly to anti-Aβ antibodies (Hock et al. 2003; Sevigny et al. 2016), peripheral administration of albumin, another Aβ-binding substance, was effective in improving cognitive function in AD patients in a Phase 2 study, and is currently undergoing a Phase 3 trial in AD patients (Boada et al. 2009, 2016).

We hypothesized that the rapid removal of Aβ from the blood by an extracorporeal system (E-BARS; extracorporeal blood Aβ removal system) may act as a peripheral Aβ sink from the brain, as shown in Fig. 10.1 (Kawaguchi et al. 2010). Smoking could affect the blood flow in the brain resulting in a change in the excretion of Aβ from the brain into the blood.

10.2 Smoking, Nicotine, and AD

Determining the exact nature of the relationship between smoking and AD or dementia has been controversial. However, a recent meta-analysis revealed that smoking is a risk factor for AD, as described below. These controversial findings may be due to the mixed effects of smoke itself and components of tobacco such as nicotine.

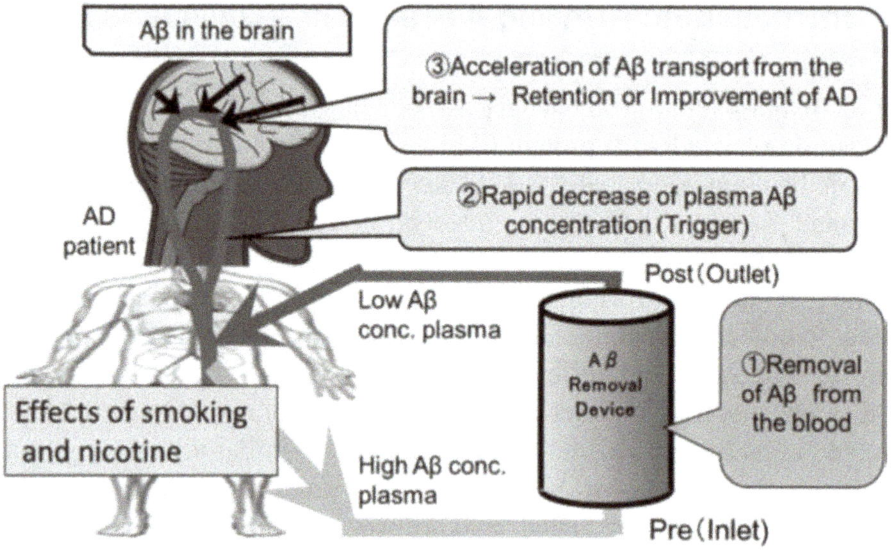

Fig. 10.1 Schema of the extracorporeal blood Aβ removal system (E-BARS) for the treatment of Alzheimer's disease (AD). Our hypothesis: the rapid reduction of Aβ concentrations in the blood by apheresis technology may act as a trigger for enhancing the excretion of Aβ from the brain, resulting in cognitive improvement. (Taken from Kawaguchi et al. 2010 and modified)

10.2.1 Smoking and AD Prevalence

Sabia et al. (2008) reported that ex-smokers had a 30% lower risk of poor vocabulary and low verbal fluency. However, the correlation between smoking history and cognitive decline was inconsistent in longitudinal analysis. Despite this ameliorative effect of smoking on memory (Sabia et al. 2008), the risk of AD was reported to be unaffected by any measure of tobacco consumption (Garcia et al. 2010). Contrary to these favorable or neutral effects of smoking on dementia, there are many reports showing that smoking has a deleterious influence on AD risk. Lower AD risk was observed in alcohol drinkers of both genders who had never smoked (OR = 0.37, 95% CI: 0.21, 0.65), regardless of the presence of apolipoprotein E4 (APOε4). Ott et al. (1998) showed that smokers had an increased risk of dementia (relative risk 2.2 [95% CI: 1.3–3.6]) and AD (relative risk 2.3 [95% CI: 1.3–4.1]) compared with never smokers, based on a study of 6870 people aged 55 years and older. Smoking was a strong risk factor for AD in individuals without the APOε4 allele (relative risk 4.6 [95% CI: 1.5–14.2]), but had no effect in participants with this allele (relative risk 0.6 [95% CI: 0.1–4.8]). By meta-analysis of 19 prospective studies with at least 12 months of follow-up, Anstey et al. (2007) concluded that elderly smokers had increased risks of dementia and cognitive decline. Current smokers at baseline, relative to never smokers, had risks of 1.79 (95% CI: 1.43, 2.23) for AD and 1.78 (95% CI: 1.28, 2.47) for vascular dementia. Compared to those who had never smoked, current smokers at baseline also showed greater yearly declines in Mini-Mental State Examination scores over the follow-up period. Compared to former smokers, current smokers at baseline showed an increased risk of AD and an increased decline in cognitive ability (Anstey et al. 2007). Furthermore, Barnes and Yaffe (2011) reported that smoking was associated with a higher risk of AD (relative risk 1.59 [95% CI: 1.15, 2.20]), and that a 10% reduction in smoking prevalence could potentially lower AD prevalence by about 412,000 cases worldwide and by almost 51,000 cases in the USA, while a 25% reduction in smoking prevalence could potentially prevent more than 1 million AD cases worldwide and 130,000 cases in the USA.

10.2.2 AD Pathology and Smoking

Recently, an interesting animal study on AD pathology was reported that used cigarette smoke rather than administration of some components of tobacco such as nicotine. When APP/PS1 transgenic mice were exposed to smoke from cigarettes, AD pathology, such as Aβ deposition and the Iba1-labeled area indicating an inflammatory response, was enhanced in the cortex and hippocampus. This enhancement was observed in the high-dose smoking group but not in the low-dose group (Moreno-Gonzalez et al. 2013).

Contrary to the animal study, it has been reported that smoking reduces both soluble and insoluble $A\beta_{1-40}$ and $A\beta_{1-42}$ in the frontal cortex and $A\beta_{1-40}$ in the temporal cortex and hippocampus in AD patients (Hellström-Lindahl et al. 2004).

10.2.3 Nicotinic Acetylcholinergic Receptors and Aβs

Regarding nicotinic acetylcholinergic receptors (nAChRs), both AD and control patients that smoked showed increased ^{3}H-cytisine (an agonist of the α4β4 nAChR) binding in the temporal cortex (Hellström-Lindahl et al. 2004). Further, Aβ levels in the brain was reduced in this study. Therefore, these authors proposed that a selective nAChR agonist could be a novel protective therapy for AD.

The α7 nAChR is also a key factor in AD pathology, particularly in relation to internalization of Aβs. Soluble Aβ is known to bind to the α7 nAChR with high affinity (Wang et al. 2000). By in vitro experimentation with SH-SY5Y cells, Yang et al. (2014) revealed that extracellular $A\beta_{1-42}$ was internalized by the cells and accumulated in endosomes/lysosomes and mitochondria. This internalization was mediated through an α7 nAChR-dependent pathway related to the activation of p38 MAPK and ERK1/2. The authors proposed that blockade of the α7 nAChR may have a beneficial effect by limiting intracellular accumulation of amyloid in the AD brain, thereby representing a potential therapeutic target for AD.

However, there are many articles showing the neuroprotective effects of nicotine. The internalization of Aβ may lead to Aβ clearance from the brain. Akaike and Shimohama's research group first demonstrated the neuroprotective effect of nicotine on Aβ toxicity (Kihara et al. 1997). Concomitant administration of nicotine with $A\beta_{25-35}$ ameliorated the death of rat cortical neurons induced by Aβ toxicity. In addition, the selective α7 nAChR antagonist, α-bungarotoxin, blocked this neuroprotective effect of nicotine. This group also revealed that stimulation of the α7 nAChR protected neurons against Aβ-enhanced glutamate neurotoxicity via PI3K (Kihara et al. 2001). Shimohama's research group reported that treatment of rat microglia with galantamine, an acetylcholinesterase inhibitor, significantly enhanced microglial Aβ phagocytosis via the nAChR pathway (Takata et al. 2010). This group also revealed early accumulation of CD68-positive microglia at Aβ deposition sites and gradual reduction of Aβ in an Aβ-injected AD mouse model, which indicates the importance of the α7 nAChR in microglia as a therapeutic target in AD (Matsumura et al. 2015).

10.3 Our Hypothesis of a Therapeutic System for AD by Removal of Blood Aβ

As described earlier, one mechanism proposed to underlie increased brain Aβ in AD is reduced Aβ clearance rather than an increase in Aβ production, particularly in sporadic AD cases. Therefore, it may be possible to treat AD by enhancing Aβ clearance from the brain. There are several known Aβ transporters such as those involved in the Aβ influx pathway from the brain into the blood; e.g., LRP1 or APOE (Donahue et al. 2006; Bell et al. 2007), and RAGE (Silverberg et al. 2010), which is also known to mediate an Aβ influx pathway into the brain. In addition, perivascular elimination of Aβ in brain capillaries has been proposed (e.g., Morris et al. 2014).

Aβ concentrations in the cerebrospinal fluid (CSF) of AD patients are almost 100 times higher than those in plasma. Aβ concentrations in the CSF in cases of AD are reported to be 7.4–42.7 ng/ml for $A\beta_{1-40}$ and 0.12–0.67 ng/ml for $A\beta_{1-42}$ (Schoonenboom et al. 2005). Concentrations in the plasma of AD patients are reported to be 190.1 ± 61.7 pg/ml for $A\beta_{1-40}$ and 23.0 ± 15.5 pg/ml for $A\beta_{1-42}$ (Lopez et al. 2008). In brief, there are large gradients with respect to Aβ concentrations between the brain and plasma. Therefore, removing Aβ from the blood could accelerate Aβ transfer from the brain, thereby reducing the Aβ burden in the brain.

Peripheral administration of Aβ-binding substances, such as anti-Aβ antibodies, non-immunogenic substances, and albumin, can reduce the Aβ burden in the brain. However, attempts to use Aβ-binding substances in the blood in a therapeutic context resulted in the formation of Aβ complexes with the binding substances inside the body, which were sometimes retained in the plasma for a long period of time (DeMattos et al. 2001). Aβ antibodies generated by passive immunization or by active immunization using synthetic Aβ peptides reduced the occurrence of senile plaques and somewhat improved cognitive impairment in AD patients (Schenk et al. 1999; Hock et al. 2003). Furthermore, non-immunogenic Aβ-binding substances, such as GM1 ganglioside or gelsolin, also decreased the Aβ burden in the brain when they were peripherally injected into mouse models of AD (Matsuoka et al. 2003). Currently, a clinical trial is in progress where AD patients are being treated using intravenous administration of albumin, an Aβ-binding substance (Boada et al. 2009). In this Phase 2 trial, plasma exchange (discard) removes the plasma of AD patients, which contains Aβ–albumin complexes, and a new albumin solution is introduced into the blood as a replacement solution; the results thus far suggest that this therapy has improved cognitive function in AD subjects. The Phase 3 trial is now also underway (Boada et al. 2016).

Based on these observations, the removal of Aβ from the blood could act as peripheral drainage and an Aβ sink from the brain. We proposed that the E-BARS, which transfers Aβ out of the body, may be useful as a therapy for AD (Kawaguchi et al. 2010) (Fig. 10.1). The rapid reduction of Aβ concentrations in the blood could act as a trigger to enhance Aβ excretion from the brain, resulting in cognitive improvement.

10.4 Definition of Aβ Removal Activities of the Devices

The Aβ removal activities assessed in our study were: (1) the removal rate for batch analysis *in vitro*, (2–1) the removal efficiency based on the concentration change at pre-/post-application of the Aβ removal device, (2–2) the reduction rate of Aβ in the whole blood circulation, and (2–3) the filtration rate. The definitions were as follows:

1. Batch analysis in vitro:

Adsorptive materials were mixed with Aβ solutions or plasma and shaken for the designated time.

$$\text{Removal Rate}(\%) = 100 \times \left(1 - \frac{A\beta\,\text{concentration with materials at the designated time}}{A\beta\,\text{concentration without adsorbents at the same time}}\right)$$

2. Flow analysis in vitro and the hemodialysis session

2-1 The Aβ removal efficiency of a dialyzer was defined as follows:

$$\text{Removal efficiency}(\%) = 100 \times \left\{1 - \frac{\text{concentration of } A\beta \text{ after leaving the dialyzer (device) at a designated time}}{\text{concentration of } A\beta \text{ before entering the dialyzer (device) at that time}}\right\}$$

2-2 The Aβ reduction rate for the experimental pool solution or the whole blood circulation was defined as follows:

$$\text{Reduction rate}\left(\%\right)=$$
$$100\times\left\{1-\frac{A\beta\,\text{concentration in the pool solution or whole blood circulation at a designated time}}{\text{Initial}\,A\beta\,\text{concentration in the pool solution or whole blood circulation}}\right\}$$

2-3 The Aβ filtration rate of a dialyzer was defined as follows:

$$\text{Filtration rate}\left(\%\right)=$$
$$100\times\left\{\frac{\text{concentration of filtrated}\,A\beta\,\text{solution at the designated time}}{\text{concentration of}\,A\beta\,\text{before the dialyzer at the same time}}\right\}$$

10.5 Adsorption Devices for Blood Aβ Removal

To obtain suitable materials for the removal of blood Aβ, we firstly investigated adsorptive materials for therapeutic blood purification (apheresis). We employed six materials: hexadecyl-alkylated cellulose particles (HDC), used to remove β_2-microglobulin in carpal tunnel syndrome; cellulose particles ligated with dextran sulfate (CLD); charcoal (CHA), which is commonly used therapeutically, for example, in hepatic failure; tryptophan-ligated polyvinyl alcohol gel (TRV), used in Guillain–Barré syndrome; and cellulose acetate particles and non-woven polyethylene terephthalate filter, used in ulcerative colitis. Among these materials, HDC and CHA demonstrated a removal rate of almost 99% for both $A\beta_{1-40}$ and $A\beta_{1-42}$ in batch analysis using synthetic Aβ peptides (Fig. 10.2) (Kawaguchi et al. 2010).

HDC is used in cases where there are complications associated with hemodialysis and, therefore, we were able to investigate Aβ concentrations before (pre, inlet of) and after (post, outlet of) HDC column in hemodialysis sessions. The high removal efficiency of HDC was maintained at approximately 50% for both $A\beta_{1-40}$ and $A\beta_{1-42}$ during a 4-h hemodialysis session, as shown in Table 10.1.

10.6 Blood Aβ Removal by Hemodialyzers in Hemodialysis

We previously reported that hemodialyzers showed high Aβ removal activity based on analyses of hemodialysis patients (Kitaguchi et al. 2011, 2015; Kato et al. 2012). Measurements of Aβ concentrations at pre (inlet of) and post (outlet of) dialyzers during hemodialysis sessions revealed that the hemodialyzers effectively removed both $A\beta_{1-40}$ and $A\beta_{1-42}$ from the plasma of non-diabetic patients. Figure 10.3 shows the Aβ concentrations at the inlet of the dialyzers (Pre) and the outlet of the dialyzers (Post) for each dialysis session (n = 57). The average removal efficiencies for

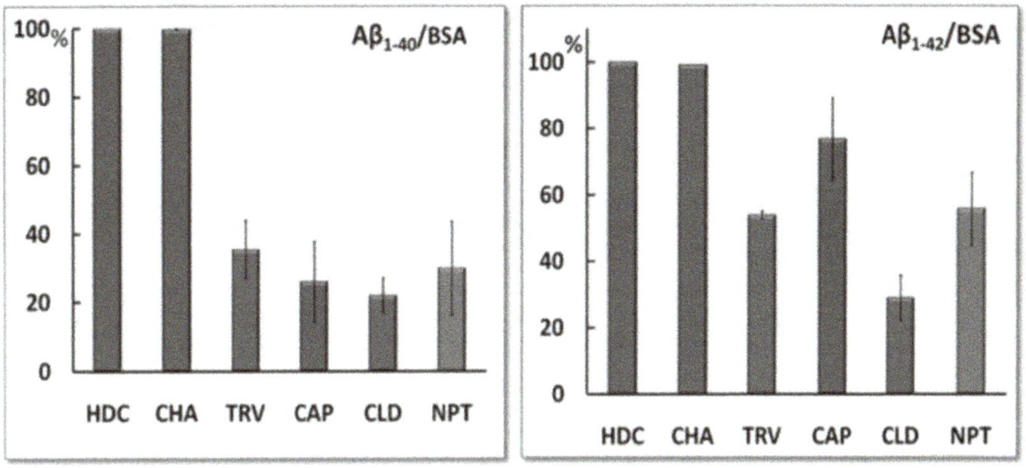

Fig. 10.2 Aβ removal rate in batch analysis with various adsorptives in a batch reaction for 16 h. *HDC* hexadecyl-alkylated cellulose particles, *CHA* charcoal, *TRV* tryptophan-ligated polyvinyl alcohol gel, *CAP* cellulose acetate particles, *CLD* cellulose particles ligated with dextran sulfate, *NPT* non-woven polyethylene terephthalate filter. HDC and CHA showed significantly higher rates than TRV ($p < 0.05$) for $A\beta_{1-40}$ removal and a higher tendency than CAP ($p < 0.1$) for $A\beta_{1-42}$ removal. (Taken from Kawaguchi et al. 2010)

Table 10.1 Removal efficiencies of HDC columns in hemodialysis

Time points during a hemodialysis session	$A\beta_{1-40}$	$A\beta_{1-42}$
1 h (n = 5)	51.1 ± 6.6%	44.9 ± 5.0%
4 h (n = 4)	46.1 ± 6.6%	38.2 ± 5.8%

Taken from Kawaguchi et al. (2010)

$A\beta_{1-40}$ were 66.0% at the 1-h point and 52.0% at the 4-h point of the hemodialysis sessions. Those for $A\beta_{1-42}$ were 61.1% and 49.2%, as shown in Fig. 10.3. The removal efficiency in for $A\beta_{1-40}$ was significantly higher than for $A\beta_{1-42}$ both at 1 h and at 4 h of each dialysis session ($p < 0.0001$ for both time points). Each dialyzer maintained its removal efficiency during the entire dialysis session. This indicates that the dialyzers had sufficient capacity for Aβ removal during the 4-h treatment.

10.7 Removal of Blood Aβs Evoked Influx of Aβs into the Blood

Due to the effective removal activity of the dialyzers during the hemodialysis sessions (Fig. 10.3), the concentrations of blood Aβs after 4-h hemodialysis would have been approximately 10% of the concentrations at the starting point if there had been no Aβ influx into the blood ("Calcd" in Fig. 10.4). However, observed

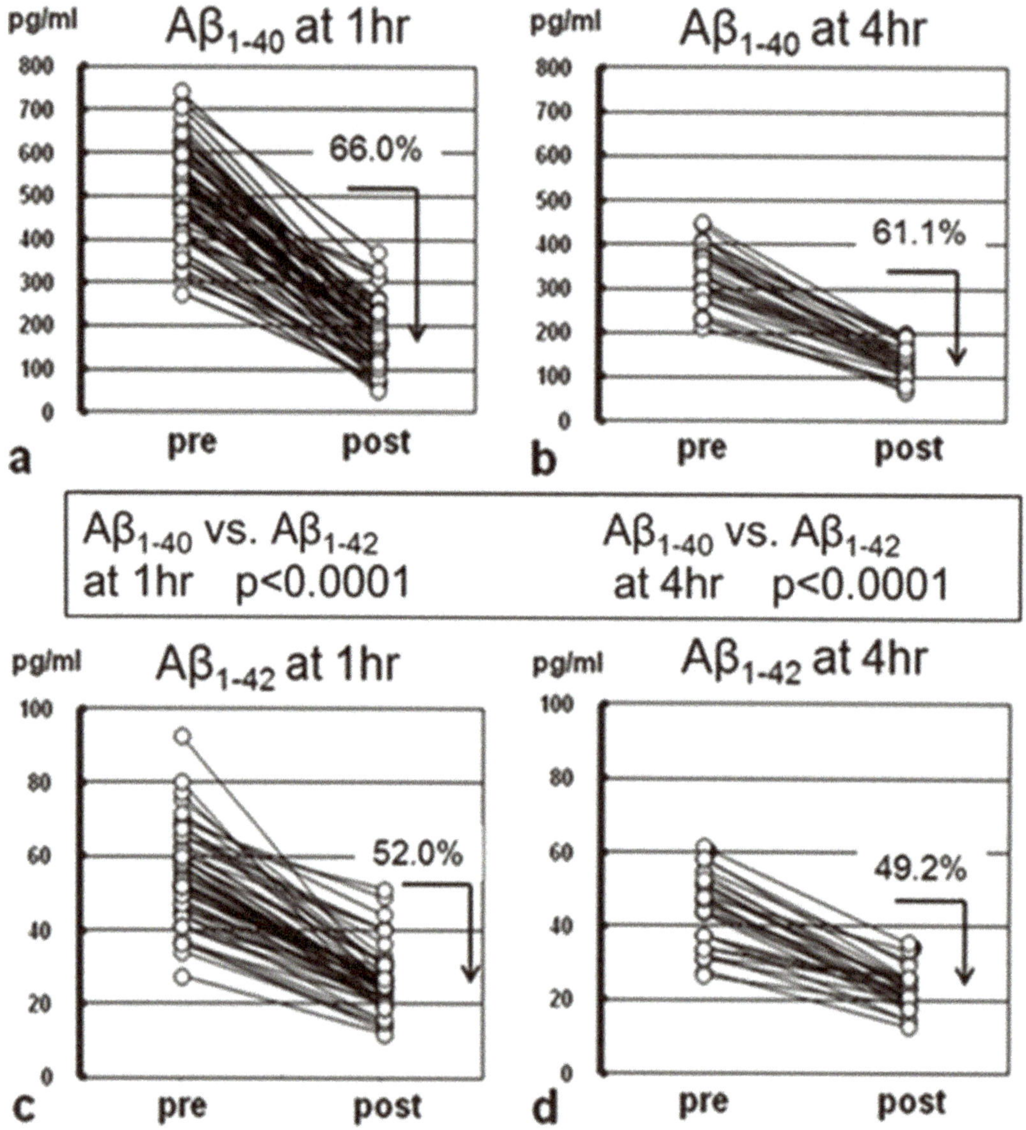

Fig. 10.3 Aβ concentrations measured at pre-/post-dialyzers at 1 and 4 h in the hemodialysis sessions. Aβ removal efficiencies for both $A\beta_{1-40}$ and $A\beta_{1-42}$ were quite high, with both being approximately 50% or greater. (**a**, **b**) $A\beta_{1-40}$; (**c**, **d**) $A\beta_{1-42}$; (**a**, **c**) at the 1-h point of the dialysis sessions; (**b**, **d**) at the 4-h point of the dialysis sessions. (Taken from Kato et al. 2012 and modified)

concentrations of blood Aβs ("Obsd" in Fig. 10.4) were not decreased compared to "Calcd." The differences between "Obsd" and "Calcd" were attributed to Aβ influx into the blood. We calculated the influx based on the differential equation described previously (Kitaguchi et al. 2011). The results of this simulation of 37 non-diabetic hemodialysis patients are shown in Fig. 10.4.

Table 10.2 shows more detailed results of the simulation of Aβ influx with 30 non-diabetic hemodialysis patients (Kitaguchi et al. 2015). The average removal efficiencies at the 1-hr point of the hemodialysis sessions were 67.3% and 51.3% for $A\beta_{1-40}$ and $A\beta_{1-42}$, respectively. Aβ influxes during 4-hr hemodialysis were calcu-

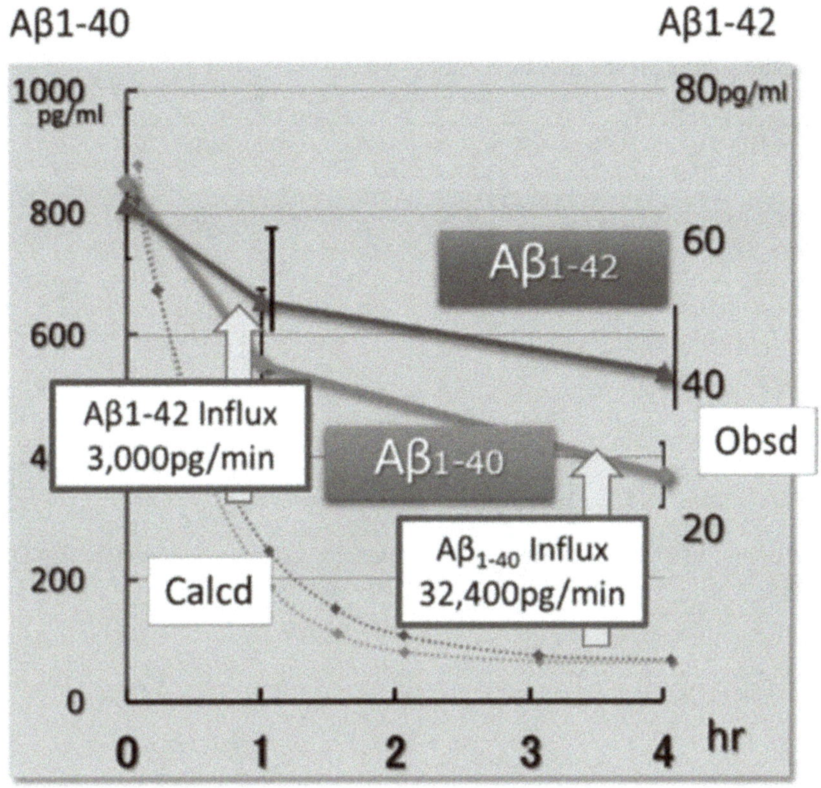

Fig. 10.4 Change in the observed plasma Aβ concentrations in the whole body circulation during hemodialysis sessions (Obsd), and, the calculated plasma Aβ concentrations based on the Aβ removal efficiencies of the dialyzers assuming no Aβ influx into the blood (Calcd). The arrows indicate Aβ influx during the hemodialysis sessions. (Taken from Kitaguchi et al. 2011 and modified)

lated as 9243 ng and 719 ng for $A\beta_{1-40}$ and $A\beta_{1-42}$, respectively, which were around five times the level of pre-existing Aβs in the blood, that is, 1952 ng and 165 ng, just before hemodialysis.

A similar Aβ influx into the blood was also observed in a rat study using HDC.

10.8 Are the Influxes of Aβs into the Blood from the Brain?

Recently, we reported that Aβ accumulation in the brains of hemodialysis (HD) patients was significantly lower than that in age-matched non-hemodialysis controls, as assessed by histopathological studies (Sakai et al. 2016). Senile plaques stained with anti-Aβ antibodies were observed more frequently in non-HD subjects and were either sparse or not seen at all in HD patients (Fig. 10.5). Regarding the ratio of senile plaques (plaque-positive/-negative subjects), there were significantly fewer neuritic and cored plaques in HD patients; only 5 of 17 HD patients showed neuritic plaques stained with 4G8 anti- Aβ antibody, whereas 12 out of 16 non-HD subjects exhibited these plaques. These findings suggest that the brain may be one origin of the Aβ influx during the hemodialysis sessions.

Table 10.2 Average Aβ influx into the blood during the hemodialysis sessions

Aβ concentrations during hemodialysis sessions (n = 30)								
	$A\beta_{1-40}$				$A\beta_{1-42}$			
Time point of HD session	0 h	1 h	4 h		0 h	1 h	4 h	
Aβ concentrations at Pre dialyzer (pg/ml)	750.7	517.7	361.8		63.3	50.0	41.5	
Removal Efficiency (%) of Pre/Post dialyzers		67.3				51.3		
Aβ removed by dialyzers (ng)		(0–1 h)	(1–4 h)	Total removed Aβ (0–4 h) (a)		(0–1 h)	(1–4 h)	Total removed Aβ (0–4 h) (a)
		3329	6925	10,254		227	549	776
Change of Aβs in the blood (ng)	1952		941	Decreased Aβ (0–4 h) (b)	165		108	Decreased Aβ (0–4 h) (b)
				1011				57
Aβ influx into the blood during hemodialysis sessions(ng) (a–b)	9243				719			

Taken from Kitaguchi et al. (2015)

10.9 Effects of Hemodialysis, One of the Blood Aβ Removal Methods, on Cognitive Function

Renal failure is well known to cause cognitive decline. In our cross-sectional study, cognitive function as measured by the MMSE was impaired in renal failure patients who did not receive hemodialysis compared to age-matched healthy controls. However, MMSE scores of hemodialysis patients were similar to those of controls (Fig. 10.6) (Kato et al. 2012).

Figure 10.7 shows the relationship between plasma Aβ concentrations, cognitive function, renal function, and hemodialysis vintage (the duration of hemodialysis) before and after initiation of hemodialysis. Before initiation of hemodialysis, plasma concentrations of both $A\beta_{1-40}$ and $A\beta_{1-42}$ increased along with a concomitant decline in renal function. However, when patients were introduced to hemodialysis (after initiation of hemodialysis), an increase in plasma Aβ concentrations was no longer apparent, but there was instead a slight tendency toward a decrease. Although the cognitive function declined along with the decline in renal function, this was maintained following initiation of hemodialysis (bottom of Fig. 10.7).

In the prospective study with 18 and 36 months follow-up, average MMSE scores did not significantly change, as shown in Fig. 10.8a, b. However, analysis of the change in individual subjects revealed that most hemodialysis patients maintained

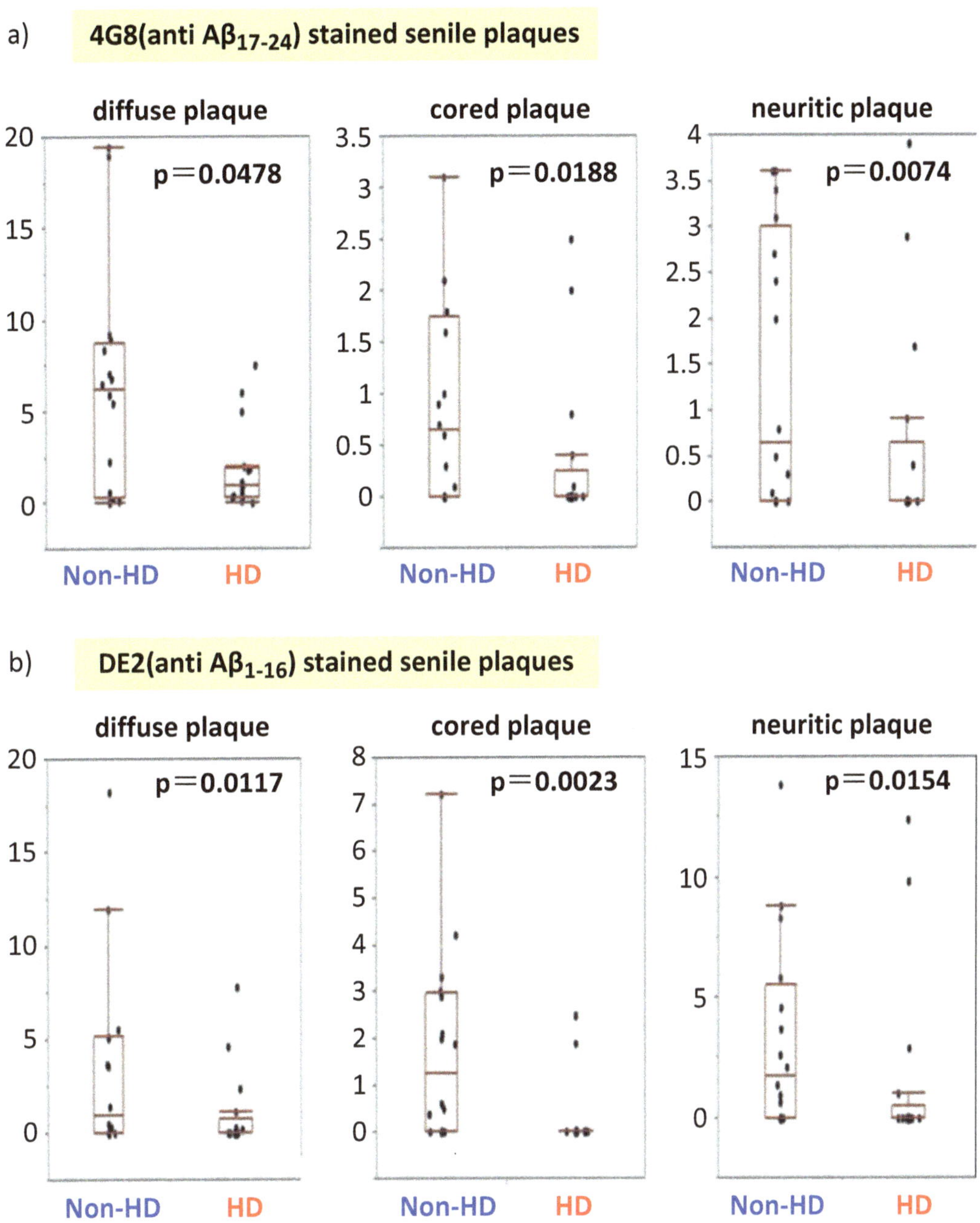

Fig. 10.5 Comparison of senile plaques in patients who had undergone hemodialysis (HD) with those who had not undergone HD (non-HD). (**a**) Stained with the anti-Aβ_{17-24} antibody 4G8; (**b**) stained with the anti-Aβ_{1-16} antibody DE2. The numbers of all types of Aβ deposition (diffuse, cored, and neuritic plaques) were significantly lower in HD patients. HD, n = 17; non-HD, n = 16. (Taken from Sakai et al. 2016 and modified)

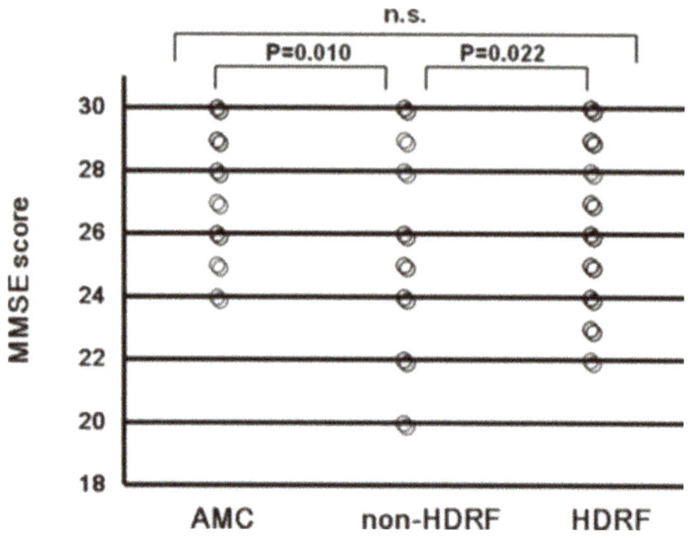

Fig. 10.6 Cognitive function deteriorated in renal failure; however, hemodialysis appeared to promote recovery or maintenance of this. AMC, age-matched healthy controls (n = 17) (66.6 ± 4.1 years old, 5 male, 12 female); non-HDRF, renal failure patients without hemodialysis (n = 26) (66.6 ± 14.7 years old, 18 male, 8 female); HDRF, renal failure patients who received hemodialysis three times a week (n = 57) (69.4 ± 3.8 years old, 29 male, 28 female). *MMSE* Mini-Mental State Examination. (Taken from Kato et al. 2012)

or improved their cognitive function, with the exception of patients that showed white matter ischemia at baseline (Fig. 10.8c). This suggests that hemodialysis, with Aβ removal from the blood three times a week, may have a positive effect on cognitive function but has almost no influence on the cognitive effects of brain ischemia.

Furthermore, using a database of over 200,000 hemodialysis patients in Japan, the risk of dementia was revealed to be significantly lower in the patient subgroup with a longer duration of hemodialysis in subjects without diabetes (Nakai et al. 2018).

10.10 Effects of Smoking on Removal of Blood Aβ

We then investigated the effects of smoking on Aβ removal efficiencies in hemodialysis. Subjects were non-diabetic hemodialysis patients; n = 57, 29 male and 28 female; age, 69.4 ± 3.8 years old (59–76 years old); duration of hemodialysis, 13.9 ± 9.4 years (1–37 years); 28 smokers and 29 non-smokers, with "smoker" defined as a patient who had ever smoked (former smokers and current smokers). Information regarding the duration of smoking, the number of cigarettes per day, and the brands of cigarettes were obtained by interview with each patient. The product of the duration and the number of cigarettes per day was also used for analysis.

Interestingly, removal efficiencies for both $A\beta_{1-40}$ and $A\beta_{1-42}$ in smokers significantly decreased during the 4-h hemodialysis sessions (Table 10.3). The efficiencies

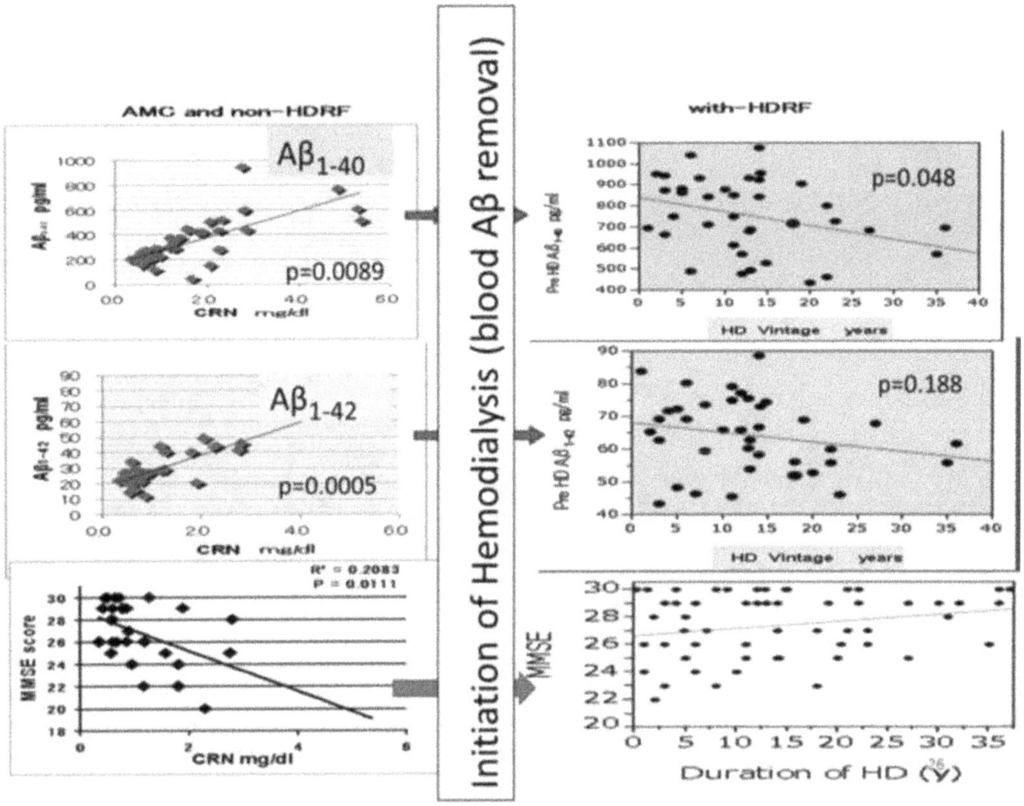

Fig. 10.7 Summary of cross-sectional study of renal failure patients before/after initiation of hemodialysis (HD). The central *box* indicates initiation of hemodialysis. Left of the central box, data from renal failure patients without hemodialysis (non-HDRF) are shown. Right of the central box, data from hemodialysis patients (with-HDRF) are shown. Vertical axis: upper, plasma $A\beta_{1-40}$ concentrations; middle, plasma $A\beta_{1-42}$ concentrations; lower, the Mini-Mental State Examination (MMSE) score (30 indicates no mistakes). Plasma for measuring Aβ concentrations after the initiation of hemodialysis was sampled at the beginning of each hemodialysis session. Horizontal axis: before initiation of hemodialysis, plasma creatinine concentrations (CRN), which indicate decline of renal function; after initiation of hemodialysis, the vintage (duration) of hemodialysis. (Data from Kato et al. 2012)

for non-smokers showed a tendency to increase, which was insignificant, rather than a decrease. The reason for this difference is unclear at present. One possibility is that Aβ species in the blood of smokers may have certain characteristics that cause saturation of Aβ adsorption or clogging of the inner surface of dialyzer membranes. A second possibility is that Aβ species flowing into the blood during hemodialysis may be more difficult to remove using a dialyzer in smokers than in non-smokers.

However, there is a limitation regarding this speculation on the effects of smoking. The ratio of male/female subjects was higher in smokers than in non-smokers. Therefore, the differences between smokers and non-smokers could be partially attributable to gender.

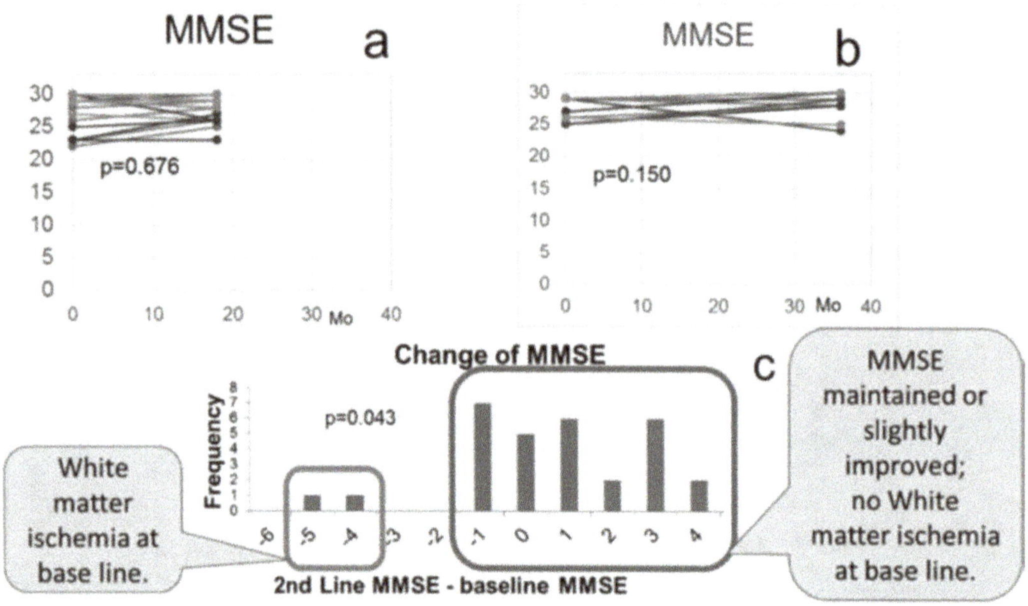

Fig. 10.8 Change in cognitive function of hemodialysis patients in prospective studies. (**a**) Mini-Mental State Examination (MMSE) changes over 18 months; (**b**) MMSE changes over 36 months; (**c**) change in MMSE from baseline for each patient. A change of −1 to 4 is regarded as maintained or improved. Patients whose MMSE declined by −4 and −5 showed white matter ischemia at baseline. (Taken from Kitaguchi et al. 2015 and modified)

Table 10.3 Effects of smoking; comparison of Aβ removal efficiencies at pre-/post dialyzers in hemodialysis sessions

Removal efficiencies %		1 h	4 h
$A\beta_{1-40}$	Smoker	70.0±9.6	60.0±8.6
		p=0.0016	
	Non-smoker	65.4 ± 9.9	70.4 ± 20.3
$A\beta_{1-42}$	Smoker	56.8±9.1	53.7±6.2
		p=0.049	
	Non-smoker	50.2 ± 11.4	55.3 ± 8.5

10.11 Effects of Smoking on Cognitive Function and Brain Atrophy in Renal Failure Patients

Figure 10.9 indicates that there appears to be no clear difference between the smoker and non-smoker cognitive function, as measured by the MMSE, in our study with a small sample size. The MMSE scores of smokers were similar to those of non-smokers in all three groups; age-matched healthy controls (AMC, seven smokers, ten non-smokers), renal failure patients who did not need hemodialysis (non-HDRF,

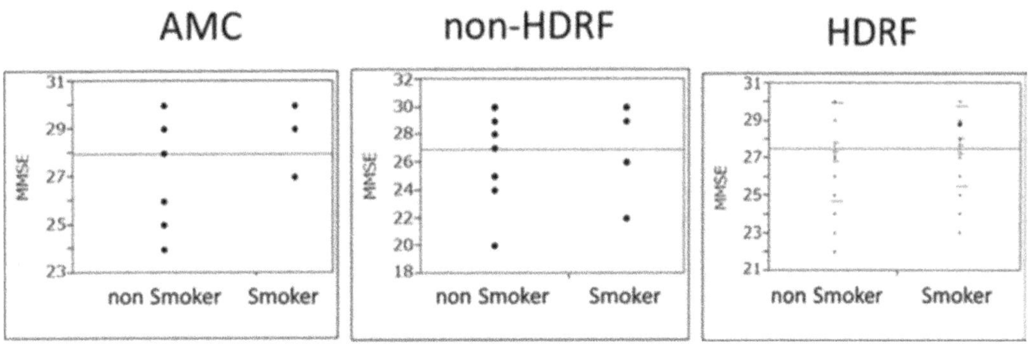

Fig. 10.9 The cognitive function of smokers and non-smokers was similar in our study. The patients were the same as those represented in Fig. 10.6 except that smoking history was obtained from only 16 non-HDRF patients. *AMC* age-matched healthy controls (seven smokers, ten non-smokers), *non-HDRF* renal failure patients without hemodialysis (seven smokers, nine non-smokers), *HDRF* severe renal failure patients who received hemodialysis three times a week (28 smokers, 29 non-smokers). *MMSE* Mini-Mental State Examination

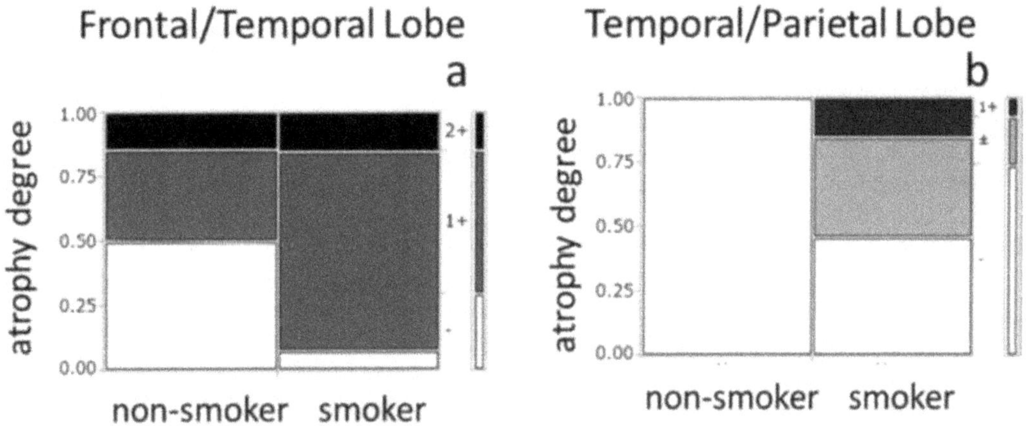

Fig. 10.10 Brain atrophy in smokers and non-smokers. Frontal/temporal atrophy and temporal/parietal atrophy was more severe in smokers than in non-smokers, as detected by brain CT scans ($p = 0.0465$ and $p = 0.0062$, respectively, by the χ^2 test). (Taken from Kitaguchi et al. 2015)

seven smokers, seven non-smokers), and severe renal failure patients who received hemodialysis three times a week (HDRF, 28 smokers, 29 non-smokers).

However, brain CT scans revealed that there were differences in brain atrophy between smokers and non-smokers. Frontal/temporal and temporal/parietal atrophies were more severe in smokers than in non-smokers, as shown in Fig. 10.10 ($p = 0.0465$ and $p = 0.0062$, respectively, by the χ^2 test). This suggests that the effects of smoking on the brain may not be sufficiently serious to affect cognitive function in our study, or that hemodialysis including Aβ removal from the blood three times a week may maintain cognitive function despite the presence of more severe atrophies in smokers.

10.12 Closing

As described above, removal of blood Aβ may enhance Aβ influx into the blood from the brain, resulting in maintenance or improvement of cognitive function. We believe that the E-BARS could contribute as a therapy for Alzheimer's disease. With respect to smoking, the patient's history in this regard may have some effect on brain atrophy and on the forms of Aβs existing in the blood. Additional study will be necessary in the future to further clarify this.

References

Anstey KJ, von Sanden C, Salim A, O'Kearney R (2007) Smoking as a risk factor for dementia and cognitive decline: a meta-analysis of prospective studies. Am J Epidemiol 166:367–378

Barnes DE, Yaffe K (2011) The projected effect of risk factor reduction on Alzheimer's disease prevalence. Lancet Neurol 10:819–828

Bell RD, Sagare AP, Friedman AE, Bedi GS, Holtzman DM, Deane R, Zlokovic BV (2007) Transport pathways for clearance of human Alzheimer's amyloid beta-peptide and apolipoproteins E and J in the mouse central nervous system. J Cereb Blood Flow Metab 27:909–918

Boada M, Ortiz P, Anaya F, Hernández I, Muñoz J, Núñez L, Olazarán J, Roca I, Cuberas G, Tárraga L, Buendia M, Pla RP, Ferrer I, Páez A (2009) Amyloid-targeted therapeutics in Alzheimer's disease: use of human albumin in plasma exchange as a novel approach for Abeta mobilization. Drug News Perspect 22:325–239

Boada M, Ramos-Fernández E, Guivernau B, Muñoz FJ, Costa M, Ortiz AM, Jorquera JI, Núñez L, Torres M, Páez A (2016) Treatment of Alzheimer disease using combination therapy with plasma exchange and haemapheresis with albumin and intravenous immunoglobulin: rationale and treatment approach of the AMBAR (Alzheimer Management By Albumin Replacement) study. Neurologia 31:473–481

DeMattos RB, Bales KR, Cummins DJ, Dodart JC, Paul SM, Holtzman DM (2001) Peripheral anti-A beta antibody alters CNS and plasma A beta clearance and decreases brain A beta burden in a mouse model of Alzheimer's disease. Proc Natl Acad Sci U S A 98:8850–8855

Donahue JE, Flaherty SL, Johanson CE, Duncan JA 3rd, Silverberg GD, Miller MC, Tavares R, Yang W, Wu Q, Sabo E, Hovanesian V, Stopa EG (2006) RAGE, LRP-1, and amyloid-beta protein in Alzheimer's disease. Acta Neuropathol 4:405–415

García AM, Ramón-Bou N, Porta M (2010) The effects of tobacco exposure before the age of onset of AD was investigated as a case-control study. Isolated and joint effects of tobacco and alcohol consumption on risk of Alzheimer's disease. J Alzheimers Dis 20:577–586

Hellström-Lindahl E, Mousavi M, Ravid R, Nordberg A (2004) Reduced levels of Abeta 40 and Abeta 42 in brains of smoking controls and Alzheimer's patients. Neurobiol Dis 15:351–360

Hock C, Konietzko U, Streffer JR, Tracy J, Signorell A, Müller-Tillmanns B, Lemke U, Henke K, Moritz E, Garcia E, Wollmer MA, Umbricht D, de Quervain DJ, Hofmann M, Maddalena A, Papassotiropoulos A, Nitsch RM (2003) Antibodies against beta-amyloid slow cognitive decline in Alzheimer's disease. Neuron 38:547–554

Hung LW, Ciccotosto GD, Giannakis E, Tew DJ, Perez K, Masters CL, Cappai R, Wade JD, Barnham KJ (2008) Amyloid-b peptide (Ab) neurotoxicity is modulated by the rate of peptide aggregation: Ab dimers and trimers correlate with neurotoxicity. J Neurosci 28:11950–11958

Kato M, Kawaguchi K, Nakai S, Murakami K, Hori H, Ohashi A, Hiki Y, Ito S, Shimano Y, Suzuki N, Sugiyama S, Ogawa H, Kusimoto H, Mutoh T, Yuzawa Y, Kitaguchi N (2012) Potential therapeutic system for Alzheimer's disease: removal of blood Abs by hemodialyzers and its effect on the cognitive functions of renal-failure patients. J Neural Transm 119:1533–1544

Kawaguchi K, Kitaguchi N, Nakai S, Murakami K, Asakura K, Mutoh T, Fujita Y, Sugiyama S (2010) Novel therapeutic approach for Alzheimer's disease by removing amyloid-β protein from the brain with an extracorporeal removal system. J Artif Organs 13:31–37

Kawaguchi K, Saigusa A, Yamada S, Gotoh T, Nakai S, Hiki Y, Hasegawa M, Yuzawa Y, Kitaguchi N (2016) Toward the treatment for Alzheimer's disease: adsorption is primary mechanism of removing amyloid β protein with hollow-fiber dialyzers of the suitable materials, Polysulfone and polymethyl methacrylate. J Artif Organs 19:149–158

Kihara T, Shimohama S, Sawada H, Kimura J, Kume T, Kochiyama H, Maeda T, Akaike A (1997) Nicotinic receptor stimulation protects neurons against beta-amyloid toxicity. Ann Neurol 42:159–163

Kihara T, Shimohama S, Sawada H, Honda K, Nakamizo T, Shibasaki H, Kume T, Akaike A (2001) Alpha 7 nicotinic receptor transduces signals to phosphatidylinositol 3-kinase to block A beta-amyloid-induced neurotoxicity. J Biol Chem 276:13541–13546

Kitaguchi N, Kawaguchi K, Nakai S, Murakami K, Ito S, Hoshino H, Hori H, Ohashi A, Shimano Y, Suzuki N, Yuzawa Y, Mutoh T, Sugiyama S (2011) Reduction of Alzheimer's disease amyloid-β in plasma by hemodialysis and its relation to cognitive functions. Blood Purif 32:57–62

Kitaguchi N, Hasegawa M, Ito S, Kawaguchi K, Hiki Y, Nakai S, Suzuki N, Shimano Y, Ishida O, Kushimoto H, Kato M, Koide S, Kanayama K, Kato T, Ito K, Takahashi H, Mutoh T, Sugiyama S, Yuzawa Y (2015) A prospective study on blood Aβ levels and the cognitive function of patients with hemodialysis: a potential therapeutic strategy for Alzheimer's disease. J Neural Transm 122:1593–1607

Kuo YM, Emmerling MR, Vigo-Pelfrey C, Kasunic TC, Kirkpatrick JB, Murdoch GH, Ball MJ, Roher AE (1996) Water-soluble Abeta (N-40, N-42) oligomers in normal and Alzheimer disease brains. J Biol Chem 271:4077–4081

Lopez OL, Kuller LH, Mehta PD, Becker JT, Gach HM, Sweet RA, Chang YF, Tracy R, DeKosky ST (2008) Plasma amyloid levels and the risk of AD in normal subjects in the Cardiovascular Health Study. Neurology 70:1664–1671

Matsumura A, Suzuki S, Iwahara N, Hisahara S, Kawamata J, Suzuki H, Yamauchi A, Takata K, Kitamura Y, Shimohama S (2015) Temporal changes of CD68 and α7 nicotinic acetylcholine receptor expression in microglia in Alzheimer's disease-like mouse models. J Alzheimers Dis 44:409–423

Matsuoka Y, Saito M, LaFrancois J, Saito M, Gaynor K, Olm V, Wang L, Casey E, Lu Y, Shiratori C, Lemere C, Duff K (2003) Novel therapeutic approach for the treatment of Alzheimer's disease by peripheral administration of agents with an affinity to β-Amyloid. J Neurosci 23:29–33

Mawuenyega KG, Sigurdson W, Ovod V, Munsell L, Kasten T, Morris JC, Yarasheski KE, Bateman RJ (2010) Decreased clearance of CNS beta-amyloid in Alzheimer's disease. Science 330:1774

Moreno-Gonzalez I, Estrada LD, Sanchez-Mejias E, Soto C (2013) Smoking exacerbates amyloid pathology in a mouse model of Alzheimer's disease. Nat Commun 4:1495

Morris AWJ, Carare RO, Schreiber S, Hawkes CA (2014) The cerebrovascular basement membrane: role in the clearance of β-amyloid and cerebral amyloid angiopathy. Front Aging Neurosci 6:1–9

Nakai S, Wakai K, Kanda E, Kawaguchi K, Sakai K, Kitaguchi N (2018) Is hemodialysis itself a risk factor for dementia? An analysis of nationwide registry data of patients on maintenance hemodialysis in Japan. Ren Replace Ther 4:12. https://doi.org/10.1186/s41100-018-0154-y

Ott A, Slooter AJ, Hofman A, van Harskamp F, Witteman JC, Van Broeckhoven C, van Duijn CM, Breteler MM (1998) Smoking and risk of dementia and Alzheimer's disease in a population-based cohort study: the Rotterdam Study. Lancet 351:1840–1843

Sabia S, Marmot M, Dufouil C, Singh-Manoux A (2008) Smoking history and cognitive function in middle age from the Whitehall II study. Arch Intern Med 168:1165–1173

Sakai K, Senda T, Hata R, Kuroda M, Hasegawa M, Kato M, Abe M, Kawaguchi K, Nakai S, Hiki Y, Yuzawa Y, Kitaguchi N (2016) Patients that have undergone hemodialysis exhibit lower amyloid deposition in the brain: evidence supporting a therapeutic strategy for Alzheimer's disease by removal of blood amyloid. J Alzheimers Dis 51:997–1002

Schenk D, Barbour R, Dunn W, Gordon G, Grajeda H, Guido T, Hu K, Huang J, Johnson-Wood K, Khan K, Kholodenko D, Lee M, Liao Z, Lieberburg I, Motter R, Mutter L, Soriano F, Shopp G, Vasquez N, Vandevert C, Walker S, Wogulis M, Yednock T, Games D, Seubert P (1999) Immunization with amyloid-beta attenuates Alzheimer-disease-like pathology in the PDAPP mouse. Nature 400:173–177

Schoonenboom NS, Mulder C, Van Kamp GJ, Mehta SP, Scheltens P, Blankenstein MA, Mehta PD (2005) Amyloid beta 38, 40, and 42 species in cerebrospinal fluid: more of the same? Ann Neurol 58:139–142

Selkoe DJ (2001) Alzheimer's disease: genes, proteins, and therapy. Physiolo Rev 81:741–766

Sevigny J, Chiao P, Bussière T, Weinreb PH, Williams L, Maier M, Dunstan R, Salloway S, Chen T, Ling Y, O'Gorman J, Qian F, Arastu M, Li M, Chollate S, Brennan MS, Quintero-Monzon O, Scannevin RH, Arnold HM, Engber T, Rhodes K, Ferrero J, Hang Y, Mikulskis A, Grimm J, Hock C, Nitsch RM, Sandrock A (2016) The antibody aducanumab reduces Aβ plaques in Alzheimer's disease. Nature 537:50–56

Silverberg GD, Miller MC, Messier AA, Majmudar S, Machan JT, Donahue JE, Stopa EG, Johanson CE (2010) Amyloid deposition and influx transporter expression at the blood-brain barrier increase in normal aging. J Neuropathol Exp Neurol 69:98–108

Takata K, Kitamura Y, Saeki M, Terada M, Kagitani S, Kitamura R, Fujikawa Y, Maelicke A, Tomimoto H, Taniguchi T, Shimohama S (2010) Galantamine-induced amyloid-{beta} clearance mediated via stimulation of microglial nicotinic acetylcholine receptors. J Biol Chem 285:40180–40191

Walsh DM, Klyubin I, Fadeeva JV, Cullen WK, Anwyl R, Wolfe MS, Rowan MJ, Selkoe DJ (2002) Naturally secreted oligomers of amyloid b protein potently inhibit hippocampal long-term potentiation in vivo. Nature 416:535–539

Wang HY, Lee DHS, D'Andrea MR, Peterson PA, Shank RP, Reitz AB (2000) Beta-amyloid(1–42) binds to α7 nicotinic acetylcholine receptor with high affinity—implications for Alzheimer's disease pathology. J Biol Chem 275:5626–5632

Yang WN, Ma KG, Chen XL, Shi LL, Bu G, Hu XD, Han H, Liu Y, Qian YH (2014) Mitogen-activated protein kinase signaling pathways are involved in regulating α7 nicotinic acetylcholine receptor-mediated amyloid-β uptake in SH-SY5Y cells. Neuroscience 278:276–290

www.ingramcontent.com/pod-product-compliance
Lightning Source LLC
LaVergne TN
LVHW082233200926
848484LV00008B/2348